Respiratory Management in Critical Care

Respiratory Management in Critical Care

Edited by

MJD Griffiths

Unit of Critical Care, Imperial College of Science, Technology and Medicine, Royal Brompton Hospital, London, UK

TW Evans

Unit of Critical Care, Imperial College of Science, Technology and Medicine, Royal Brompton Hospital, London, UK

First published in 2004
by BMJ Books, BMA House, Tavistock Square,
London WC1H 9JR

www.bmjbooks.com

British Library Cataloguing in Publication Data

A catalogue record for this book is available from the British Library

ISBN 0 7279 1729 3

Typeset by BMJ Electronic Production
Printed and bound in Spain by GraphyCems, Navarra

Contents

Contributors

K Atabai
Lung Biology Center, Department of Medicine, University of California, San Francisco, USA

SV Baudoin
Department of Anaesthesia, Royal Victoria Infirmary, Newcastle upon Tyne, UK

GJ Bellingan
Department of Intensive Care Medicine, University College London Hospitals, The Middlesex Hospital, London, UK

RM du Bois
Interstitial Lung Disease Unit, Royal Brompton Hospital, London, UK

RJ Boyton
Host Defence Unit, Royal Brompton Hospital, London, UK

S Brett
Department of Anaesthesia and Intensive Care, Hammersmith Hospital, London, UK

JJ Cordingley
Department of Anaesthesia and Intensive Care, Royal Brompton Hospital, London, UK

PA Corris
Department of Respiratory Medicine, Cardiothoracic Block, Freeman Hospital, Newcastle upon Tyne, UK

J Cranshaw
Unit of Critical Care, NHLI Division, Imperial College of Science, Technology and Medicine, Royal Brompton Hospital, London, UK

J Dakin
Unit of Critical Care, NHLI Division, Imperial College of Science, Technology and Medicine
Royal Brompton Hospital, London, UK

AC Davidson
Departments of Critical Care and Respiratory Support (Lane Fox Unit), Guys & St Thomas' Hospital, London, UK

SC Davies
Department of Haematology and Sickle Cell Unit, Central Middlesex Hospital, London, UK

J Dunning
Pulmonary Vascular Diseases Unit, Papworth Hospital, Cambridge and Department of Medicine, University of Cambridge School of Clinical Medicine, Addenbrooke's Hospital, Cambridge, UK

TW Evans
Unit of Critical Care, NHLI Division, Imperial College of Science, Technology and Medicine, Royal Brompton Hospital, London, UK

S Ewig
Institut Clinic De Pneumologia i Cirurgia Toracica, Hospital Clinic, Servei de Pneumologia i Al.lergia Respiratoria, Barcelona, Spain

CS Garrard
Intensive Care Unit, John Radcliffe Hospital, Oxford, UK

A Gascoigne
Department of Respiratory Medicine and Intensive Care, Royal Victoria Infirmary, Newcastle upon Tyne, UK

J Goldstone
Department of Intensive Care Medicine, University College London Hospitals, The Middlesex Hospital, London, UK

P Goldstraw
Department of Thoracic Surgery, Royal Brompton Hospital, London, UK.

JT Granton
University Health Network, Mount Sinai Hospital and the Interdepartmental Division of Critical Care, University of Toronto, Toronto, Ontario, Canada

ME Griffith
Department of Renal Failure, St Mary's Hospital NHS Trust, London, UK

MJD Griffiths
Unit of Critical Care, NHLI Division, Imperial College of Science, Technology and Medicine, Royal Brompton Hospital, London, UK

N Hart
Sleep and Ventilation Unit, Royal Brompton and Harefield NHS Trust, London, UK

AT Jones
Adult Intensive Care Unit, Royal Brompton Hospital, London, UK

BF Keogh
Department of Anaesthesia and Intensive Care, Royal Brompton Hospital, London, UK

OM Kon
Chest and Allergy Department, St Mary's Hospital NHS Trust, London, UK

SE Lapinsky
Mount Sinai Hospital and the Interdepartmental Division of Critical Care, University of Toronto, Toronto, Ontario, Canada

RM Leach
Department of Intensive Care, Guy's & St Thomas' NHS Trust, London, UK

JL Lordan
Department of Respiratory Medicine, Cardiothoracic Block, Freeman Hospital, Newcastle upon Tyne, UK

V Mak
Department of Respiratory and Critical Care Medicine, Central Middlesex Hospital, London, UK

MA Matthay
Cardiovascular Research Institute and Departments of Medicine and Anesthesia, University of California, San Francisco, USA

K McNeil
Pulmonary Vascular Diseases Unit, Papworth Hospital, Cambridge and Department of Medicine, University of Cambridge School of Clinical Medicine, Addenbrooke's Hospital, Cambridge, UK

DM Mitchell
Chest and Allergy Department, St Mary's Hospital NHS Trust, London, UK

ED Moloney
Imperial College School of Medicine at the National Heart and Lung Institute,
Royal Brompton Hospital, London, UK

NW Morrell
Pulmonary Vascular Diseases Unit, Papworth Hospital, Cambridge and Department of Medicine, University of Cambridge School of Clinical Medicine, Addenbrooke's Hospital, Cambridge, UK

P Phipps
Department of Intensive Care, Royal Prince Alfred Hospital, Sydney, Australia

AK Simonds
Sleep and Ventilation Unit, Royal Brompton and Harefield NHS Trust, London, UK

AS Slutsky
Department of Critical Care and Department of Medicine, St MichaelÆs Hospital, Interdepartmental Division of Critical Care, University of Toronto, Toronto, Ontario, Canada

SR Thomas
Department of Respiratory Medicine, St George's Hospital, London, UK

A Torres
Institut Clinic De Pneumologia i Cirurgia Toracica, Hospital Clinic, Servei de Pneumologia i Al.lergia Respiratoria, Barcelona, Spain

DF Treacher
Department of Intensive Care, Guy's & St Thomas' NHS Trust, London, UK

AU Wells
Interstitial Lung Disease Unit, Royal Brompton Hospital, London, UK

T Whitehead
Department of Respiratory Medicine, Central Middlesex Hospital, London, UK

Introduction

M J D Griffiths, T W Evans

The care of the critically ill has changed radically during the past 10 years. Technological advances have improved monitoring, organ support, and data collection, while small steps have been made in the development of drug therapies. Conversely, new challenges (e.g. severe acute respiratory syndrome [SARS], multiple antimicrobial resistance, bioterrorism) continue to arise and public expectations are elevated, sometimes to an unreasonable level. In this book we summarize some of the most important medical advances that have emerged, concentrating particularly on those relevant to the growing numbers of respiratory physicians who pursue a subspecialty interest in this clinical arena.

EVOLUTION OF INTENSIVE CARE MEDICINE AS A SPECIALTY

In Europe intensive care medicine (ICM) has been one of the most recent clinical disciplines to emerge. During a polio epidemic in Denmark in the early 1950s mortality was dramatically reduced by the application of positive pressure ventilation to patients who had developed respiratory failure and by concentrating them in a designated area with medical staff in constant attendance. This focus on airway care and ventilatory management led to the gradual introduction of intensive care units (ICU), principally by anaesthesiologists, throughout Western Europe. The development of sophisticated physiological monitoring equipment in the 1960s facilitated the diagnostic role of the intensivist, extending their skill base beyond anaesthesiology and attracting clinicians trained in general internal medicine into the ICU. Moreover, because respiratory failure was (and still is) the most common cause of ICU admission, pulmonary physicians, particularly in the USA, were frequently involved in patient care.

ARE INTENSIVE CARE UNITS EFFECTIVE?

Does intensive care work and does the way in which it is provided affect patients' outcomes? A higher rate of attributable mortality has been documented in patients who are refused intensive care, particularly on an emergency basis.[1] Clinical outcome is improved by the conversion of so-called "open" ICU to closed facilities in which patient management is directed primarily by intensive care specialists.[2][3] Superior organisational practices emphasising strong medical and nursing leadership can also improve outcome.[4] The emergence of intermediate care, high dependency, or step down facilities has attempted to fill the growing gap between the level of care that may be provided in the ICU and that in the general wards. Worryingly, the time at which patients are discharged from ICU in the UK has a demonstrable effect on their outcome.[5] Early identification of patients at risk of death—both before admission and after discharge from the ICU—may decrease mortality.[6] Patients can be identified who have a low risk of mortality and who are likely to benefit from a brief period of more intensive supervision and care.[7] Designated teams that are equipped to transfer critically ill patients between specialist units have a crucial role to play in ensuring that patient care and the use of resources are optimized.[8] Finally, long term follow up of the critically ill as outpatients following discharge from hospital may identify problems of chronic ill health that require active management and rehabilitation.[9]

TRAINING IN INTENSIVE CARE MEDICINE

Improved training of medical and nursing staff and organisational changes have undoubtedly played their part in improving the outcome of critical illness. ICM is now a recognised specialty in two European Union member states, namely Spain and the UK. Where available, training in ICM is of variable duration and is accessible variably to clinicians of differing base specialties. In Spain 5 years of training are required to achieve specialist status, 3 years of which are in ICM. In France, Germany, Greece, and the UK, 2 years of training in ICM are required, in addition to thos needed for the base specialty (usually anaesthesiology, respiratory or general internal medicine). In Italy, only anaesthesiologists may practice ICM. There is considerable variation between members states of the European Union regarding the amount of exposure to ICM in the training of pulmonary physicians as a mandatory (M) or optional (O) requirement: France and Greece 6 months (O), Germany 6 months (M, as part of general internal medicine), UK 3 months (O), and Italy and Spain none.

TRAINING IN INTENSIVE CARE MEDICINE IN THE UK

An increasing number of appointments in ICM are now available to trainees in general internal medicine at senior house officer level, usually for a period of 3 months. For specialist registrars, a number of options have emerged. First, in some specialties (e.g. respiratory medicine, infectious diseases) specialist registrars are already encouraged to undertake a period of training in ICM. Second, 6 months of training in anaesthesia plus 6 months of ICM (in addition to 3 months of experience as a senior house officer) in approved programmes confers intermediate accreditation by the Inter-Collegiate Board for Training in ICM (http://www.ics.ac.uk/ibticm_board.html). Finally a further 12 months of experience in recognised units can lead to the award of a Certificate of Completion of Specialist Training (CCST) combined with base specialty. Importantly, up to 12 months of such experience can be substituted for 6 months in general internal medicine (for anaesthesia) and respiratory medicine (for ICM).

Table 1   Proposed classification of critical illness[10]

Level 0	Patients whose needs can be met through normal ward care in an acute hospital
Level 1	Patients at risk of their condition deteriorating, or those recently relocated from higher levels of care, whose needs can be met on an acute ward with additional advice and support from the critical care team
Level 2	Patients requiring more detailed observations or intervention including support for a single failing organ system or postoperative care and those "stepping down" from higher levels of care
Level 3	Patients requiring advanced respiratory support alone or basic respiratory support together with support of at least two organ systems. This level includes all complex patients requiring support for multiorgan failure

Thus, a period of 5 years is needed for intermediate accreditation in ICM plus a CCST in general internal and respiratory medicine, and 6 for the award of a treble CCST. Programmes are now becoming available in all regions to enable trainees with National Training Numbers from all base specialties to achieve these training requirements and the proscribed competencies in ICM.

THE FUTURE FOR INTENSIVE CARE MEDICINE: A UK PERSPECTIVE

The changing requirements and increased need for provision of intensive care were recognised in the UK in the late 1990s by the Department of Health which commissioned the report entitled *"Comprehensive Critical Care"* produced by an expert group to provide a blue print for the future development of ICM within the NHS.[10] A central tenet of the report is the idea that the service should extend to the provision of critical care throughout the hospital, and not merely to patients located within the traditional confines of the ICU. To this end, the adoption of a new classification of illness severity based on dependency rather than location was recommended. Traditionally, the critically ill were defined according to their need for intensive care (delivered at a ratio of one nurse to one patient) and those requiring high dependency care (delivered at a ratio of one nurse to two or more patients). The new classification is based on the severity of the patient's illness and on the level of care needed (table 1). The report therefore represents a "whole systems" approach encompassing the provision of care, both before and after the acute episode within an integrated system.

To initiate and oversee the implementation of this policy, 29 local "networks" have been established, with an administrative and clinical infrastructure. Networks will be used to pilot national initiatives and enable groups of hospitals to establish locally agreed practices and protocols. Critically ill patients will be transferred between network hospitals if facilities or expertise within a single institution are inadequate to provide the necessary care, thereby obviating the problems associated with moving such patients over long distances to access a suitable bed.

CONCLUSION

How should the respiratory physician react to these developments? We suggest that an attachment in ICM for all respiratory trainees is necessary. Indeed, specialty recognition and the increased availability of training opportunities should encourage some trainees from respiratory medicine to seek a CCST combined with ICM. Second, we suggest that changes in the organisational and administrative structure of intensive care services heralded by the publication of *"Comprehensive Critical Care"* are likely to impact most heavily on respiratory physicians. For example, respiratory support services using non-invasive ventilation are particularly attractive in providing both "step up" (from the general wards) and "step down" (from the ICU) facilities. In the USA, respiratory physicians have for a long time been the major providers of critical care. In the UK and the rest of Europe, given appropriate resources and training, the pulmonary physician is ideally suited to become an integral component of the critical care service within all hospitals.

REFERENCES

1 **Metcalfe MA**, Sloggett A, McPherson K. Mortality among appropriately referred patients refused admission to intensive-care units. *Lancet* 1997;**350**:7–11.
2 **Carson SS**, Stocking C, Podsadecki T, *et al.* Effects of organizational change in the medical intensive care unit of a teaching hospital: a comparison of 'open' and 'closed' formats. *JAMA* 1996;**276**:322–8.
3 **Ghorra S**, Reinert SE, Cioffi W, *et al.* Analysis of the effect of conversion from open to closed surgical intensive care unit. *Ann Surg* 1999;**229**:163–71.
4 **Zimmerman JE**, Shortell SM, Rousseau DM, *et al.* Improving intensive care: observations based on organizational case studies in nine intensive care units: a prospective, multicenter study. *Crit Care Med* 1993;**21**:1443–51.
5 **Goldfrad C**, Rowan K. Consequences of discharges from intensive care at night. *Lancet* 2000;**355**:1138–42.
6 **Jakob SM**, Rothen HU. Intensive care 1980–1995: change in patient characteristics, nursing workload and outcome. *Intensive Care Med* 1997;**23**:1165–70.
7 **Kilpatrick A**, Ridley S, Plenderleith L. A changing role for intensive therapy: is there a case for high dependency care? *Anaesthesia* 1994;**49**:666–70.
8 **Bellingan G**, Olivier T, Batson S, Webb A. Comparison of a specialist retrieval team with current United Kingdom practice for the transport of critically ill patients. *Intensive Care Med* 2000;**26**:740–4.
9 **Angus DC**, Musthafa AA, Clermont G, *et al.* Quality-adjusted survival in the first year after the acute respiratory distress syndrome. *Am J Respir Crit Care Med* 2001;**163**:1389–94.
10 **Department of Health**. *Comprehensive critical care: review of adult critical care services*. London: Department of Health, 2000.

1 Pulmonary investigations for acute respiratory failure

J Dakin, MJD Griffiths

Patients with acute respiratory failure (ARF) commonly require intensive care, either for mechanical ventilatory support or because adequate investigation of the precipitating illness is impossible without endotracheal intubation. Similarly, respiratory complications such as nosocomial infection, pulmonary oedema, and pneumothorax frequently develop as a complication of life threatening illness . Here we discuss the investigation of the respiratory system of patients who are mechanically ventilated with emphasis on those presenting with ARF and diffuse pulmonary infiltrates.

STRATEGY FOR INVESTIGATING ACUTE RESPIRATORY FAILURE AND DIFFUSE PULMONARY INFILTRATES

The syndrome of ARF and diffuse pulmonary infiltrates consistent with pulmonary oedema excluding haemodynamic causes is termed lung injury and can be defined as acute lung injury (ALI) or acute respiratory distress syndrome (ARDS) if the oxygenation defect is sufficiently severe.[1] Identifying the conditions that precipitate ARDS or that cause a pulmonary disease with a different pathology but a similar clinical presentation is crucial because many have specific treatments or prognostic significance (table 1.1). A simple scheme for investigating ARF and diffuse pulmonary infiltrates is presented in figure 1.1, although investigations not specifically targeting the lung may be equally important (e.g. serological tests in the diagnosis of diffuse alveolar haemorrhage).

Many patients develop ARDS while they are being treated for presumed community-acquired pneumonia. High permeability pulmonary oedema is diagnosed by excluding cardiac and haemodynamic causes because there is no simple and reproducible bedside method for assessing permeability of the alveolar–capillary membrane (for review[2]). In the majority of cases major cardiac pathology may be excluded on the basis of the history, electrocardiogram, and the results of an echocardiogram or data from a pulmonary artery catheter. Rarely, unsuspected intermittent haemodynamic compromise (caused, for example, by ischaemia with or without associated mitral regurgitation or dynamic left ventricular outflow tract obstruction) may be detected at the bedside by continuous cardiac output monitoring with (stress) echocardiography (fig 1.2).

Where possible we perform thoracic computed tomography (CT), bronchoscopy, and broncho-alveolar lavage (BAL) in patients with lung injury in order to diagnose underlying pulmonary conditions and their complications (e.g. abscess, empyema, pneumothorax; fig 1.3). Repeating these investigations should be considered at any time it is felt that the patient is not recovering as predicted. Occasionally, in patients who fail to improve or those whose primary cause of ARF

remains obscure, histological analysis of lung tissue may be required. CT may help to guide the operator in determining the sites to biopsy and, where the pathology is bronchocentric, the choice between surgical and transbronchial lung biopsy (TBB). In our practice, lung biopsies in selected patients have revealed a variety of pulmonary pathologies that have altered management, including herpetic pneumonia, organizing pneumonia, bronchoalveolar cell carcinoma, and disseminated malignancy.

BRONCHOSCOPY

The British Thoracic Society recommends that fibreoptic bronchoscopy (FOB) should be available for use in all intensive care units (ICUs).[3] In patients presenting with ARF of unknown cause, FOB is used primarily as a means of collecting samples in patients who have failed to respond to first line antimicrobial therapy or those in whom an atypical micro-organism or non-infectious aetiology is suspected. Alternative indications for FOB in the ICU include the relief of endobronchial obstruction, the facilitation of endotracheal tube placement, and the localization of a site of trauma or of a source of bleeding (see chapter 22).

Table 1.1 Conditions that mimic and/or cause the acute respiratory distress syndrome (ARDS) may have a specific treatment

Condition		Specific treatment
Pneumonia		
Bacterial	Miliary tuberculosis	Yes
Viral	Cytomegalovirus	Yes
	Herpes simplex	Yes
	Hantavirus	
	SARS	
Fungal	Pneumocystis carinii	Yes
Others	Strongyloidiasis	Yes
	Acute interstitial	
Cryptogenic	pneumonia	Yes
	Cryptogenic organising pneumonia	Yes
	Acute eosinophilic pneumonia	Yes
	Bronchoalveolar cell	
Malignancy	carcinoma	
	Lymphangitis	
	Acute leukaemia	Yes
	Lymphoma	Yes
Pulmonary vascular disease	Diffuse alveolar haemorrhage	Yes
	Veno-occlusive disease	
	Pulmonary embolism	Yes
	Sickle lung	Yes

There is a considerable overlap between conditions that cause ARDS and those that are also associated with a distinct pathology that may have a specific treatment.

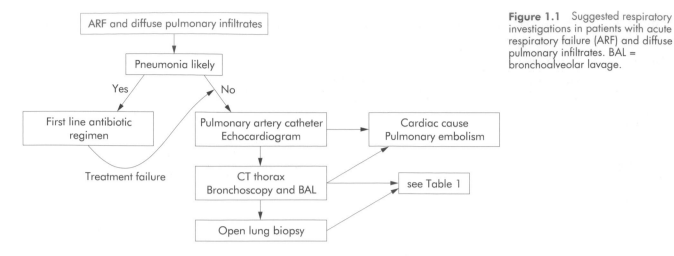

Figure 1.1 Suggested respiratory investigations in patients with acute respiratory failure (ARF) and diffuse pulmonary infiltrates. BAL = bronchoalveolar lavage.

Bronchoscopy procedure in patients who are mechanically ventilated

The inspired oxygen concentration (Fio_2) should be raised to 1.0 before the bronchoscope is introduced through a modified catheter mount incorporating an airtight seal around the suction port of an endotracheal or tracheostomy tube. The resultant increased resistance to expiration results in gas trapping and increased positive end expiratory pressure (PEEP). An 8 mm endotracheal tube is the smallest that should be used with an adult instrument because with smaller diameter tubes the level of PEEP may exceed 20 cm H_2O.[4] Paediatric bronchoscopes may be passed through smaller endotracheal tubes at the cost of a smaller visual field and significantly less suction capability.[5] In patients with ARF requiring mechanical ventilation, adequate sedation and paralysis facilitate not only effective oxygenation but also obviate the risk of damage to the instrument should the patient bite the endotracheal tube. Finally, limiting the duration of instrumentation by intermittently withdrawing the bronchoscope during the operation helps to maintain adequate alveolar ventilation and to limit the rise in $Paco_2$ which may be particularly relevant in those with head trauma. When prolonged instrumentation of the airway is expected—for example, during bronchoscopic surveillance of percutaneous tracheostomy—monitoring of end tidal CO_2 is recommended.[6]

Complications are few. Malignant cardiac arrhythmia occurred in about 2% of cases in an early series in which FOB was performed in patients soon after cardiopulmonary arrest.[7] In a subsequent series no serious complications were reported.[8]

Specimen retrieval techniques have been reviewed recently elsewhere.[9] There is little difference in sensitivity and specificity between FOB directed BAL and protected specimen brush (PSB) in establishing a microbiological diagnosis.[10 11] In order to obtain samples for cellular analysis (table 1.2), repeated aliquots of 50–60 ml to a total of 250–300 ml should be instilled, of which about 50% should be retrieved. In ventilated patients a lower volume is commonly used to reduce ventilatory disturbance, although there is no standard recommendation. Bacteriological analysis requires collection of only 5 ml fluid, although larger volumes are more commonly used. Blind (non-bronchoscopic) tracheobronchial aspiration is routine practice in all ventilated patients to provide upper airway toilet. Blind sampling of lower respiratory tract secretions (aspiration or mini-BAL using various catheter or brush devices to obtain specimens for quantitative cultures) has been extensively examined as an alternative diagnostic method in cases of suspected ventilator associated pneumonia (VAP). Generally, these have compared favourably with bronchoscope guided methods in trials on critically ill patients.[12 13]

Transbronchial (TBB) versus surgical lung (SLB) biopsy

TBB carries a substantial risk of pneumothorax which afflicts 8–14% of ventilated patients.[14 15] For this reason, TBB is rarely performed in these circumstances except in patients after lung transplantation where the sensitivity for detection of acute or chronic rejection is 70–90%, with a specificity of 90–100% when performed in an appropriate clinical context.[16–18] The Lung Rejection Study Group recommends collecting at least

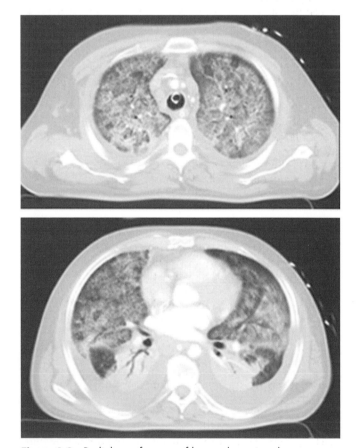

Figure 1.2 Radiology of a case of haemodynamic pulmonary oedema and histological non-specific interstitial pneumonia masquerading as community-acquired pneumonia and ARDS. Prominent septal lines (upper panel) and large pleural effusions (lower panel) suggest a cardiac cause of pulmonary oedema in this man aged 30 years of no fixed abode. Having failed to respond to antibiotics and corticosteroids, he improved following two vessel coronary angioplasty, mitral valve replacement with one coronary artery bypass graft, and finally a further course of high dose steroids. The diagnosis of ischaemic mitral valve regurgitation was made by stress echocardiography. Subsequently, pulmonary diagnosis was made by an open lung biopsy taken at the time of his cardiac surgery.

Table 1.2 Typical bronchoalveolar lavage differential cell counts in conditions associated with acute respiratory failure and diffuse pulmonary infiltrates

Condition	Cell differential counts				Comments
	Macrophage	Lymphocyte	Neutrophil	Eosinophil	
Normal	90%	10%	<4%	<1%	Neutrophils usually <2% in non-smokers
Acute interstitial pneumonia		↑	↑	↑	Eosinophils or neutrophils each raised in about 70% of cases of CFA; both being raised is characteristic. Neutrophils may be raised in isolation but this is more typical of infection. Lymphocytes raised in about 10%
Alveolar haemorrhage	↑				BAL fluid may be bloody. Haemosiderin-laden macrophages appear after 48 hours and are diagnostic
ARDS			↑		Neutrophils commonly around 70% of differential count
Bacterial pneumonia			↑		Neutrophils >50% in ventilated patients with bacterial pneumonia
Eosinophilic pneumonia				↑↑	Eosinophils typically 40%, range 20–90%. Neutrophils may also be raised, but always lower than eosinophils

CFA = cryptogenic fibrosing alveolitis; BAL = bronchoalveolar lavage; ARDS = acute respiratory distress syndrome.

five pieces of lung parenchyma to get an adequate sample of small bronchioles and to diagnose bronchiolitis obliterans.[19] Widespread pulmonary infiltrates developing within 72 hours of lung transplantation are more likely to represent alveolar oedema caused by ischaemia-reperfusion injury than rejection or infection.[20 21]

A recent study retrospectively examined the strategy of performing BAL and TBB simultaneously rather than as staged procedures in mechanically ventilated patients with unexplained pulmonary infiltrates.[22] Pneumothorax occurred in nine out of 38 patients, six requiring intercostal tube drainage; four out of 38 suffered significant bleeding that was self limiting or terminated with instillation of adrenaline. Diagnostic yields were estimated at 74% for BAL/TBB, whereas those for TBB and BAL alone were 63% and 29%, respectively. Patients in the later phases of ARDS represented 11 of 38 patients and experienced a relatively high incidence of complications and lower diagnostic value, in part because BAL alone could adequately diagnose infection.

A 10 year retrospective review of 24 mechanically ventilated patients undergoing SLB found that a diagnosis was made histologically in 46%.[23] Intraoperative complications were generally well tolerated, although 17% had persistent air leaks and two patients died as a consequence of the procedure. Complication rates in other series have been lower and the estimates of diagnostic usefulness have been considerably higher.[24–27] For example, in 27 patients with ARF, persistent air leak occurred in six following SLB but there were no perioperative deaths.[27] In a retrospective review of 27 OLBs in patients with ARF, persistent air leak occurred in six but there were no perioperative deaths.[27] In a retrospective series of 80 patients,[26] many of whom were immunosuppressed, eight had a persistent air leak with one perioperative myocardial infarction.

Bronchoscopy in specific conditions
Pneumonia
The microbiological yield from bronchoscopy is low (13–48%) in ventilated patients with community acquired pneumonia (CAP), possibly because of the frequency of antibiotic administration before admission to the ICU.[28–30] By contrast, patients who have been mechanically ventilated for several days generally have extensive colonisation even of the lower respiratory tract. In these patients with suspected VAP, negative microbiological culture predicts the absence of pneumonia but false positives arise frequently. Invasive investigation has not been shown in patients with either CAP or VAP to alter treatment and outcome significantly[11 29 31–33] and may be reserved for patients failing first line treatment or those from whom specimens are not readily obtainable by blind tracheobronchial aspiration (see chapters 3 and 4). Patients with common causes of immunosuppression, such as the acquired immune deficiency syndrome (AIDS) and malignancy, have a poor prognosis when admitted to the ICU with ARF (see chapter 20). For example, bone marrow transplant recipients requiring mechanical ventilation have an in-hospital mortality in excess of 95%.[34] Although these data have deterred referral of such patients to the ICU, temporary endotracheal intubation may be required for sedation and FOB to be performed safely.

The sensitivity of BAL in the detection of AIDS related pneumocystis pneumonia (PCP) is high (86–97%).[35–37] Fewer organisms may be recovered by BAL from patients using nebulised pentamidine prophylaxis[38 39] or with non-AIDS related PCP, but the yield may be increased by taking samples from two lobes and targeting the area of greatest radiological abnormality.[40] Cytomegalovirus (CMV) pneumonia is a common cause of death after transplantation, particularly in recipients of allogeneic bone marrow and lung grafts.[41] The definitive diagnosis of CMV pneumonitis is made by the finding of typical cytomegalic cells with inclusions on BAL or TBB,[42] the latter being more sensitive. Detection of early antigen fluorescent foci (DEAFF)[43] performed on virus cultured from BAL fluid allows a presumptive diagnosis to be made.

Invasive pulmonary aspergillosis occurs predominantly in neutropenic patients[44] in whom early diagnosis and treatment are essential.[45] The incidence of aspergillosis may be rising in this patient group, probably secondary to more aggressive chemotherapy regimens and more widespread use of prophylactic broad spectrum antibiotics and anticandidal agents. The sensitivity of BAL is high in the presence of diffuse radiological changes.[46] A positive culture has a specificity of 90% but results may take up to 3 weeks.[47] The sensitivity of culture alone (23–40%) is greatly increased by the addition of microscopic examination for hyphae (58–64%).[48 49] Galactomannan antigen testing of blood provides an early warning of infection[50] and may prove useful in BAL fluid.

Respiratory failure due to non-infectious lung disease
Patients presenting with ARF and pulmonary infiltrates are generally assumed to have pneumonia and further investigation is prompted by treatment failure. Analysis of BAL fluid may distinguish the differential diagnoses and/or pulmonary risk factors for ARDS, many of which have specific treatments (table 1.1). The BAL white cell differential provides information that may be diagnostically helpful (table 1.2).[51] A moderate eosinophilia (>15%) implicates a relatively small number of conditions including Churg-Strauss syndrome, AIDS related infection, eosinophilic pneumonia, drug induced lung disease, or helminthic infection.[52 53]

Apart from helping to uncover a cause or differential diagnosis for ARDS, the BAL fluid cell profile may give prognostic information. In patients with ARDS secondary to sepsis a BAL fluid neutrophilia had adverse prognostic significance while a higher macrophage count was associated with a better outcome.[54] The fibroproliferative phase of ARDS may be amenable to treatment with steroids[55] and it is recommended that either BAL or PSB is performed before starting treatment to exclude infection.

For patients with suspected or confirmed ARDS a sensitive and specific marker of disease would have several benefits. Firstly, it might improve the ability to predict which patients with risk factors develop ARDS[56] so that potentially protective measures could be assessed and developed. Secondly, it may help to quantify the severity of disease and to predict complications such as fibrosis and superadded infection. Most studies have involved assays on plasma samples or BAL fluid.[56] Analysis may provide information about soluble inflammatory mediators and by-products of inflammation (such as shed adhesion molecules, elastase, peroxynitrite) in the distal airways and air spaces. Analysis of samples from patients at risk has revealed increased alveolar levels of the potent neutrophil chemokine interleukin 8 (IL-8) in those patients who progress to ARDS.[57] The development of established fibrosis conveys a poor prognosis in ARDS.[58] Type III procollagen peptide is present from the day of tracheal intubation in the pulmonary oedema fluid of patients with incipient lung injury, and the concentration correlates with mortality.[59] Less invasive methods of sampling distal lung lining fluid using exhaled breath[60 61] or exhaled breath condensates[62 63] are being examined in critically ill patients. The assay of potential biomarkers is currently used exclusively as a research tool.

RADIOLOGY
Chest radiography[64 65]
The cost effectiveness of a daily chest radiograph in the mechanically ventilated patient has been debated[66 67] but is recommended by the American College of Radiology[68] based on series highlighting the incidence (15–18%) of unsuspected findings leading directly to changes in management.[69–71] Film acquisition in the ICU is technically demanding but guidelines have been published.[72] Digital imaging techniques permit the use of lower radiation doses and manipulate images to produce, in effect, a standard exposure as well as an edge enhanced image to facilitate visualisation of, for example, intravenous lines and pneumothoraces.

Endotracheal tubes and central venous catheters[73]
A radiograph is recommended after placement or repositioning of all central venous catheters, pleural drains, nasogastric, and endotracheal tubes.[68] The tip of the endotracheal tube may move up to 4 cm with neck flexion and extension,[74] and the end should be 5–7 cm from the carina or project on a plain chest radiograph to the level of T3–T4.[75] Tracheal rupture may be reflected in radiological evidence of overdistension of the endotracheal tube or tracheostomy balloon to a greater diameter than that of the trachea. Surprisingly, the presentation of this potentially catastrophic complication is often gradual, with surgical emphysema and pneumomediastinum developing over 24 hours.[76]

Central venous catheters should be positioned in the superior vena cava (SVC) at the level of or slightly above the azygos vein. Caudal to this, the SVC lies within the pericardium making tamponade likely if the atrial wall is perforated. Positioning of left sided lines with their ends abutting the wall of the SVC is a risk factor for perforation. Encroachment of lines into the atrium may cause arrhythmia and be associated with a higher incidence of endocarditis.[77] The ideal radiological placement of pulmonary artery catheters has not been studied. To minimize the risk of infarction or perforation, the balloon should be sited routinely in the largest diameter pulmonary artery that will provide a wedge trace on inflation, and

placement should be reviewed frequently to prevent migration of the catheter tip more away from the hilum.[78]

Radiographic appearances in ARF
The radiographic appearance of ARDS is a cornerstone of its diagnosis (see chapter 5). However, distinguishing between cardiogenic and high permeability pulmonary oedema on radiographic signs alone is unreliable.[79] The cardiac size and vascular pedicle width reflect the haemodynamic state of the patient,[80] but this sign relies on exact and often unachievable patient positioning. Pleural effusions and Kerley's lines reflecting lymphatic engorgement are not characteristic of ARDS because the high protein content and viscosity of the oedema fluid prevents it from spreading into the peripheral interstitial and pleural spaces. Air bronchograms are seen in up to one third of cases as the airways remain dry in ARDS, thereby contrasting with the surrounding parenchyma.

In contrast to hydrostatic pulmonary oedema, the radiographic signs of ARDS are frequently not visible on the plain chest radiograph for 24 hours after the onset of symptoms. Early changes comprise patchy ill defined densities that become confluent to form ground glass shadowing. In ventilated patients air space shadowing commonly results from pneumonia or atelectasis; other causes are ARDS, haemorrhage, and lung contusion. The detection and quantification of pleural fluid by the supine chest radiograph is inaccurate.[81 82]

Thoracic ultrasound
The presence of fluid within the pleural space has an adverse effect on ventilation-perfusion matching[83]; removal improves oxygenation and pulmonary compliance.[83 84] Drainage may be performed safely by ultrasound guided thoracocentesis in the ventilated patient.[85 86]

Thoracic computed tomography (CT)
Transportation to and monitoring of a critically ill patient for CT scanning involves a team effort from medical, nursing, and technical support staff. There are no published data describing the risks and benefits of this investigation in a well defined group of critically ill patients. However, in a retrospective review of 108 thoracic CT scans performed on patients in a general ICU, at least one new clinically significant finding (most commonly abscess, malignancy, unsuspected pneumonia, or pleural effusion) was identified in 30% of cases and in 22% led to a change in management.[87] The normal standards and precautions for transporting critically ill patients apply,[88] including a period of stabilisation on the transport ventilator prior to movement. Despite the added risk of complications such as pneumothorax, haemodynamic instability and lung derecruitment associated with transportation, we routinely scan patients with ARDS if their gas exchange on the transport ventilator is acceptable. Portable CT scanners provide mediastinal images of comparable quality to those obtained in the radiology department, but the images of the lung parenchyma are inferior.[89]

Thoracic CT in specific conditions
ARDS
Insight into the nature of ARDS has been obtained from CT scanning, for example, by defining the disease distribution and demonstrating ventilator induced lung injury (see chapter 8).[90] CT scans of the lung parenchyma show that the diffuse opacification on the plain radiograph is not homogenous; classically, there is a gradient of decreasing aeration passing from ventral to dorsal dependent regions.[91] Tidal volume is therefore directed exclusively to the overlying anterior regions which are consequently overdistended. This may account for the anterior distribution of reticular damage seen on CT scans in survivors.[92] The improvement in oxygenation of patients with

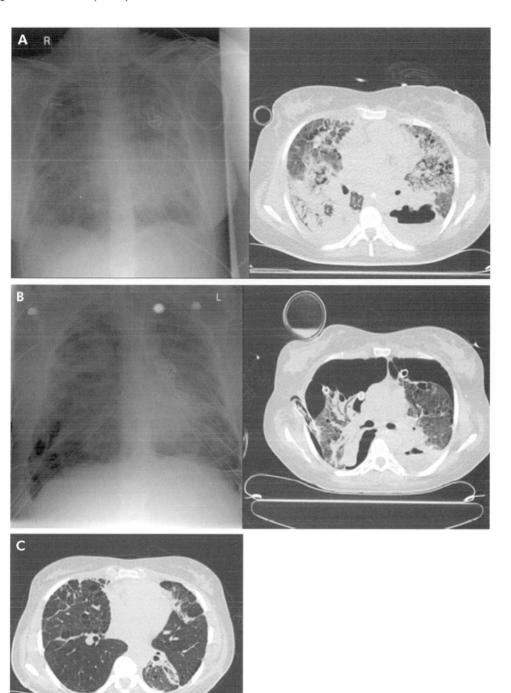

Figure 1.3. Radiology of a case of left lower lobe pneumonia complicated by ARDS. (A) Chest radiograph and CT scan taken on the same day 3 weeks after the onset of respiratory failure. An abscess is obvious in the apical segment of the left lower lobe on the CT scan. There is dense dependent consolidation bilaterally but elsewhere the lungs are affected in a patchy distribution. (B) Chest radiograph and CT scan taken on the same day 5 months after the onset of respiratory failure. Bilateral loculated pneumothoraces are evident despite the placement of several intercostal chest drains on both sides. (C) Chest CT scan taken 6 months after discharge from hospital showing diffuse emphysema and patchy areas of fibrosis.

ARDS following prone positioning suggests improved ventilation-perfusion matching. However, microsphere CT studies in animal models of ARDS have failed to demonstrate redirection of perfusion with prone positioning[93]; redirection of ventilation to the consolidated dorsal regions may therefore be the mechanism responsible.

Recovery from ARDS is commonly complicated by pneumothoraces which are often loculated. If a pneumothorax does not extend to the lateral thoracic wall, it will not be readily apparent on a chest radiograph. Its presence may be inferred from a range of indirect signs such as a vague radiolucency or undue clarity of the diaphragm, but this gives no information as to whether the collection of air is located anteriorly or posteriorly. Similarly,

empyema and abscess formation may cause treatment failure in patients with pneumonia and ARDS and are not infrequently missed on the plain film (fig 1.3).[94] CT guided percutaneous drainage may be required for loculated pneumothoraces and may be an alternative to surgery for lung abscesses.

Pulmonary embolus
Massive pulmonary embolus is a treatable cause of rapid cardiorespiratory deterioration which is frequently not diagnosed before death (see chapter 14). Radionuclide scanning has a long image acquisition time and assays for detecting D-dimers are unduly sensitive in this setting, making both unsuitable for the critically ill patient. CT pulmonary angiography is the

investigation of choice and may provide an alternative diagnosis to account for the presentation.

Trauma
Routine CT scanning of all victims of serious trauma uncovers lesions (pneumothorax, haemothorax, pulmonary contusion) not detected on clinical examination and plain radiography.[95] However, there is no evidence to suggest that a better patient outcome follows routine scanning. Different trauma centres favour aggressive[96] and conservative[97][98] management of small pneumothoraces in the ventilated patient.

LUNG FUNCTION

Formal assessment of lung function is most commonly required for patients who experience difficulty in weaning where measurements of peak flow, vital capacity, and respiratory muscle strength may be useful (see chapters 11 and 19). An airtight connection between the endotracheal tube and a hand held spirometer can give accurate and reproducible results. A vital capacity of 10 ml/kg is usually required to sustain spontaneous ventilation. If respiratory muscle weakness is suspected, measurements should be performed sitting and supine. A supine reduction of 25% or more indicates diaphragm weakness. Direct measurement of diaphragm strength is useful where borderline results are obtained from spirometric testing, in uncooperative patients, or in those with lung disease that impairs spirometric measurements. Transdiaphragmatic pressure, an index of the strength of diaphragmatic contractility, is measured by peroral passage of balloon manometers into the oesophagus and stomach. A volitional measurement is made by asking the patient to sniff forcefully from functional residual capacity. A non-volitional measurement can be made reproducibly by magnetic stimulation of the phrenic nerves using a coil directly applied to the skin of the neck.[99] A low maximal inspiratory pressure (PI_{max}) predicts failure to wean, although it is insensitive in predicting success.[100]

In the mechanically ventilated patient gas exchange and ventilation are assessed routinely by arterial blood gas analysis and continuous oxygen saturation monitoring. Refractory hypoxia that is characteristic of ARDS is almost entirely caused by intrapulmonary shunting.[101] Oxygenation is quantified in the American-European Consensus Conference (AECC) definition of ARDS and ALI by the ratio of the arterial partial pressure and the inspired oxygen concentration (Pao_2/Fio_2).[1] This initial value does not predict survival[102] but is a reasonable predictor of shunt fraction[103] and has epidemiological importance as it is used to distinguish patients with severe (ARDS) and less severe (ALI) lung injury. The Pao_2/Fio_2 ratio is simple to calculate but does not take into account other factors that affect oxygenation such as the mean airway pressure (mPaw).[104] The oxygenation index (OI = mPaw × Fio_2 × 100/Pao_2) benefits from including this variable; similarly, the respiratory severity index (Po_2alveolar − Po_2arterial/Po_2alveolar + 0.014PEEP) is more cumbersome but the value in the first 24 hours did distinguish survivors and non-survivors in a study of 56 consecutive patients with ARDS defined using the AECC criteria.[105] As a compromise the Pao_2/Fio_2 ratio may be calculated at a standardised level of PEEP.

Assessment of respiratory physiology has undergone a recent resurgence as novel adjuncts to ventilator therapy (e.g. prone positioning and inhaled vasodilators) have been investigated and the importance of mitigating ventilator induced lung injury has been recognised.[106] Most ventilators continuously display airway pressures, delivered and exhaled volumes, and compliance. The compliance of the respiratory system is defined by the relationship:

$$\text{change in volume/change in elastic recoil pressure} =$$
$$\text{tidal volume/plateau pressure} - \text{PEEP (ml/cm H}_2\text{O)}$$

This gives the total compliance of the lung and chest wall assuming that the patient is making no spontaneous respiratory effort. Values are commonly halved or lower in ARDS (normal range 50–80 ml/cm H_2O), although measurement of this variable is not required by the standard definition.[1] Studying pressure-volume curves of patients with ARDS highlighted the risk of overdistension at what would be considered a "normal" tidal volume,[107] and the results of the recent ARDS network study confirmed the benefit of ventilation at a restricted volume.[106] While the optimum balance between PEEP and Fio_2 and the role of the pressure-volume curve in setting the optimum level of PEEP remain to be determined, we cannot recommend that generating pressure-volume curves in patients with lung injury is required other than for research.[108]

SUMMARY

When investigating patients with ARF and pulmonary infiltrates, one must achieve a balance between the necessity of rapid diagnosis and the early instigation of effective therapy, against the potential harm caused by invasive techniques in patients with very limited reserves. Because of the pressure on intensive care beds in the UK, our facilities and expertise in providing temporary support are probably under-used in the investigation of such cases before mechanical ventilation is mandatory. We suggest a scheme for the investigation of patients presenting with ARF and discuss the effects of mechanical ventilation and critical illness on commonly used investigations of the respiratory system.

REFERENCES

1 **Bernard GR**, Artigas A, Brigham KL, *et al.* The American-European Consensus Conference on ARDS. Definitions, mechanisms, relevant outcomes, and clinical trial coordination. *Am J Respir Crit Care Med* 1994;**149**(3 Pt 1):818–24.

2 **Macnaughton P**, Evans T. Pulmonary function in the intensive care unit. In: Hughes J, Pride N, eds. *Lung function tests. Physiological principles and clinical applications, 1st ed.* London: Saunders, 1999:185–201.

3 **British Thoracic Society**. British Thoracic Society guidelines on diagnostic flexible bronchoscopy. *Thorax* 2001;**56**(Supplement 1):i1–22.

4 **Lindholm CE**, Ollman B, Snyder JV, *et al.* Cardiorespiratory effects of flexible fiberoptic bronchoscopy in critically ill patients. *Chest* 1978;**74**:362–8.

5 **Jolliet P**, Chevrolet JC. Bronchoscopy in the intensive care unit. *Intensive Care Med* 1992;**18**:160–9.

6 **Marx WH**, Ciaglia P, Graniero KD. Some important details in the technique of percutaneous dilatational tracheostomy via the modified Seldinger technique. *Chest* 1996;**110**:762–6.

7 **Barrett CR Jr.** Flexible fiberoptic bronchoscopy in the critically ill patient. Methodology and indications. *Chest* 1978;**73**(5 Suppl):746–9.

8 **Olopade CO**, Prakash UB. Bronchoscopy in the critical-care unit. *Mayo Clin Proc* 1989;**64**:1255–63.

9 **Niederman M**, Torres A. Bronchospopy for pneumonia: indications, methodology and applications. In: Feinsilver SFA, ed. *Textbook of bronchoscopy.* Baltimore: Williams and Wilkins, 1995:221–41.

10 **Jimenez P**, Saldias F, Meneses M, *et al.* Diagnostic fiberoptic bronchoscopy in patients with community-acquired pneumonia. Comparison between bronchoalveolar lavage and telescoping plugged catheter cultures. *Chest* 1993;**103**:1023–7.

11 **Ruiz M**, Torres A, Ewig S, *et al.* Noninvasive versus invasive microbial investigation in ventilator-associated pneumonia: evaluation of outcome. *Am J Respir Crit Care Med* 2000;**162**:119–25.

12 **Papazian L**, Thomas P, Garbe L, *et al.* Bronchoscopic or blind sampling techniques for the diagnosis of ventilator-associated pneumonia. *Am J Respir Crit Care Med* 1995;**152**(6 Pt 1):1982–91.

13 **Marik PE**, Brown WJ. A comparison of bronchoscopic vs blind protected specimen brush sampling in patients with suspected ventilator-associated pneumonia. *Chest* 1995;**108**:203–7.

14 **Papin TA**, Grum CM, Weg JG. Transbronchial biopsy during mechanical ventilation. *Chest* 1986;**89**:168–70.

15 **Pincus PS**, Kallenbach JM, Hurwitz MD, *et al.* Transbronchial biopsy during mechanical ventilation. *Crit Care Med* 1987;**15**:1136–9.

16 **Trulock EP**, Ettinger NA, Brunt EM, *et al.* The role of transbronchial lung biopsy in the treatment of lung transplant recipients. An analysis of 200 consecutive procedures. *Chest* 1992;**102**:1049–54.

17 **Scott JP**, Fradet G, Smyth RL, *et al.* Prospective study of transbronchial biopsies in the management of heart-lung and single lung transplant patients. *J Heart Lung Transplant* 1991;**10**(5 Pt 1):626–36; discussion 636–7.

18 **Higenbottam T**, Stewart S, Penketh A, *et al.* Transbronchial lung biopsy for the diagnosis of rejection in heart-lung transplant patients. *Transplantation* 1988;**46**:532–9.

19 **Yousem SA**, Berry GJ, Cagle PT, et al. Revision of the 1990 working formulation for the classification of pulmonary allograft rejection: Lung Rejection Study Group. *J Heart Lung Transplant* 1996;**15**(1 Pt 1):1–15.

20 **McGregor CG**, Daly RC, Peters SG, et al. Evolving strategies in lung transplantation for emphysema. *Ann Thorac Surg* 1994;**57**:1513–20; discussion 1520–1.

21 **Trulock EP**. Management of lung transplant rejection. *Chest* 1993;**103**:1566–76.

22 **Bulpa PA**, Dive AM, Mertens L, et al. Combined bronchoalveolar lavage and transbronchial lung biopsy: safety and yield in ventilated patients. *Eur Respir J* 2003;**21**:489–94.

23 **Flabouris A**, Myburgh J. The utility of open lung biopsy in patients requiring mechanical ventilation. *Chest* 1999;**115**:811–7.

24 **Papazian L**, Thomas P, Bregeon F, et al. Open-lung biopsy in patients with acute respiratory distress syndrome. *Anesthesiology* 1998;**88**:935–44.

25 **Nelems JM**, Cooper JD, Henderson RD, et al. Emergency open lung biopsy. *Ann Thorac Surg* 1976;**22**:260–4.

26 **Warner DO**, Warner MA, Divertie MB. Open lung biopsy in patients with diffuse pulmonary infiltrates and acute respiratory failure. *Am Rev Respir Dis* 1988;**137**:90–4.

27 **Canver CC**, Mentzer RM Jr. The role of open lung biopsy in early and late survival of ventilator-dependent patients with diffuse idiopathic lung disease. *J Cardiovasc Surg* 1994;**35**:151–5.

28 **Moine P**, Vercken JB, Chevret S, et al. Severe community-acquired pneumonia. Etiology, epidemiology, and prognosis factors. French Study Group for Community-Acquired Pneumonia in the Intensive Care Unit. *Chest* 1994;**105**:1487–95.

29 **Sorensen J**, Forsberg P, Hakanson E, et al. A new diagnostic approach to the patient with severe pneumonia. *Scand J Infect Dis* 1989;**21**:33–41.

30 **Potgieter PD**, Hammond JM. Etiology and diagnosis of pneumonia requiring ICU admission. *Chest* 1992;**101**:199–203.

31 **Pachon J**, Prados MD, Capote F, et al. Severe community-acquired pneumonia. Etiology, prognosis, and treatment. *Am Rev Respir Dis* 1990;**142**:369–73.

32 **Torres A**, Serra-Batlles J, Ferrer A, et al. Severe community-acquired pneumonia. Epidemiology and prognostic factors. *Am Rev Respir Dis* 1991;**144**:312–8.

33 **Sole Violan J**, Fernandez JA, Benitez AB, et al. Impact of quantitative invasive diagnostic techniques in the management and outcome of mechanically ventilated patients with suspected pneumonia. *Crit Care Med* 2000;**28**:2737–41.

34 **Crawford SW**, Petersen FB. Long-term survival from respiratory failure after marrow transplantation for malignancy. *Am Rev Respir Dis* 1992;**145**:510–4.

35 **Gal AA**, Klatt EC, Koss MN, et al. The effectiveness of bronchoscopy in the diagnosis of Pneumocystis carinii and cytomegalovirus pulmonary infections in acquired immunodeficiency syndrome. *Arch Pathol Lab Med* 1987;**111**:238–41.

36 **Golden JA**, Hollander H, Stulbarg MS, et al. Bronchoalveolar lavage as the exclusive diagnostic modality for Pneumocystis carinii pneumonia. A prospective study among patients with acquired immunodeficiency syndrome. *Chest* 1986;**90**:18–22.

37 **Broaddus C**, Dake MD, Stulbarg MS, et al. Bronchoalveolar lavage and transbronchial biopsy for the diagnosis of pulmonary infections in the acquired immunodeficiency syndrome. *Ann Intern Med* 1985;**102**:747–52.

38 **Jules-Elysee KM**, Stover DE, Zaman MB, et al. Aerosolized pentamidine: effect on diagnosis and presentation of Pneumocystis carinii pneumonia. *Ann Intern Med* 1990;**112**:750–7.

39 **Levine SJ**, Kennedy D, Shelhamer JH, et al. Diagnosis of Pneumocystis carinii pneumonia by multiple lobe, site-directed bronchoalveolar lavage with immunofluorescent monoclonal antibody staining in human immunodeficiency virus-infected patients receiving aerosolized pentamidine chemoprophylaxis. *Am Rev Respir Dis* 1992;**146**:838–43.

40 **Yung RC**, Weinacker AB, Steiger DJ, et al. Upper and middle lobe bronchoalveolar lavage to diagnose Pneumocystis carinii pneumonia. *Am Rev Respir Dis* 1993;**148**(6 Pt 1):1563–6.

41 **Salomon N**, Perlman DC. Cytomegalovirus pneumonia. *Semin Respir Infect* 1999;**14**:353–8.

42 **Clelland C**, Higenbottam T, Stewart S, et al. Bronchoalveolar lavage and transbronchial lung biopsy during acute rejection and infection in heart-lung transplant patients. Studies of cell counts, lymphocyte phenotypes, and expression of HLA-DR and interleukin-2 receptor. *Am Rev Respir Dis* 1993;**147**(6 Pt 1):1386–92.

43 **Rawlinson WD**. Diagnosis of human cytomegalovirus infection and disease. *Pathology* 1999;**31**:109–15.

44 **Denning DW**. Invasive aspergillosis. *Clin Infect Dis* 1998;**26**:781–803; quiz 804–5.

45 **Stevens DA**, Kan VL, Judson MA, et al. Practice guidelines for diseases caused by Aspergillus. Infectious Diseases Society of America. *Clin Infect Dis* 2000;**30**:696–709.

46 **McWhinney PH**, Kibbler CC, Hamon MD, et al. Progress in the diagnosis and management of aspergillosis in bone marrow transplantation: 13 years' experience. *Clin Infect Dis* 1993;**17**:397–404.

47 **Denning DW**, Evans EG, Kibbler CC, et al. Guidelines for the investigation of invasive fungal infections in haematological malignancy and solid organ transplantation. British Society for Medical Mycology. *Eur J Clin Microbiol Infect Dis* 1997;**16**:424–36.

48 **Kahn FW**, Jones JM, England DM. The role of bronchoalveolar lavage in the diagnosis of invasive pulmonary aspergillosis. *Am J Clin Pathol* 1986;**86**:518–23.

49 **Levy H**, Horak DA, Tegtmeier BR, et al. The value of bronchoalveolar lavage and bronchial washings in the diagnosis of invasive pulmonary aspergillosis. *Respir Med* 1992;**86**:243–8.

50 **Maertens J**, Verhaegen J, Demuynck H, et al. Autopsy-controlled prospective evaluation of serial screening for circulating galactomannan by a sandwich enzyme-linked immunosorbent assay for hematological patients at risk for invasive aspergillosis. *J Clin Microbiol* 1999;**37**:3223–8.

51 **Klech H**, Hutter C. Clinical guidelines and indications for bronchoalveolar lavage (BAL): report of the European Society of Pneumonology Task Group on BAL. *Eur Respir J* 1990;**3**:938–69.

52 **Allen JN**, Davis WB, Pacht ER. Diagnostic significance of increased bronchoalveolar lavage fluid eosinophils. *Am Rev Respir Dis* 1990;**142**:642–7.

53 **Velay B**, Pages J, Cordier JF, et al. Hypereosinophilia in bronchoalveolar lavage. Diagnostic value and correlations with blood eosinophilia. *Rev Mal Respir* 1987;**4**:257–60.

54 **Steinberg KP**, Milberg JA, Martin TR, et al. Evolution of bronchoalveolar cell populations in the adult respiratory distress syndrome. *Am J Respir Crit Care Med* 1994;**150**:113–22.

55 **Meduri GU**, Headley AS, Golden E, et al. Effect of prolonged methylprednisolone therapy in unresolving acute respiratory distress syndrome: a randomized controlled trial. *JAMA* 1998;**280**:159–65.

56 **Pittet JF**, Mackersie RC, Martin TR, et al. Biological markers of acute lung injury: prognostic and pathogenetic significance. *Am J Respir Crit Care Med* 1997;**155**:1187–205.

57 **Donnelly SC**, Strieter RM, Kunkel SL, et al. Interleukin-8 and development of adult respiratory distress syndrome in at-risk patient groups. *Lancet* 1993;**341**:643–7.

58 **Martin C**, Papazian L, Payan MJ, et al. Pulmonary fibrosis correlates with outcome in adult respiratory distress syndrome. A study in mechanically ventilated patients. *Chest* 1995;**107**:196–200.

59 **Chesnutt AN**, Matthay MA, Tibayan FA, et al. Early detection of type III procollagen peptide in acute lung injury. Pathogenetic and prognostic significance. *Am J Respir Crit Care Med* 1997;**156**(3 Pt 1):840–5.

60 **Adrie C**, Monchi M, Tuan Dinh-Xuan A, et al. Exhaled and nasal nitric oxide as a marker of pneumonia in ventilated patients. *Am J Respir Crit Care Med* 2001;**163**:1143–9.

61 **Brett SJ**, Evans TW. Measurement of endogenous nitric oxide in the lungs of patients with the acute respiratory distress syndrome. *Am J Respir Crit Care Med* 1998;**157**(3 Pt 1):993–7.

62 **Carpenter CT**, Price PV, Christman BW. Exhaled breath condensate isoprostanes are elevated in patients with acute lung injury or ARDS. *Chest* 1998;**114**:1653–9.

63 **Schubert JK**, Muller WP, Benzing A, et al. Application of a new method for analysis of exhaled gas in critically ill patients. *Intensive Care Med* 1998;**24**:415–21.

64 **Tocino I**. Chest imaging in the intensive care unit. *Eur J Radiol* 1996;**23**:46–57.

65 **Maffessanti M**, Berlot G, Bortolotto P. Chest roentgenology in the intensive care unit: an overview. *Eur Radiol* 1998;**8**:69–78.

66 **Helfaer M**. To chest x-rays and beyond. *Crit Care Med* 1999;**27**:1676–7.

67 **Price MB**, Grant MJ, Welkie K. Financial impact of elimination of routine chest radiographs in a pediatric intensive care unit. *Crit Care Med* 1999;**27**:1588–93.

68 **American College of Radiology**. ACR appropriateness criteria: routine portable daily X-ray. 1999.

69 **Bekemeyer WB**, Crapo RO, Calhoon S, et al. Efficacy of chest radiography in a respiratory intensive care unit. A prospective study. *Chest* 1985;**88**:691–6.

70 **Greenbaum DM**, Marschall KE. The value of routine daily chest x-rays in intubated patients in the medical intensive care unit. *Crit Care Med* 1982;**10**:29–30.

71 **Strain DS**, Kinasewitz GT, Vereen LE, et al. Value of routine daily chest x-rays in the medical intensive care unit. *Crit Care Med* 1985;**13**:534–6.

72 **American College of Radiology**. ACR standards for the performance of pediatric and adult bedside (portable) chest radiography. 1997.

73 **Dunbar RD**. Radiologic appearance of compromised thoracic catheters, tubes, and wires. *Radiol Clin North Am* 1984;**22**:699–722.

74 **Conrardy PA**, Goodman LR, Lainge F, et al. Alteration of endotracheal tube position. Flexion and extension of the neck. *Crit Care Med* 1976;**4**:7–12.

75 **Goodman LR**, Conrardy PA, Laing F, et al. Radiographic evaluation of endotracheal tube position. *AJR* 1976;**127**:433–4.

76 **Satyadas T**, Nasir N, Erel E, Mudan SS. Iatrogenic tracheal rupture: a novel approach to repair and a review of the literature. *J Trauma* 2003;**54**:369–71.

77 **Tsao MM**, Katz D. Central venous catheter-induced endocarditis: human correlate of the animal experimental model of endocarditis. *Rev Infect Dis* 1984;**6**:783–90.

78 **Gomez CM**, Palazzo MG. Pulmonary artery catheterization in anaesthesia and intensive care. *Br J Anaesth* 1998;**81**:945–56.

79 **Thomason JW**, Ely EW, Chiles C, et al. Appraising pulmonary edema using supine chest roentgenograms in ventilated patients. *Am J Respir Crit Care Med* 1998;**157**(5 Pt 1):1600–8.

80 **Milne EN**, Pistolesi M, Miniati M, et al. The radiologic distinction of cardiogenic and noncardiogenic edema. *AJR* 1985;**144**:879–94.

81 **Emamian SA**, Kaasbol MA, Olsen JF, et al. Accuracy of the diagnosis of pleural effusion on supine chest X-ray. *Eur Radiol* 1997;**7**:57–60.

82 **Eibenberger KL**, Dock WI, Ammann ME, et al. Quantification of pleural effusions: sonography versus radiography. *Radiology* 1994;**191**:681–4.

83 **Agusti AG**, Cardus J, Roca J, *et al.* Ventilation-perfusion mismatch in patients with pleural effusion: effects of thoracentesis. *Am J Respir Crit Care Med* 1997;**156**(4 Pt 1):1205–9.

84 **Talmor M**, Hydo L, Gershenwald JG, *et al.* Beneficial effects of chest tube drainage of pleural effusion in acute respiratory failure refractory to positive end-expiratory pressure ventilation. *Surgery* 1998;**123**:137–43.

85 **Lichtenstein D**, Hulot JS, Rabiller A, *et al.* Feasibility and safety of ultrasound-aided thoracentesis in mechanically ventilated patients. *Intensive Care Med* 1999;**25**:955–8.

86 **Keske U**. Ultrasound-aided thoracentesis in intensive care patients. *Intensive Care Med* 1999;**25**:896–7.

87 **Miller WT Jr**, Tino G, Friedburg JS. Thoracic CT in the intensive care unit: assessment of clinical usefulness. *Radiology* 1998;**209**:491–8.

88 **Intensive Care Society**. *Guidelines for the transport of the critically ill adult.* 1997.

89 **White CS**, Meyer CA, Wu J, *et al.* Portable CT: assessing thoracic disease in the intensive care unit. *AJR* 1999;**173**:1351–6.

90 **Gattinoni L**, Presenti A, Torresin A, *et al.* Adult respiratory distress syndrome profiles by computed tomography. *J Thorac Imaging* 1986;**1**:25–30.

91 **Desai SR**, Wells AU, Suntharalingam G, *et al.* Acute respiratory distress syndrome caused by pulmonary and extrapulmonary injury: a comparative CT study. *Radiology* 2001;**218**:689–93.

92 **Pelosi P**, Crotti S, Brazzi L, *et al.* Computed tomography in adult respiratory distress syndrome: what has it taught us? *Eur Respir J* 1996;**9**:1055–62.

93 **Wiener CM**, Kirk W, Albert RK. Prone position reverses gravitational distribution of perfusion in dog lungs with oleic acid-induced injury. *J Appl Physiol* 1990;**68**:1386–92.

94 **Snow N**, Bergin KT, Horrigan TP. Thoracic CT scanning in critically ill patients. Information obtained frequently alters management. *Chest* 1990;**97**:1467–70.

95 **Guerrero-Lopez F**, Vazquez-Mata G, Alcazar-Romero PP, *et al.* Evaluation of the utility of computed tomography in the initial assessment of the critical care patient with chest trauma. *Crit Care Med* 2000;**28**:1370–5.

96 **Enderson BL**, Abdalla R, Frame SB, *et al.* Tube thoracostomy for occult pneumothorax: a prospective randomized study of its use. *J Trauma-Injury Infect Crit Care* 1993;**35**:726–9; discussion 729–30.

97 **Wolfman NT**, Gilpin JW, Bechtold RE, *et al.* Occult pneumothorax in patients with abdominal trauma: CT studies. *J Comput Assist Tomogr* 1993;**17**:56–9.

98 **Garramone RR Jr**, Jacobs LM, Sahdev P. An objective method to measure and manage occult pneumothorax. *Surg Gynecol Obstet* 1991;**173**:257–61.

99 **Watson AC**, Hughes PD, Louise Harris M, *et al.* Measurement of twitch transdiaphragmatic, esophageal, and endotracheal tube pressure with bilateral anterolateral magnetic phrenic nerve stimulation in patients in the intensive care unit. *Crit Care Med* 2001;**29**:1325–31.

100 **Yang KL**, Tobin MJ. A prospective study of indexes predicting the outcome of trials of weaning from mechanical ventilation. *N Engl J Med* 1991;**324**:1445–50.

101 **Dantzker DR**, Brook CJ, Dehart P, *et al.* Ventilation-perfusion distributions in the adult respiratory distress syndrome. *Am Rev Respir Dis* 1979;**120**:1039–52.

102 **Krafft P**, Fridrich P, Pernerstorfer T, *et al.* The acute respiratory distress syndrome: definitions, severity and clinical outcome. An analysis of 101 clinical investigations. *Intensive Care Med* 1996;**22**:519–29.

103 **Covelli HD**, Nessan VJ, Tuttle WK 3rd. Oxygen derived variables in acute respiratory failure. *Crit Care Med* 1983;**11**:646–9.

104 **Marini JJ**, Ravenscraft SA. Mean airway pressure: physiologic determinants and clinical importance – part 2: clinical implications. *Crit Care Med* 1992;**20**:1604–16.

105 **Villar J**, Perez-Mendez L, Kacmarek RM. Current definitions of acute lung injury and the acute respiratory distress syndrome do not reflect their true severity and outcome. *Intensive Care Med* 1999;**25**:930–5.

106 **The Acute Respiratory Distress Syndrome Network**. Ventilation with lower tidal volumes as compared with traditional tidal volumes for acute lung injury and the acute respiratory distress syndrome. *N Engl J Med* 2000;**342**:1301–8.

107 **Roupie E**, Dambrosio M, Servillo G, *et al.* Titration of tidal volume and induced hypercapnia in acute respiratory distress syndrome. *Am J Respir Crit Care Med* 1995;**152**:121–8.

108 **Dreyfuss D**, Saumon G. Pressure-volume curves. Searching for the grail or laying patients with adult respiratory distress syndrome on Procrustes' bed? *Am J Respir Crit Care Med* 2001;**163**:2–3.

2 Oxygen delivery and consumption in the critically ill

R M Leach, D F Treacher

Although traditionally interested in conditions affecting gas exchange within the lungs, the respiratory physician is increasingly, and appropriately, involved in the care of critically ill patients and therefore should be concerned with systemic as well as pulmonary oxygen transport. Oxygen is the substrate that cells use in the greatest quantity and upon which aerobic metabolism and cell integrity depend. Since the tissues have no storage system for oxygen, a continuous supply at a rate that matches changing metabolic requirements is necessary to maintain aerobic metabolism and normal cellular function. Failure of oxygen supply to meet metabolic needs is the feature common to all forms of circulatory failure or "shock". Prevention, early identification, and correction of tissue hypoxia are therefore necessary skills in managing the critically ill patient and this requires an understanding of oxygen transport, delivery, and consumption.

OXYGEN TRANSPORT

Oxygen transport describes the process by which oxygen from the atmosphere is supplied to the tissues as shown in fig 2.1 in which typical values are quoted for a healthy 75 kg individual. The phases in this process are either convective or diffusive: (1) the convective or "bulk flow" phases are alveolar ventilation and transport in the blood from the pulmonary to the systemic microcirculation: these are energy requiring stages that rely on work performed by the respiratory and cardiac "pumps"; and (2) the diffusive phases are the movement of oxygen from alveolus to pulmonary capillary and from systemic capillary to cell: these stages are passive and depend on the gradient of oxygen partial pressures, the tissue capillary density (which determines diffusion distance), and the ability of the cell to take up and use oxygen.

This chapter will not consider oxygen transport within the lungs but will focus on transport from the heart to non-pulmonary tissues, dealing specifically with global and regional oxygen delivery, the relationship between oxygen delivery and consumption, and some of the recent evidence relating to the uptake and utilisation of oxygen at the tissue and cellular level.

OXYGEN DELIVERY

Global oxygen delivery (Do_2) is the total amount of oxygen delivered to the tissues per minute irrespective of the distribution of blood flow. Under resting conditions with normal distribution of cardiac output it is more than adequate to meet the total oxygen requirements of the tissues (Vo_2) and ensure that aerobic metabolism is maintained.

Recognition of inadequate global Do_2 can be difficult in the early stages because the clinical features are often non-specific. Progressive metabolic acidosis, hyperlactataemia, and falling mixed venous oxygen saturation (Svo_2), as well as organ specific features such as oliguria and impaired level of consciousness, suggest inadequate Do_2. Serial lactate measurements can indicate both progression of the underlying problem and the response to treatment. Raised lactate levels (>2 mmol/l) may be caused by either increased production or reduced hepatic metabolism. Both mechanisms frequently apply in the critically ill patient since a marked reduction in Do_2 produces global tissue ischaemia and impairs liver function.

Table 2.1 illustrates the calculation of Do_2 from the oxygen content of arterial blood (Cao_2) and cardiac output (Qt) with examples for a normal subject and a patient presenting with hypoxaemia, anaemia, and a reduced Qt. The effects of providing an increased inspired oxygen concentration, red blood cell transfusion, and increasing cardiac output are shown. This emphasises that: (1) Do_2 may be compromised by anaemia, oxygen desaturation, and a low cardiac output, either singly or in combination; (2) global Do_2 depends on oxygen saturation rather than partial pressure and there is therefore little extra benefit in increasing Pao_2 above 9 kPa since, due to the sigmoid shape of the oxyhaemoglobin dissociation curve, over 90% of haemoglobin (Hb) is already saturated with oxygen at that level. This does not apply to the diffusive component of oxygen transport that does depend on the gradient of oxygen partial pressure.

Although blood transfusion to polycythaemic levels might seem an appropriate way to increase Do_2, blood viscosity increases markedly above 100 g/l. This impairs flow and oxygen delivery, particularly in smaller vessels and when the perfusion pressure is reduced, and will therefore exacerbate tissue hypoxia.[1] Recent evidence suggests that even the traditionally accepted Hb concentration for critically ill patients of approximately 100 g/l may be too high since an improved outcome was observed if Hb was maintained between 70 and 90 g/l with the exception of patients with coronary artery disease in whom a level of 100 g/l remains appropriate.[2] With the appropriate Hb achieved by transfusion, and since the oxygen saturation (Sao_2) can usually be maintained above 90% with supplemental oxygen (or if necessary by intubation and mechanical ventilation), cardiac output is the variable that is most often manipulated to achieve the desired global Do_2 levels.

Abbreviations: So_2, oxygen saturation (%); Po_2, oxygen partial pressure (kPa); Pio_2, inspired Po_2; Peo_2, mixed expired Po_2; $Peco_2$, mixed expired Pco_2; Pao_2, alveolar Po_2; Pao_2, arterial Po_2; Sao_2, arterial So_2; Svo_2, mixed venous So_2; Qt, cardiac output; Hb, haemoglobin; Cao_2, arterial O_2 content; Cvo_2, mixed venous O_2 content; Vo_2, oxygen consumption; Vco_2, CO_2 production; O_2R, oxygen return; Do_2, oxygen delivery; Vi/e, minute volume, inspiratory/expiratory.

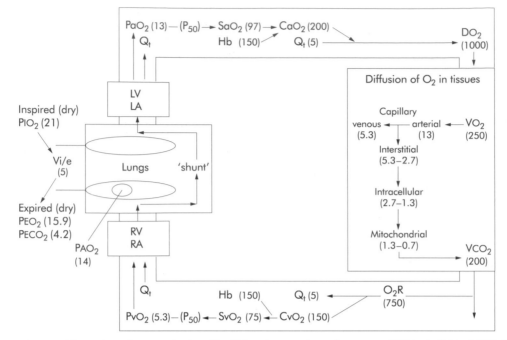

Figure 2.1 Oxygen transport from atmosphere to mitochondria. Values in parentheses for a normal 75 kg individual (BSA 1.7 m²) breathing air (FiO₂ 0.21) at standard atmospheric pressure (P_B 101 kPa). Partial pressures of O₂ and CO₂ (PO₂, PCO₂) in kPa; saturation in %; contents (CaO₂, CvO₂) in ml/l; Hb in g/l; blood/gas flows (Qt, Vi/e) in l/min. P₅₀ = position of oxygen haemoglobin dissociation curve; it is PO₂ at which 50% of haemoglobin is saturated (normally 3.5 kPa). DO₂ = oxygen delivery; VO₂ = oxygen consumption, VCO₂ = carbon dioxide production; PIO₂, PEO₂ = inspired and mixed expired PO₂; PECO₂ = mixed expired PCO₂; PAO₂ = alveolar PO₂.

OXYGEN CONSUMPTION

Global oxygen consumption (VO₂) measures the total amount of oxygen consumed by the tissues per minute. It can be measured directly from inspired and mixed expired oxygen concentrations and expired minute volume, or derived from the cardiac output (Qt) and arterial and venous oxygen contents:

$$VO_2 = Qt \times (CaO_2 - CvO_2)$$

Directly measured VO₂ is slightly greater than the derived value that does not include alveolar oxygen consumption. It is important to use the directly measured rather than the derived value when studying the relationship between VO₂ and DO₂ to avoid problems of mathematical linkage.[3]

The amount of oxygen consumed (VO₂) as a fraction of oxygen delivery (DO₂) defines the oxygen extraction ratio (OER):

$$OER = VO_2/DO_2$$

In a normal 75 kg adult undertaking routine activities, VO₂ is approximately 250 ml/min with an OER of 25% (fig 2.1), which increases to 70–80% during maximal exercise in the well trained athlete. The oxygen not extracted by the tissues returns to the lungs and the mixed venous saturation (SvO₂) measured in the pulmonary artery represents the pooled venous saturation from all organs. It is influenced by changes in both global DO₂ and VO₂ and, provided the microcirculation

and the mechanisms for cellular oxygen uptake are intact, a value above 70% indicates that global DO₂ is adequate.

A mixed venous sample is necessary because the saturation of venous blood from different organs varies considerably. For example, the hepatic venous saturation is usually 40–50% but the renal venous saturation may exceed 80%, reflecting the considerable difference in the balance between the metabolic requirements of these organs and their individual oxygen deliveries.

CLINICAL FACTORS AFFECTING METABOLIC RATE AND OXYGEN CONSUMPTION

The cellular metabolic rate determines VO₂. The metabolic rate increases during physical activity, with shivering, hyperthermia and raised sympathetic drive (pain, anxiety). Similarly, certain drugs such as adrenaline[4] and feeding regimens containing excessive glucose increase VO₂. Mechanical ventilation eliminates the metabolic cost of breathing which, although normally less than 5% of the total VO₂, may rise to 30% in the catabolic critically ill patient with respiratory distress. It allows the patient to be sedated, given analgesia and, if necessary, paralysed, further reducing VO₂.

Table 2.1 Relative effects of changes in PaO₂, haemoglobin (Hb), and cardiac output (Qt) on oxygen delivery (DO₂)

	FiO₂	PaO₂ (kPa)	SaO₂ (%)	Hb (g/l)	Dissolved O₂ (ml/l)	CaO₂ (ml/l)	Qt (l/min)	DO₂ (ml/min)	DO₂ (% change)‡
Normal*	0.21	13.0	96	130	3.0	170	5.3	900	0
Patient†	0.21	6.0	75	70	1.4	72	4.0	288	− 68
↑FiO₂	0.35	9.0	92	70	2.1	88	4.0	352	+ 22
↑↑FiO₂	0.60	16.5	98	70	3.8	96	4.0	384	+ 9
↑Hb	0.60	16.5	98	105	3.8	142	4.0	568	+48
↑Qt	0.60	16.5	98	105	3.8	142	6.0	852	+50

DO₂ = CaO₂ × Qt ml/min, CaO₂ = (Hb × SaO₂ × 1.34) + (PaO₂ × 0.23) ml/l where FiO₂ = fractional inspired oxygen concentration; PaO₂, SaO₂, CaO₂ = partial pressure, saturation and content of oxygen in arterial blood; Qt = cardiac output. 1.34 ml is the volume of oxygen carried by 1 g of 100% saturated Hb. PaO₂ (kPa) × 0.23 is the amount of oxygen in physical solution in 1 l of blood, which is less than <3% of total CaO₂ for normal PaO₂ (ie <14 kPa). *Normal 75 kg subject at rest. †Patient with hypoxaemia, anaemia, reduced cardiac output, and evidence of global tissue hypoxia. ‡Change in DO₂ expressed as a percentage of the preceding value.

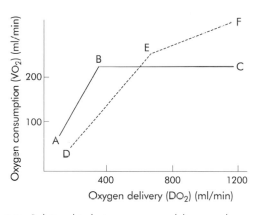

Figure 2.2 Relationship between oxygen delivery and consumption.

RELATIONSHIP BETWEEN OXYGEN CONSUMPTION AND DELIVERY

The normal relationship between Vo_2 and Do_2 is illustrated by line ABC in fig 2.2. As metabolic demand (Vo_2) increases or Do_2 diminishes (C–B), OER rises to maintain aerobic metabolism and consumption remains independent of delivery. However, at point B—called critical Do_2 (cDo_2)—the maximum OER is reached. This is believed to be 60–70% and beyond this point any further increase in Vo_2 or decline in Do_2 must lead to tissue hypoxia.[5] In reality there is a family of such Vo_2/Do_2 relationships with each tissue/organ having a unique Vo_2/Do_2 relationship and value for maximum OER that may vary with stress and disease states. Although the technology currently available makes it impracticable to determine these organ specific relationships in the critically ill patient, it is important to realise that conclusions drawn about the genesis of individual organ failure from the "global" diagram are potentially flawed.

In critical illness, particularly in sepsis, an altered global relationship is believed to exist (broken line DEF in fig 2.2). The slope of maximum OER falls (DE *v* AB), reflecting the reduced ability of tissues to extract oxygen, and the relationship does not plateau as in the normal relationship. Hence consumption continues to increase (E–F) to "supranormal" levels of Do_2, demonstrating so called "supply dependency" and the presence of a covert oxygen debt that would be relieved by further increasing Do_2.[6]

The relationship between global Do_2 and Vo_2 in critically ill patients has received considerable attention over the past two decades. Shoemaker and colleagues demonstrated a relationship between Do_2 and Vo_2 in the early postoperative phase that had prognostic implications such that patients with higher values had an improved survival.[7] A subsequent randomised placebo controlled trial in a similar group of patients showed improved survival if the values for Do_2 (>600 ml/min/m²) and Svo_2 (>70%) that had been achieved by the survivors in the earlier study were set as therapeutic targets ("goal directed therapy").[8]

This evidence encouraged the use of "goal directed therapy" in patients with established ("late") septic shock and organ dysfunction in the belief that this strategy would increase Vo_2 and prevent multiple organ failure. Do_2 was increased using vigorous intravenous fluid loading and inotropes, usually dobutamine. The mathematical linkage caused by calculating both Vo_2 and Do_2 using common measurements of Qt and Cao_2[3] and the "physiological" linkage resulting from the metabolic effects of inotropes increasing both Vo_2 and Do_2 were confounding factors in many of these studies.[9] This approach was also responsible for a considerable increase in the use of pulmonary artery catheters to direct treatment. However, after a decade of conflicting evidence from numerous small, often methodologically flawed studies, two major randomised

controlled studies finally showed that there was no benefit and possibly harm from applying this approach in patients with established "shock".[10 11] Interestingly, these studies also found that those patients who neither increased their Do_2 spontaneously nor in response to treatment had a particularly poor outcome. This suggested that patients with late "shock" had "poor physiological reserve" with myocardial and other organ failure caused by fundamental cellular dysfunction. These changes would be unresponsive to Shoemaker's goals that had been successful in "early" shock. Indeed, one might predict that, in patients with the increased endothelial permeability and myocardial dysfunction that typifies late "shock", aggressive fluid loading would produce widespread tissue oedema impairing both pulmonary gas exchange and tissue oxygen diffusion. The reported increase in mortality associated with the use of pulmonary artery catheters[12] may reflect the adverse effects of their use in attempting to achieve supranormal levels of Do_2.

SHOULD GOAL DIRECTED THERAPY BE ABANDONED?

Recent studies examining perioperative "optimisation" in patients, many of whom also had significant pre-existing cardiopulmonary dysfunction, have confirmed that identifying and treating volume depletion and poor myocardial performance at an early stage is beneficial.[13-16] This was the message from Shoemaker's studies 20 years ago, but unfortunately it was overinterpreted and applied to inappropriate patient populations causing the confusion that has only recently been resolved. Thus, adequate volume replacement in relatively volume depleted perioperative patients is entirely appropriate. However, the strategy of using aggressive fluid replacement and vasoactive agents in pursuit of supranormal "global" goals does not improve survival in patients presenting late with incipient or established multiorgan failure.

This saga highlights the difference between "early" and "late" shock and the concept well known to traumatologists as the "golden hour". Of the various forms of circulatory shock, two distinct groups can be defined: those with hypovolaemic, cardiogenic, and obstructive forms of shock (group 1) have the primary problem of a low cardiac output impairing Do_2; those with septic, anaphylactic, and neurogenic shock (group 2) have a problem with the distribution of Do_2 between and within organs—that is, abnormalities of regional Do_2 in addition to any impairment of global Do_2. Sepsis is also associated with cellular/metabolic defects that impair the uptake and utilisation of oxygen by cells. Prompt effective treatment of "early" shock may prevent progression to "late" shock and organ failure. In group 1 the peripheral circulatory response is physiologically appropriate and, if the global problem is corrected by intravenous fluid administration, improvement in myocardial function or relief of the obstruction, the peripheral tissue consequences of prolonged inadequacy of global Do_2 will not develop. However, if there is delay in instituting effective treatment, then shock becomes established and organ failure supervenes. Once this late stage has been reached, manipulation of the "global" or convective components of Do_2 alone will be ineffective. Global Do_2 should nonetheless be maintained by fluid resuscitation to correct hypovolaemia and inotropes to support myocardial dysfunction.

REGIONAL OXYGEN DELIVERY

Hypoxia in specific organs is often the result of disordered regional distribution of blood flow both between and within organs rather than inadequacy of global Do_2.[17] The importance of regional factors in determining tissue oxygenation should not be surprising since, under physiological conditions of metabolic demand such as exercise, alterations in local vascular tone ensure the necessary increase in regional and overall

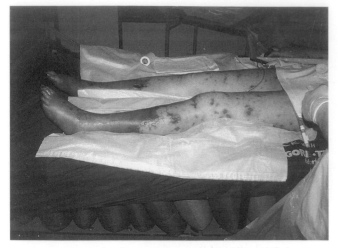

Figure 2.3 Example of tissue ischaemia and necrosis from extensive microvascular and macrovascular occlusion in a patient with severe meningococcal sepsis.

blood flow—that is, "consumption drives delivery". It is therefore important to distinguish between global and regional Do_2 when considering the cause of tissue hypoxia in specific organs. Loss of normal autoregulation in response to humoral factors during sepsis or prolonged hypotension can cause severe "shunting" and tissue hypoxia despite both global Do_2 and Svo_2 being normal or raised.[18] In these circumstances, improving peripheral distribution and cellular oxygen utilisation will be more effective than further increasing global Do_2. Regional and microcirculatory distribution of cardiac output is determined by a complex interaction of endothelial, neural, metabolic, and pharmacological factors. In health, many of these processes have been intensively investigated and well reviewed elsewhere.[19]

Until recently the endothelium had been perceived as an inert barrier but it is now realised that it has a profound effect on vascular homeostasis, acting as a dynamic interface between the underlying tissue and the many components of flowing blood. In concert with other vessel wall cells, the endothelium not only maintains a physical barrier between the blood and body tissues but also modulates leucocyte migration, angiogenesis, coagulation, and vascular tone through the release of both constrictor (endothelin) and relaxing factors (nitric oxide, prostacyclin, adenosine).[20] The differential release of such factors has an important role in controlling the distribution of regional blood flow during both health and critical illness. The endothelium is both exposed to and itself produces many inflammatory mediators that influence vascular tone and other aspects of endothelial function. For example, nitric oxide production is increased in septic shock following induction of nitric oxide synthase in the vessel wall. Inhibition of nitric oxide synthesis increased vascular resistance and systemic blood pressure in patients with septic shock, but no outcome benefit could be demonstrated.[21] Similarly, capillary microthrombosis following endothelial damage and neutrophil activation is probably a more common cause of local tissue hypoxia than arterial hypoxaemia (fig 2.3). Manipulation of the coagulation system, for example, using activated protein C may reduce this thrombotic tendency and improve outcome as shown in a recent randomised, placebo controlled, multicentre study in patients with severe sepsis.[22]

The clinical implications of disordered regional blood flow distribution vary considerably with the underlying pathological process. In the critically ill patient splanchnic perfusion is reduced by the release of endogenous vasoconstrictors and the gut mucosa is frequently further compromised by failure to maintain enteral nutrition. In sepsis and experimental endotoxaemia the oxygen extraction ratio is reduced and the critical Do_2 increased to a greater extent in splanchnic tissue than

in skeletal muscle.[23] This tendency to splanchnic ischaemia renders the gut mucosa "leaky", allowing translocation of endotoxin and possibly bacteria into the portal circulation. This toxic load may overwhelm hepatic clearance producing widespread endothelial damage. Treatment aimed at maintaining or improving splanchnic perfusion reduces the incidence of multiple organ failure and mortality.[24]

Although increasing global Do_2 may improve blood flow to regionally hypoxic tissues by raising blood flow through all capillary beds, this is an inefficient process and, if achieved using vasoactive drugs, may adversely affect regional distribution, particularly to the kidneys and splanchnic beds. The potent α receptor agonist noradrenaline is frequently used to counteract sepsis induced vasodilation and hypotension. The increase in blood pressure may improve perfusion to certain hypoxia sensitive vital organs but may also compromise blood flow to other organs, particularly the splanchnic bed. The role of vasodilators is less well defined: tissue perfusion is frequently already compromised by systemic hypotension and a reduced systemic vascular resistance, and their effect on regional distribution is unpredictable and may impair blood flow to vital organs despite increasing global Do_2. In a group of critically ill patients prostacyclin increased both Do_2 and Vo_2 and this was interpreted as indicating that there was a previously unidentified oxygen debt. However, there is no convincing evidence that vasodilators improve outcome in critically ill patients. An alternative strategy that attempts to redirect blood flow from overperfused non-essential tissues such as skin and muscle tissues to underperfused "vital" organs by exploiting the differences in receptor population and density between different arteries is theoretically attractive. While dobutamine may reduce splanchnic perfusion, dopexamine hydrochloride has dopaminergic and β-adrenergic but no α-adrenergic effects and may selectively increase renal and splanchnic blood flow.[25]

OXYGEN TRANSPORT FROM CAPILLARY BLOOD TO INDIVIDUAL CELLS

The delivery of oxygen from capillary blood to the cell depends on:

- factors that influence diffusion (fig 2.4);
- the rate of oxygen delivery to the capillary (Do_2);
- the position of the oxygen-haemoglobin dissociation relationship (P_{50});
- the rate of cellular oxygen utilisation and uptake (Vo_2).

The sigmoid oxygen-haemoglobin dissociation relationship is influenced by various physicochemical factors and its position is defined by the Pao_2 at which 50% of the Hb is saturated (P_{50}), normally 3.5 kPa. An increase in P_{50} or rightward shift in this relationship reduces the Hb saturation (Sao_2) for any given Pao_2, thereby increasing tissue oxygen availability. This is caused by pyrexia, acidosis, and an increase in intracellular phosphate, notably 2,3-diphosphoglycerate (2,3-DPG). The importance of correcting hypophosphataemia, often found in diabetic ketoacidosis and sepsis, is frequently overlooked.[26]

Mathematical models of tissue hypoxia show that the fall in cellular oxygen resulting from an increase in intercapillary distance is more severe if the reduction in tissue Do_2 is caused by "hypoxic" hypoxia (a fall in Pao_2) rather than "stagnant" (a fall in flow) or "anaemic" hypoxia (fig 2.5).[27] Studies in patients with hypoxaemic respiratory failure have also shown that it is Pao_2 rather than Do_2—that is, diffusion rather than convection—that has the major influence on outcome.[9]

Thus, tissue oedema due to increased vascular permeability or excessive fluid loading may result in impaired oxygen diffusion and cellular hypoxia, particularly in clinical situations associated with arterial hypoxaemia. In these situations, avoiding tissue oedema may improve tissue oxygenation.

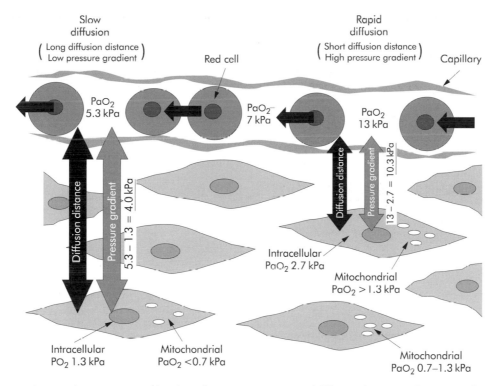

Figure 2.4 Diagram showing the importance of local capillary oxygen tension and diffusion distance in determining the rate of oxygen delivery and the intracellular Po₂. On the left there is a low capillary Po₂ and pressure gradient for oxygen diffusion with an increased diffusion distance resulting in low intracellular and mitochondrial Po₂. On the right the higher Po₂ pressure gradient and the shorter diffusion distance result in significantly higher intracellular Po₂ values.

OXYGEN DELIVERY AT THE TISSUE LEVEL

Individual organs and cells vary considerably in their sensitivity to hypoxia.[28] Neurons, cardiomyocytes, and renal tubular cells are exquisitely sensitive to a sudden reduction in oxygen supply and are unable to survive sustained periods of hypoxia, although ischaemic preconditioning does increase tolerance to hypoxia. Following complete cessation of cerebral perfusion, nuclear magnetic resonance (NMR) measurements show a 50% decrease in cellular adenosine triphosphate (ATP) within 30 seconds and irreversible damage occurs within 3 minutes. Mechanisms have developed in other tissues to survive longer without oxygen: the kidneys and liver can tolerate 15–20 minutes of total hypoxia, skeletal muscle 60–90 minutes, and vascular smooth muscle 24–72 hours. The most extreme example of hypoxic tolerance is that of hair and nails which continue to grow for several days after death.

Variation in tissue tolerance to hypoxia has important clinical implications. In an emergency, maintenance of blood flow to the most hypoxia sensitive organs should be the primary goal. Hypoxic brain damage after cardiorespiratory collapse will leave a patient incapable of independent life even if the other organ systems survive. Although tissue death may not occur as rapidly in less oxygen sensitive tissues, prolonged failure to make the diagnosis has equally serious consequences. For example, skeletal muscle may survive severe ischaemia for several hours but failure to remove the causative arterial embolus will result in muscle necrosis with the release into the circulation of myoglobin and other toxins and activation of the inflammatory response.

Tolerance to hypoxia differs in health and disease. In a septic patient inhibition of enzyme systems and oxygen utilisation reduces hypoxic tolerance.[29] Methods aimed at enhancing metabolic performance including the use of alternative substrates, techniques to inhibit endotoxin induced cellular damage, and drugs to reduce oxidant induced intracellular damage are currently under investigation. Ischaemic preconditioning of the heart and skeletal muscle is recognised both in vivo and in experimental models. Progressive or repeated exposure to hypoxia enhances tissue tolerance to oxygen deprivation in much the same way as altitude acclimatisation. An acclimatised mountaineer at the peak of Mount Everest can tolerate a Pao₂ of 4–4.5 kPa for several hours, which would result in loss of consciousness within a few minutes in a normal subject at sea level.

What is the critical level of tissue oxygenation below which cellular damage will occur? The answer mainly depends on the patient's circumstances, comorbid factors, and the duration of hypoxia. For example, young previously healthy patients with the acute respiratory distress syndrome tolerate prolonged hypoxaemia with saturations as low as 85% and can recover completely. In the older patient with widespread atheroma, however, prolonged hypoxaemia at such levels would be unacceptable.

RECOGNITION OF INADEQUATE TISSUE OXYGEN DELIVERY

The blood lactate concentration is an unreliable indicator of tissue hypoxia. It represents a balance between tissue production and consumption by hepatic and, to a lesser extent, by cardiac and skeletal muscle.[30] It may be raised or normal during hypoxia because the metabolic pathways utilising glucose during aerobic metabolism may be blocked at several points.[31] Inhibition of phosphofructokinase blocks glucose utilisation without an increase in lactate concentration. In contrast, endotoxin and sepsis may inactivate pyruvate dehydrogenase, preventing pyruvate utilisation in the Krebs cycle resulting in lactate production in the absence of hypoxia.[32] Similarly, a normal Do₂ with an unfavourable cellular redox state may result in a high lactate concentration, whereas compensatory reductions in energy state [ATP]/[ADP][Pi] or [NAD⁺]/[NADH] may be associated with a low lactate concentration during hypoxia.[33] Thus, the value of a single lactate measurement in the assessment of tissue hypoxia is limited.[34] The suggestion that pathological supply dependency occurs only when blood lactate concentrations are raised is incorrect as the

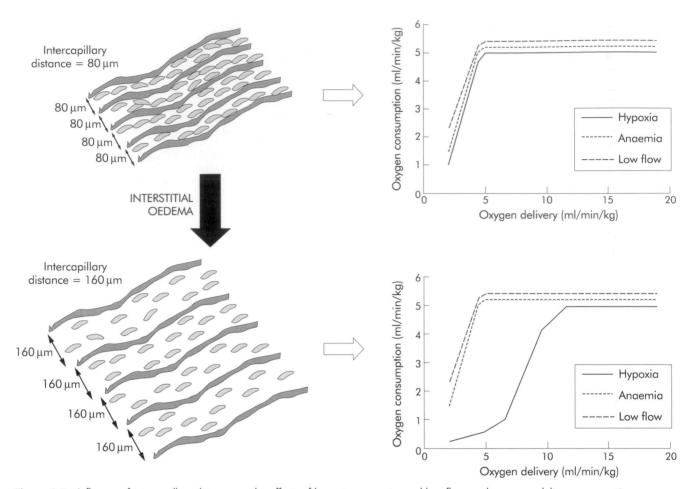

Figure 2.5 Influence of intercapillary distance on the effects of hypoxia, anaemia, and low flow on the oxygen delivery-consumption relationship. With a normal intercapillary distance illustrated in the top panels the DO_2/VO_2 relationship is the same for all interventions. However, in the lower panels an increased intercapillary distance, as would occur with tissue oedema, reducing DO_2 by progressive falls in arterial oxygen tension results in a change in the DO_2/VO_2 relationship with VO_2 falling at much higher levels of global DO_2. This altered relationship is not seen when DO_2 is reduced by anaemia or low blood flow.

same relationship may be found in patients with normal lactate concentrations.[35] Serial lactate measurements, particularly if corrected for pyruvate, may be of greater value.

Measurement of individual organ and tissue oxygenation is an important goal for the future. These measurements are difficult, require specialised techniques, and are not widely available. At present only near infrared spectroscopy and gastric tonometry have clinical applications in the detection of organ hypoxia.[24] In the future NMR spectroscopy may allow direct non-invasive measurement of tissue energy status and oxygen utilisation.[36]

CELLULAR OXYGEN UTILISATION

In general, eukaryotic cells are dependent on aerobic metabolism as mitochondrial respiration offers greater efficiency for extraction of energy from glucose than anaerobic glycolysis. The maintenance of oxidative metabolism is dependent on complex but poorly understood mechanisms for microvascular oxygen distribution and cellular oxygen uptake. Teleologically, the response to reduced blood flow in a tissue is likely to have evolved as an energy conserving mechanism when substrates, particularly molecular oxygen, are scarce. Pathways that use ATP are suppressed and alternative anaerobic pathways for ATP synthesis are induced.[37] This process involves oxygen sensing and transduction mechanisms, gene activation, and protein synthesis.

CELLULAR METABOLIC RESPONSE TO HYPOXIA

Although cellular metabolic responses to hypoxia remain poorly understood, the importance of understanding and

modifying the cellular responses to acute hypoxia in the critically ill patient has recently been appreciated. In isolated mitochondria the partial pressure of oxygen required to generate high energy phosphate bonds (ATP) that maintain aerobic cellular biochemical functions is only about 0.2–0.4 kPa.[17 28] However, in intact cell preparations hypoxia induced damage may result from failure of energy dependent membrane ion channels with subsequent loss of membrane integrity, changes in cellular calcium homeostasis, and oxygen dependent changes in cellular enzyme activity.[28] The sensitivity of an enzyme to hypoxia is a function of its PO_2 in mm Hg at which the enzyme rate is half maximum (Kmo_2),[28] and the wide range of values for a variety of cellular enzymes is shown in table 2.2, illustrating that certain metabolic functions are much more sensitive to hypoxia than others. Cellular tolerance to hypoxia may involve "hibernation" strategies that reduce metabolic rate, increased oxygen extraction from surrounding tissues, and enzyme adaptations that allow continuing metabolism at low partial pressures of oxygen.[37]

Anaerobic metabolism is important for survival in some tissues despite its inherent inefficiency: skeletal muscle increases glucose uptake by 600% during hypoxia and bladder smooth muscle can generate up to 60% of total energy requirement by anaerobic glycolysis.[38] In cardiac cells anaerobic glucose utilisation protects cell membrane integrity by maintaining energy dependent K^+ channels.[39] During hypoxic stress endothelial and vascular smooth muscle cells increase glucose transport through the expression of membrane glucose transporters (GLUT-1 and GLUT-4) and the production of glycolytic enzymes, thereby increasing anaerobic glycolysis and maintaining energy production.[38] High energy functions like ion

Table 2.2 Oxygen affinities of cellular enzymes expressed as the partial pressure of oxygen in mm Hg at which the enzyme rate is half maximum (Km_{O_2})

Enzyme	Substrate	Km_{O_2}
Glucose oxidase	Glucose	57
Xanthine oxidase	Hypoxanthine	50
Tryptophan oxygenase	Tryptophan	37
Nitric oxide synthase	L-arginine	30
Tyrosine hydroxylase	Tyrosine	25
NADPH oxidase	Oxygen	23
Cytochrome aa3	Oxygen	0.05

Key points

- Restoration of global oxygen delivery is an important goal in early resuscitation but thereafter circulatory manipulation to sustain "supranormal" oxygen delivery does not improve survival and may be harmful.
- Regional distribution of oxygen delivery is vital: if skin and muscle receive high blood flows but the splanchnic bed does not, the gut may become hypoxic despite high global oxygen delivery.
- Microcirculatory, tissue diffusion, and cellular factors influence the oxygen status of the cell and global measurements may fail to identify local tissue hypoxaemia.
- Supranormal levels of oxygen delivery cannot compensate for diffusion problems between capillary and cell, nor for metabolic failure within the cell.
- When assessing D_{O_2}/V_{O_2} relationships, direct measurements should be used to avoid errors due to mathematical linkage.
- Strategies to reduce metabolic rate to improve tissue oxygenation should be considered.

transport and protein production are downregulated to balance supply and demand.

Cellular oxygen utilisation is inhibited by metabolic poisons (cyanide) and toxins associated with sepsis such as endotoxin and other cytokines, thereby reducing energy production.[29] It is yet to be established whether there are important differences in the response to tissue hypoxia resulting from damage to mitochondrial and other intracellular functions as occurs in poisoning and sepsis, as opposed to situations such as exercise and altitude when oxygen consumption exceeds supply.

OXYGEN SENSING AND GENE ACTIVATION

The molecular basis for oxygen sensing has not been established and may differ between tissues. Current evidence suggests that, following activation of a "hypoxic sensor", the signal is transmitted through the cell by second messengers which then activate regulatory protein complexes termed transcription factors.[40 41] These factors translocate to the nucleus and bind with specific DNA sequences, activating various genes with the subsequent production of effector proteins. It has long been postulated that the "hypoxic sensor" may involve haem-containing proteins, redox potential or mitochondrial cytochromes.[42] Recent evidence from vascular smooth muscle suggests that hypoxia induced inhibition of electron transfer at complex III in the electron transport chain may act as the "hypoxic sensor".[43] This sensing mechanism is associated with the production of oxygen free radicals (ubiquinone cycle) that may act as second messengers in the activation of transcription factors.

Several transcription factors play a role in the response to tissue hypoxia including hypoxia inducible factor 1 (HIF-1), early growth response 1 (Erg-1), activator protein 1 (AP-1), nuclear factor kappa-B (NF-κB), and nuclear factor IL-6 (NF-IL-6). HIF-1 influences vascular homeostasis during hypoxia by activating the genes for erythropoietin, nitric oxide synthase, vascular endothelial growth factor, and glycolytic enzymes and glucose transport thereby altering metabolic function.[40] Erg-1 protein is also rapidly induced by hypoxia leading to transcription of tissue factor, which triggers prothrombotic events.[41]

REFERENCES

1 **Harrison MJG**, Kendall BE, Pollock S, et al. Effect of haematocrit on carotid stenosis and cerebral infarction. Lancet 1981;ii:114–5.
2 **Hebert PC**, Wells G, Blajchman MA, et al. A multicentre, randomized, controlled clinical trial of transfusion requirements in critical care. N Engl J Med 1999;**340**:409–17.
3 **Archie JP**. Mathematic coupling of data. A common source of error. Ann Surg 1981;**193**:296–303.
4 **Fellows IW**, Bennett T, MacDonald IA. The effects of adrenaline upon cardiovascular and metabolic functions in man. Clin Sci 1985;**69**:215–22.
5 **Schumacker PT**, Cain SM. The concept of a critical DO_2. Intensive Care Med 1987;**13**:223.
6 **Bihari D**, Smithies M, Gimson A, et al. The effect of vasodilation with prostacyclin on oxygen delivery and uptake in critically ill patients. N Engl J Med 1987;**317**:397–403.
7 **Shoemaker WC**, Appel PL, Waxman K, et al. Clinical trial of survivors' cardiorespiratory patterns as therapeutic goals in critically ill postoperative patients. Crit Care Med 1982;**10**:398–403.
8 **Shoemaker WC**, Appel PL, Kram HB, et al. Prospective trial of supranormal values of survivors as therapeutic goals in high-risk surgical patients. Chest 1988;**94**:1176–86.
9 **Leach RM**, Treacher DF. The relationship between oxygen delivery and consumption. Disease-a-Month 1994;**40**:301–68.
10 **Hayes MA**, Timmins AC, Yau E, et al. Elevation of systemic oxygen delivery in the treatment of critically ill patients. N Engl J Med 1994;**330**:1712–22.
11 **Gattinoni L**, Brazzi L, Pelosi P, et al. A trial of goal-orientated haemodynamic therapy in critically ill patients. N Engl J Med 1995;**333**:1025–32.
12 **Connors AF**, Speroff T, Dawson NV, et al. The effectivenss of right heart catheterisation in the initial care of critically ill patients. JAMA 1996;**276**:889–97.
13 **Boyd O**, Grounds M, Bennett ED. A randomised clinical trial of the effect of deliberate peri-operative increase of oxygen delivery on mortality in high-risk surgical patients. JAMA 1993;**270**:2699–708.
14 **Sinclair S**, James S, Singer M. Intraoperative intravascular volume optimisation and length of hospital stay after repair of proximal femoral fracture; randomised control trial. BMJ 1997;**315**:909–12.
15 **Wilson J**, Woods I, Fawcett J, et al. Reducing the risk of major elective surgery: randomised control trial of preoperative optimising of oxygen delivery. BMJ 1999;**318**:1099–103.
16 **Lobo SMA**, Salgado PF, Castillo VGT, et al. Effects of maximizing oxygen delivery on morbidity and mortality in high-risk surgical patients. Crit Care Med 2000;**28**:3396–404.
17 **Duling BR**. Oxygen, metabolism, and microcirculatory control. In: Kaley G, Altura BM, eds. Microcirculation. Volume 2. Baltimore: University Park Press, 401–29.
18 **Curtis SE**, Cain SM. Regional and systemic oxygen delivery/uptake relations and lactate flux in hyperdynamic, endotoxin-treated dogs. Am Rev Respir Dis 1992;**145**:348–54.
19 **Mulvany MJ**, Aalkjaer C, Heagerty AM, et al, eds. Resistance arteries, structure and function. Amsterdam: Elsevier Science, 1991.
20 **Karimova A**, Pinsky DJ. The endothelial response to oxygen deprivation: biology and clinical implications. Intensive Care Med 2001;**27**:19–31.
21 **Petros A**, Bennett A, Vallance P. Effect of nitric oxide synthase inhibitors on hypotension in patients with septic shock. Lancet 1991;**338**:1557–8.
22 **Bernard GR**, Vincent J-L, Laterre P-F, et al. Efficacy and safety of recombinant human activated protein C for severe sepsis. N Engl J Med 2001;**344**:699–709.
23 **Nelson DP**, Samsel RW, Wood LDH, et al. Pathological supply dependence of systemic and intestinal O_2 uptake during endotoxaemia. J Appl Physiol 1988;**64**:2410–9.
24 **Gutierrez G**, Palizas F, Doglio G, et al. Gastric intramucosal pH as a therapeutic index of tissue oxygenation in critically ill patients. Lancet 1992;**339**:195–9.
25 **Stephan H**, Sonntag H, Henning H, et al. Cardiovascular and renal haemodynamic effects of dopexamine: comparison with dopamine. Br J Anaesth 1990;**65**:380–7.
26 **Clebaux T**, Detry B, Reynaert M, et al. Re-estimation of the effects of inorganic phosphates on the equilibrium between oxygen and hemoglobin. Intensive Care Med 1992;**18**:222–5.
27 **Schumacker PT**, Samsel RW. Analysis of oxygen delivery and uptake relationships in the Krogh tissue model. J Appl Physiol 1989;**67**:1234–44.
28 **Robin ED**. Of men and mitochondria: coping with hypoxic dysoxia. Am Rev Respir Dis 1980;**122**:517–31.
29 **Bradley SG**. Cellular and molecular mechanisms of action of bacterial endotoxins. Ann Rev Microbiol 1979;**33**:67–94.

30 **Vincent J-L**, Roman A, De Backer D, *et al.* Oxygen uptake/supply dependency. *Am Rev Respir Dis* 1990;**142**:2–7.

31 **Cain SM**, Curtis SE. Experimental models of pathologic oxygen supply dependence. *Crit Care Med* 1991;**19**:603–11.

32 **Vary TC**, Siegel JH, Nakatani T, *et al.* Effects of sepsis on activity of pyruvate dehydrogenase complex in skeletal muscle and liver. *Am J Physiol* 1986;**250**:E634–9.

33 **Wilson DF**, Erecinska M, Drown C, *et al.* Effect of oxygen tension on cellular energetics. *Am J Physiol* 1973;**233**:C135–40.

34 **Silverman HJ**. Lack of a relationship between induced changes in oxygen consumption and changes in lactate levels. *Chest* 1991;**100**:1012–5.

35 **Mohsenifar Z**, Amin D, Jasper AC, *et al.* Dependence of oxygen consumption on oxygen delivery in patients with chronic congestive heart failure. *Chest* 1987;**92**:447–56.

36 **Leach RM**, Sheehan DW, Chacko VP, *et al.* Energy state, pH, and vasomotor tone during hypoxia in precontracted pulmonary and femoral arteries. *Am J Physiol* 2000;**278**:L294–304.

37 **Hochachka PW**, Buck LT, Doll CJ, *et al.* Unifying theory of hypoxia tolerance: molecular/metabolic defense and rescue mechanisms for surviving oxygen lack. *Proc Natl Acad Sci USA* 1996;**93**:9493–8.

38 **Cartee GD**, Dounen AG, Ramlai T, *et al.* Stimulation of glucose transport in skeletal muscle by hypoxia. *J Appl Physiol* 1991;**70**:1593–600.

39 **Paul RJ**. Smooth muscle energetics. *Ann Rev Physiol* 1989;**51**:331–49.

40 **Semenza GL**. Hypoxia-inducible factor 1: master regulator of O_2 homeostasis. *Curr Opin Genet Dev* 1998;**8**:588–94.

41 **Yan S-F**, Lu J, Zou YS, *et al.* Hypoxia-associated induction of early growth response-1 gene expression. *J Biol Chem* 1999;**274**:15030–40.

42 **Archer SL**, Weir EK, Reeve HL, *et al.* Molecular identification of O_2 sensors and O_2-sensitive potassium channels in the pulmonary circulation. *Adv Exp Med Biol* 2000;**475**:219–40.

43 **Leach RM**, Hill HS, Snetkov VA, *et al.* Divergent roles of glycolysis and the mitochondrial electron transport chain in hypoxic pulmonary vasoconstriction of the rat: identity of the hypoxic sensor. *J Physiol* 2001;**536**:211–24.

3 Critical care management of community acquired pneumonia

S V Baudouin

Community acquired pneumonia (CAP) is a common illness with an estimated incidence of 2–12 cases/1000 population per year.[1 2] The majority of cases of CAP are successfully managed outside hospital, but approximately 20% require hospital admission. Out of this group about 10% develop severe CAP and need treatment in an intensive care unit (ICU). The mortality of these patients can exceed 50%, and the purpose of this chapter is to review the management of severe CAP. Excellent guidelines for the management of CAP have been produced by several organisations including the British Thoracic Society (BTS), the American Thoracic Society (ATS), European and Infectious Disease Working Groups.[3–6] Revised BTS guidelines have recently been published[4] and previous ATS recommendations are being revised. Any practitioner who is responsible for patients with CAP should consult one of these documents. This chapter will discuss both general approaches to CAP and also highlight specific areas of critical care management.

ASSESSMENT OF SEVERITY

For the purposes of epidemiological studies, the definition of severe CAP as "CAP needing ICU admission" is adequate. In practical management terms, however, a more detailed method of assessment is needed. Severe CAP is almost always a multiorgan disease and patients with severe CAP at presentation will either already have, or will be rapidly developing, multiple organ failure. It is important that respiratory and other "front line" physicians appreciate this aspect of the disease. Apparent stability on high flow oxygen can rapidly change to respiratory, circulatory, and renal failure. Progressive loss of tissue oxygenation needs to be anticipated, recognised quickly, and rapid action taken to prevent its progression to established organ failure.

The BTS guidelines define severe pneumonia ("rule 1") as the presence of two or more of the following features on hospital admission[4]:

- Respiratory rate $\geq$30/minute
- Diastolic blood pressure $\leq$60 mm Hg
- Urea >7 mmol/l

The guidelines include three additional assessment recommendations. The presence of any one of these approximately doubles the rate of death:

- Altered mental status, confusion or an Abbreviated Mental Test score of <8/10
- Hypoxaemia (Po_2 <8 kPa or O_2 saturation <90%), with or without a raised Fio_2
- Bilateral or multilobar (more than two lobes) shadowing on the chest radiograph

In a number of studies, use of BTS "rule 1" identifies a group of inpatients with a greater than 20% mortality from CAP.[7]

The ATS guidelines on CAP include minor and major criteria for severity assessment. Minor criteria on admission include:

- Respiratory rate >30/minute
- Severe respiratory failure (Pao_2/Fio_2 <250 mm Hg)
- Bilateral involvement on chest radiograph
- Multilobe involvement on chest radiograph
- Systolic blood pressure <90 mm Hg
- Diastolic blood pressure <60 mm Hg

Major criteria at or following admission include:

- Need for mechanical ventilation
- Increase in the size of radiographic infiltrates $\geq$50% in the presence or absence of a clinical response or deterioration
- Need for vasopressor support for >4 hours
- Worsening renal function as defined by a serum creatinine of $\geq$180 mmol/l

Using the need for ICU admission as the end point, various combinations of minor and major criteria give different combinations of specificity and sensitivity.[1] In the presence of at least one of the ATS criteria sensitivity was 98% but specificity only 32%. Positive predictive power was much improved using a combination of two of three major criteria and multilobar involvement. Sensitivity was 78% and specificity 94%.

More than a decade ago the BTS performed a ground breaking study on severe CAP.[8] In their series 60 patients from 25 hospitals required ICU care in a 12 month period. One of the more striking findings was that eight patients were admitted to the ICU only after suffering cardiorespiratory arrest on general medical wards. In retrospect, six of these eight could have been identified using the BTS "rule 1" severity guide. In a related study CAP related deaths over 3 years in patients aged <65 years in the Nottingham area of the UK were retrospectively audited.[9] They found evidence of suboptimum care in a number of cases, including a lack of appreciation of disease severity, lack of input from senior doctors, and lack of suitable investigations including arterial blood gas measurements. These and other studies provided evidence of suboptimal management of patients with severe CAP in the late 1980s and early 1990s. They also produced clear and simple assessment tools and guidelines to improve practice. Unfortunately, recent reports suggest that these important lessons have not been learnt. McQuillan and coworkers recently performed a confidential inquiry into the quality of care before admission to the ICU[10] which covered a wide range of both medical and surgical admissions including patients with severe CAP. The study found that suboptimal care had been given to 54% and, importantly, that hospital mortality in this group was significantly higher than in those managed well (56% v 35%). Errors in the management of the airway, breathing, circulation, monitoring, and oxygen therapy were common.

Correct management of severe CAP before admission to the ICU is therefore essential. Recognition of the severity of illness is the first vital step, in which application of the BTS severity rules and screening pulse oximetry are useful tools. Repeated regular assessment by the same observer in the initial stages of the illness is necessary and rapid review by a critical care practitioner should be arranged for any patient who meets the BTS or similar severity criteria or who is deteriorating. The need for increasing F_{IO_2}, altered mental state (confusion, aggression), and the onset of either respiratory or metabolic acidosis are all signs of disease progression and the need for further intervention.

In the UK the recent publication of the Department of Health document "*Comprehensive Critical Care*"[11] suggests expanding high dependency or—in the new terminology—level 2 care. This would provide a suitable environment for the initial treatment of patients with severe CAP who do not need immediate mechanical ventilation. These patients are likely to benefit from more intensive monitoring (arterial line, central venous line, urinary catheter) and treatment (rapid correction of hypovolaemia, inotropic support, continuous positive airway pressure (CPAP), non-invasive ventilation (NIV)). Level 2 care also allows the rapid initiation of invasive mechanical ventilation when needed.

CO-MORBIDITY

The original BTS study on severe CAP pointed to the importance of pre-existing co-morbidity[8]: 63% of this group had serious pre-morbid conditions including chronic obstructive pulmonary disease (COPD, 32%), asthma (13%), and cardiac problems (15%). Other significant conditions included diabetes, chronic liver disease, chronic renal failure, and alcohol dependency. Immunosuppression was also a risk factor for severe CAP. The incidence of severe CAP increases with age and increasing age probably adversely affects outcome; analysis of 11 studies of CAP in the elderly[12] showed that more than 90% of pneumonia deaths occurred in patients over the age of 70.

MICROBIOLOGY

In the last decade a number of important facts have been established about the microbiology of CAP[1 2]: (1) a relatively small number of pathogens account for the majority of infections; (2) *Streptococcus pneumoniae* has been consistently shown to be the commonest pathogen in Europe and North America; and (3) in at least one third of cases no definite causative pathogen can be isolated. However, the relative importance of pathogens varies considerably worldwide. For example, in a report from Singapore, *Burkholderia pseudomallei* was the most common cause of severe CAP.[13]

In addition to *S pneumoniae*, other important pathogens in CAP include *Haemophilus influenza*, *Legionella* species, *Staphylococcus aureus*, Gram negative organisms, *Mycoplasma*, *Coxiella* species, and respiratory viruses. European and North American studies have found similar incidences of specific pathogens. In a survey of 16 studies of severe CAP the following pathogens were isolated: *S pneumoniae* 12–38%; *Legionella* spp 0–30%; *Staph aureus* 1–18%; and Gram negative enteric bacilli 2–34%.[1] There is an important change in the frequency of these pathogens depending on the severity of the illness (fig 3.1). In the UK there is a high relative frequency of *Legionella* and *Staph aureus* in severe CAP compared with cases cared for

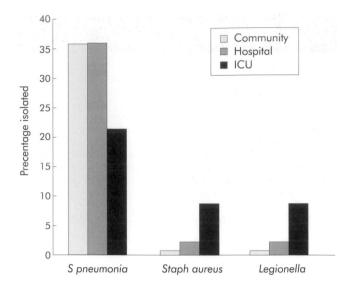

Figure 3.1 Percentage isolation of *S pneumoniae*, *Staph aureus*, and *Legionella* species from patients with CAP treated in the community, general medical wards, and intensive care units. *S pneumoniae* remains the commonest pathogen isolated in the critically ill but the frequency of *Staph aureus* and *Legionella* infections significantly increases in this group. Data adapted from the BTS guidelines.[4]

in the community or the general wards. The relative frequency of *S pneumoniae* is reduced in severe CAP, but it remains the most frequent pathogen isolated.

MICROBIOLOGICAL INVESTIGATION AND DIAGNOSIS

At least three strategies have been used in the microbiological diagnosis of severe CAP. These can be summarised as (1) the syndrome approach; (2) the laboratory based approach; and (3) the empirical approach.[1] The strengths or weaknesses of each of these strategies will be reviewed in the following sections.

The syndrome approach

This is based on the assumption that different pathogens cause distinct and non-overlapping clinical syndromes. The terms "typical" and "atypical" pneumonia were adopted to describe these syndromes. Typical pneumonia was caused by the pneumococcus and was said to present with pyrexia of greater than 39°C, pleuritic chest pain, a lobar distribution of consolidation, and an increase in immature granulocytes. Features of atypical pneumonia included a more gradual onset and a diffuse interstitial or alveolar pattern on the plain chest radiograph.

Numerous studies, however, have shown that clinical overlap between the different pathogens is great and that no single or combination of symptoms and plain chest radiology will reliably differentiate between the different pathogens.[1] In severe CAP the situation is even more difficult; case series of severe pneumococcal, staphylococcal, and legionella pneumonia show no reliable distinguishing features. In a recent series of 84 patients requiring ICU admission for severe legionella pneumonia, 39% had only unilateral radiographic changes at presentation.[14] Hyponatraemia is often quoted as a sign of legionella pneumonia but in this series[14] hyponatraemia was strongly associated with poor outcome, suggesting that it is a marker of disease severity rather than disease type.

The laboratory based approach

There are a number of reasons for attempting to identify precisely the pathogen in severe CAP: to confirm the diagnosis, to guide antibiotic choice, to define antibiotic sensitivities, and to provide epidemiological information. All current guidelines

Box 3.1 BTS guidelines for routine investigations in hospital for all patients with severe CAP

- Blood cultures
- Sputum or lower respiratory tract sample for Gram stain, routine culture, and sensitivity tests
- Pleural fluid analysis, if present
- Pneumococcal antigen test on sputum, blood, or urine
- Investigations for legionella pneumonia including (a) urine for legionella antigen, (b) sputum or lower respiratory tract samples for legionella culture and direct immunofluorescence, and (c) initial and follow up legionella serology
- Respiratory samples for direct immunofluorescence to respiratory viruses, Chlamydia species, and possibly Pneumocystis
- Initial and follow up serology for atypical pathogens

recommend intensive microbiological investigation. The BTS recommendations for routine investigations in severe CAP are summarised in box 3.1.[4] While it is difficult to disagree with this thorough approach to diagnosis, a number of practical problems require discussion. Firstly, there is no good evidence that this strategy alters the outcome of severe CAP and retrospective studies disagree about the impact of laboratory based microbiological testing on outcome.[15 16] In at least 30% of cases no pathogen can be isolated and this group has as good a prognosis. Outcome in severe CAP is also strongly related to secondary factors including the number of failed organs and co-morbidities. For these reasons the precise identification of the respiratory pathogen may have little impact on recovery. Secondly, current diagnostic tests are neither sensitive nor specific in severe CAP.[17] One difficulty is that isolation of a pathogen in severe CAP does not necessarily indicate causation unless the pathogen is never isolated from healthy individuals—for example, Mycobacterium tuberculosis. Respiratory tract specimens containing few squamous epithelial cells, numerous neutrophils, and large numbers of Gram positive, lancet-shaped diplococci are highly specific for pneumococcal pneumonia. However, sensitivity is much lower. Poorly obtained or processed specimens and lack of observer experience can dramatically alter the yield. Sputum culture suffers from similar problems of low sensitivity and specificity, with the quality of the sample and prior antibiotic treatment having a major impact on yield. Blood cultures are positive in only 4–18% of hospitalised patients with CAP.[17] Pneumococcus is the most common pathogen isolated but prior antibiotic treatment significantly reduces yield.

Pneumococcal polysaccharide antigen can be detected in respiratory or other fluids by a variety of methods. It has the advantage of being less strongly influenced by prior antibiotics, but sensitivity and specificity are very variable between studies. Urinary antigen testing for legionella serogroup 1 is more than 95% specific for infection, but sensitivity is low and the test does not detect other Legionella species. There is current interest in the detection of specific microbiological nucleic acids by amplification techniques such as reverse transcriptase polymerase chain reaction (RT-PCR). These techniques are likely to suffer from similar sensitivity and specificity problems that affect conventional tests.

Most patients with severe CAP require endotracheal intubation and mechanical ventilatory support. In these circumstances, fibreoptic bronchoscopy becomes relatively straightforward and safe. Should all intubated patients with severe but microbiologically undiagnosed CAP be bronchoscoped? An evidence based approach cannot be taken as randomised controlled trials have not been performed. The advantages are that other pathology such as endobronchial obstruction may be discovered and that a targeted sample of lower respiratory tract secretions may be obtained. However,

samples obtained using standard techniques are always contaminated by upper airway flora and are probably no better than standard sputum samples. Protected specimen brush (PSB) and bronchoalveolar lavage (BAL) are techniques which attempt to overcome some of these obstacles. PSB techniques use a telescoped plugged catheter that is passed through the bronchoscope. It contains a brush protected by a plug which is used to obtain the sample and then placed in culture medium. Quantification of the subsequent culture is usually performed to improve diagnosis. Studies on nonintubated patients with CAP report potential pathogens in 54–85% of cases. However, the yield in three series of intubated patients with severe CAP already receiving antibiotics was reduced to 13–48%.[18–20] BAL samples a larger lung volume than PSB and the yield appears to be comparable to PSB, although the evidence is very limited. In patients with CAP who fail to respond to initial treatment, BAL identifies pathogens in 12–30%.[21 22] Hence, while the yield in severe CAP is relatively low, it is recommended that bronchoscopy is performed where the diagnosis is not established or where treatment is failing.

Empirical approach to microbiological treatment

All major guidelines take the view that clinical syndromes are non-specific and that diagnostic tests are either too slow or insufficiently reliable to help in the initial choice of treatment. An empirical approach relies on a good knowledge of the range of likely local pathogens and the fact that a small number of antibiotics (or a single agent) will usually be effective. It has the added advantage of preventing long delays in treatment while the results of laboratory tests are awaited. The performance of diagnostic tests is encouraged as a guide to modify antibiotic treatment if a pathogen is identified.

ANTIMICROBIAL TREATMENT

Detailed reviews of candidate antibiotics for the treatment of severe CAP are available in recently published articles.[23 24] If the specific pathogen has been isolated, then the choice is relatively straightforward. The optimal choice of antibiotics for the empirical treatment of severe CAP is less clear. This will be determined by local surveillance data but in Europe and North America must include effective treatment for S pneumoniae, Legionella spp, Haemophilus spp and Staphylococcus spp. Gram negative bacilli are a rare cause of severe CAP in most series, although they may be found in patients with pre-existing lung disease or on steroid therapy.

Antibiotic resistance is becoming an increasing problem with a number of reports of penicillin resistant S pneumoniae. In the UK, however, clinically relevant S pneumoniae resistance is rare and the BTS guidelines continue to recommend amoxicillin alone for non-severe home based CAP treatment.

The severely ill patient with CAP requires a broader antibiotic coverage that must include the pathogens most commonly causing severe CAP. The BTS guidelines[4] recommend the combination of amoxicillin/clavulanate with clarithromycin and the optional addition of rifampicin. The amoxicillin/clavulanate combination will cover both the pneumococcus and beta-lactamase producing pathogens such as H influenzae. Clarithromycin is a macrolide antibiotic that is effective against "atypical" organisms including Legionella spp and against S pneumoniae. Rifampicin is effective against Legionella spp and provides antistaphylococcal cover. Other antibiotic regimens have been suggested for the empirical treatment of severe CAP but there is little objective evidence to support one approach over another. Alternatives for patients intolerant of the preferred combination include:

- Substitution of cefuroxime, cefotaxime, or ceftriaxone for amoxicillin/clavulanate; clarithromycin and rifampicin remain

- Use of a single fluoroquinolone with Gram positive cover (e.g. levofloxacin)

INTENSIVE CARE TREATMENT

Published case series of severe CAP emphasise that the ICU treatment of this group of patients involves the support of multiple failing organ systems. Most patients die of the complications of multiorgan failure rather than from respiratory failure alone. In the BTS severe CAP study 32% developed acute renal failure and 55% septic shock; 25% developed central nervous system problems including vascular events and convulsions.[8]

Patients with severe CAP have sepsis from a respiratory source and are optimally managed by a team with experience of the complications of sepsis. These patients often require haemofiltration for renal replacement therapy, invasive circulatory monitoring, and the use of vasopressors and inotropes. Survivors of severe CAP tend to have prolonged ICU admissions and complications are frequent. In the BTS study 12 of the 18 patients who still required ventilatory support at 14 days ultimately survived. Most patients who need prolonged ventilatory support will require a tracheostomy to wean from ventilation.

RESPIRATORY MANAGEMENT

All patients with severe CAP require high flow oxygen therapy. In all except those with a background of chronic respiratory failure, FIO_2 can be rapidly titrated against non-invasive SaO_2 measurements with regular arterial blood gas analysis used to check calibration. Hypercapnia is a sign of ventilatory failure and indicates the need for more intensive support (usually intubation and mechanical ventilation). Increasing metabolic acidosis indicates the development of circulatory shock and the requirement for fluid resuscitation and inotropic support.

CPAP can improve oxygenation in diffuse lung disease by recruiting and stabilising collapsed alveolar units. It is a standard treatment in severe pneumocystis pneumonia and a few case reports describe its successful use in severe CAP.[25] However, a recent randomised controlled trial of CPAP in patients at high risk of developing acute respiratory distress syndrome (ARDS) was negative.[26] In the study 123 consecutive adult patients with marked impairment of gas exchange (PaO_2/FIO_2 <300 mm Hg) were randomised to either standard treatment or standard treatment and facial CPAP. The group was heterogeneous but 52 patients had pneumonia. There was no significant difference in intubation rates (34% v 39% in the standard group) or hospital mortality. Of concern was the occurrence of four cardiorespiratory arrests in the CPAP group, probably due to delayed endotracheal intubation.

NIV is a further treatment option in severe CAP. Its use in exacerbations of COPD is supported by a number of randomised clinical trials.[27] A recent randomised trial of NIV in severe CAP has also been reported.[28] Fifty eight consecutive patients with severe CAP were randomised to either conventional treatment or conventional treatment and NIV. Both the intubation rate (50% v 21%) and length of stay in the ICU (6 v 1.8 days) were significantly reduced by NIV. However, subgroup analysis shows that the benefit only occurred in patients with COPD. Of concern was the trend to higher mortality in the NIV treated patients without COPD. Similarly, a small randomised study of NIV given in the emergency room for pneumonia had a higher mortality in the NIV group.[29] One explanation for the higher mortality in NIV treated patients is delay in intubation which was demonstrated in the emergency room study. The message is clear. Non-invasive respiratory support (CPAP or NIV) should only be given to patients with severe CAP in designated and properly staffed critical care areas. In addition, enthusiasm for non-invasive support should not delay intubation, particularly in patients without COPD.

Most patients with severe CAP (88% in the BTS study) will require intubation and mechanical ventilation. A number of these will develop diffuse lung injury and should be managed in a manner identical to others with ARDS (see chapter 9). In occasional cases with focal pneumonia massive shunt across the diseased lobe is the cause of severe hypoxaemia. The use of positioning and differential lung ventilation has been described in this situation.[30-32] Placing the "good lung down" may increase PaO_2 by 1.5–2.0 kPa as blood flow increases to the well ventilated lung. Differential lung ventilation requires the placement of a double lumen tube. The correct placement of such tubes can be difficult in the stable patient and requires great expertise in the severely ill. Following placement, each lung can be separately ventilated and the effects of different ventilatory strategies assessed.

The optimal ventilatory strategy for most patients with severe CAP has not been established. Both volume controlled and pressure controlled modes are used with varying levels of positive end expiratory pressure (PEEP). The recent multicentre ARDS study on ventilation suggests that a volume limited strategy should be adopted to reduce ventilator associated lung injury.[33] Although the approach of limiting tidal volume and airway pressure and allowing a controlled degree of hypercapnia is appealing, this strategy has not been examined in patients with severe CAP without ARDS.

FAILURE TO IMPROVE

Lack of clinical response at 48–72 hours is usually taken as an indication of probable treatment failure, although improvement in the elderly may take longer. The diagnosis should be reviewed and conditions such as cardiac failure and pulmonary infarction excluded. Culture results will be available by this stage and may necessitate a change in antibiotics. Pulmonary and extrapulmonary complications of infection should be investigated and treated. These include lung abscess and necrosis, empyema, meningitis, endocarditis, and nosocomial infections (including pneumonia and line infections). A recent multicentre study on the management of ventilator associated pneumonia suggested that bronchoscopy and lavage may be useful at this stage.[34] The possibility of immunosuppression should be considered and a history of recent foreign travel excluded. Pathogens that are very unusual in the UK are common causes of CAP in some countries[13] and tuberculosis still occasionally presents as overwhelming pneumonia.

OUTCOME AND PROGNOSIS

The mortality of patients with CAP needing ICU admission is high. A meta-analysis found a mortality of 36.5% in ICU admissions with a range of 21.7–57.3%.[35] In the early 1970s Knaus and coworkers developed a predictive model of ICU outcome known as the APACHE (acute physiology and chronic health evaluation) scoring system.[36] This model has been refined and alternative models produced. All these systems indicate that outcome in ICU is related to the initial severity of illness (as measured by abnormal physiology on admission), the type of illness, and the pre-admission health status of the patient. Increasing age also has a negative impact on outcome. A number of studies have confirmed that these variables are important determinants of outcome in severe CAP.[1] The independent impact of individual pathogens on survival is more difficult to determine. S pneumoniae, Staph aureus, Legionella spp, and Gram negative bacilli have all been reported in different studies to be independently associated with death.

REFERENCES

1 **Ewig S**, Torres A. Severe community-acquired pneumonia. *Clin Chest Med* 1999;**20**:575–87.
2 **Brown PD**, Lerner SA. Community-acquired pneumonia. *Lancet* 1998;**352**:1295–302.

3 **European Respiratory Society Task Force Report**. Guidelines for management of adult community-acquired lower respiratory tract infections. *Eur Respir J* 1998;**11**:986–91.

4 **British Thoracic Society**. BTS guidelines for the management of community acquired pneumonia in adults. *Thorax* 2001;**56**(Suppl IV):iv1–64.

5 **Niederman MS**, Bass JB, Campbell GD, *et al*. Guidelines for the initial management of adults with community-acquired pneumonia: diagnosis, assessment of severity, and initial antimicrobial therapy. American Thoracic Society. *Am Rev Respir Dis* 1993;**148**:1418–26.

6 **Mandell LA**, Marrie TJ, Grossman RF, *et al*. Canadian guidelines for the initial management of community-acquired pneumonia: an evidence-based update by the Canadian Infectious Diseases Society and the Canadian Thoracic Society. The Canadian Community-Acquired Pneumonia Working Group. *Clin Infect Dis* 2000;**31**:383–421.

7 **Woodhead M**. Predicting death from pneumonia. *Thorax* 1996;**51**:970.

8 **British Thoracic Society Research Committee and The Public Health Laboratory Service**. The aetiology, management and outcome of severe community-acquired pneumonia on the intensive care unit. *Respir Med* 1992;**86**:7–13.

9 **Tang CM**, Macfarlane JT. Early management of younger adults dying of community acquired pneumonia. *Respir Med* 1993;**87**:289–94.

10 **McQuillan P**, Pilkington S, Allan A, *et al*. Confidential inquiry into quality of care before admission to intensive care. *BMJ* 1998;**316**:1853–8.

11 **Department of Health**. *Comprehensive critical care. A review of adult critical care services*. London: Department of Health, 2000.

12 **Woodhead M**. Pneumonia in the elderly. *J Antimicrob Chemother* 1994;**34**(Suppl A):85–92.

13 **Tan YK**, Khoo KL, Chin SP, *et al*. Aetiology and outcome of severe community-acquired pneumonia in Singapore. *Eur Respir J* 1998;**12**:113–5.

14 **El Ebiary M**, Sarmiento X, Torres A, *et al*. Prognostic factors of severe Legionella pneumonia requiring admission to ICU. *Am J Respir Crit Care Med* 1997;**156**:1467–72.

15 **Leroy O**, Santre C, Beuscart C, *et al*. A five-year study of severe community-acquired pneumonia with emphasis on prognosis in patients admitted to an intensive care unit. *Intensive Care Med* 1995;**21**:24–31.

16 **Torres A**, Serra-Batlles J, Ferrer A, *et al*. Severe community-acquired pneumonia. Epidemiology and prognostic factors. *Am Rev Respir Dis* 1991;**144**:312–8.

17 **Skerrett SJ**. Diagnostic testing for community-acquired pneumonia. *Clin Chest Med* 1999;**20**:531–48.

18 **Moine P**, Vercken JB, Chevret S, *et al*. Severe community-acquired pneumonia. Etiology, epidemiology, and prognosis factors. French Study Group for Community-Acquired Pneumonia in the Intensive Care Unit. *Chest* 1994;**105**:1487–95.

19 **Sorensen J**, Forsberg P, Hakanson E, *et al*. A new diagnostic approach to the patient with severe pneumonia. *Scand J Infect Dis* 1989;**21**:33–41.

20 **Potgieter PD**, Hammond JM. Etiology and diagnosis of pneumonia requiring ICU admission. *Chest* 1992;**101**:199–203.

21 **Feinsilver SH**, Fein AM, Niederman MS, *et al*. Utility of fiberoptic bronchoscopy in nonresolving pneumonia. *Chest* 1990;**98**:1322–6.

22 **Ortqvist A**, Kalin M, Lejdeborn L, *et al*. Diagnostic fiberoptic bronchoscopy and protected brush culture in patients with community-acquired pneumonia. *Chest* 1990;**97**:576–82.

23 **Mandell LA**. Antibiotic therapy for community-acquired pneumonia. *Clin Chest Med* 1999;**20**:589–98.

24 **Ortqvist A**. In-hospital management of adults who have community-acquired pneumonia. *Semin Respir Infect* 1999;**14**:135–50.

25 **Brett A**, Sinclair DG. Use of continuous positive airway pressure in the management of community acquired pneumonia. *Thorax* 1993;**48**:1280–1.

26 **Delclaux C**, L'Her E, Alberti C, *et al*. Treatment of acute hypoxemic nonhypercapnic respiratory insufficiency with continuous positive airway pressure delivered by a face mask: a randomized controlled trial. *JAMA* 2000;**284**:2352–60.

27 **Plant PK**, Elliott MW. Non-invasive positive pressure ventilation. *J R Coll Physicians Lond* 1999;**33**:521–5.

28 **Confalonieri M**, Potena A, Carbone G, *et al*. Acute respiratory failure in patients with severe community-acquired pneumonia. A prospective randomized evaluation of noninvasive ventilation. *Am J Respir Crit Care Med* 1999;**160**:1585–91.

29 **Wood KA**, Lewis L, Von Harz B, *et al*. The use of noninvasive positive pressure ventilation in the emergency department: results of a randomized clinical trial. *Chest* 1998;**113**:1339–46.

30 **Hillman KM**, Barber JD. Asynchronous independent lung ventilation (AILV). *Crit Care Med* 1980;**8**:390–5.

31 **Carlon GC**, Ray C, Klein R, *et al*. Criteria for selective positive end-expiratory pressure and independent synchronized ventilation of each lung. *Chest* 1978;**74**:501–7.

32 **Dreyfuss D**, Djedaini K, Lanore JJ, *et al*. A comparative study of the effects of almitrine bismesylate and lateral position during unilateral bacterial pneumonia with severe hypoxemia. *Am Rev Respir Dis* 1992;**146**:295–9.

33 **The Acute Respiratory Distress Syndrome Network**. Ventilation with lower tidal volumes as compared with traditional tidal volumes for acute lung injury and the acute respiratory distress syndrome. *N Engl J Med* 2000;**342**:1301–8.

34 **Fagon JY**, Chastre J, Wolff M, *et al*. Invasive and noninvasive strategies for management of suspected ventilator-associated pneumonia. A randomized trial. *Ann Intern Med* 2000;**132**:621–30.

35 **Fine MJ**, Smith MA, Carson CA, *et al*. Prognosis and outcomes of patients with community-acquired pneumonia. A meta-analysis. *JAMA* 1996;**275**:134–41.

36 **Knaus WA**, Draper EA, Wagner DP, *et al*. APACHE II: a severity of disease classification system. *Crit Care Med* 1985;**13**:818–29.

4 Nosocomial pneumonia

S Ewig, A Torres

Nosocomial pneumonia is the second most frequent hospital acquired infection and the most frequently acquired infection in the intensive care unit (ICU). The incidence is age dependent, with about 5/1000 cases in hospitalised patients aged under 35 and up to 15/1000 in those over 65 years of age.[1-3] Death from nosocomial pneumonia in ventilated patients reaches 30–50%, with an estimated attributable mortality of 10–50%.[4-9] Increasing microbial resistance worldwide imposes an additional challenge for prevention and antimicrobial treatment strategies.[10]

In the last two decades efforts have been made to improve outcomes by establishing valid diagnostic and therapeutic strategies. Nevertheless, controversy persists in many issues regarding the management of nosocomial pneumonia. This chapter focuses on the main controversies in diagnosis and treatment.

DEFINITIONS

Nosocomial pneumonia usually affects mechanically ventilated patients, hence the term "ventilator associated pneumonia (VAP)" is used synonymously. However, nosocomial pneumonia may occur in non-ventilated patients, creating a distinct entity (table 4.1). Notably, all concepts of nosocomial pneumonia refer to the non-immunosuppressed host, with absence of "immunosuppression" defined as absence of risk for infection with opportunistic pathogens.

Dividing patients with VAP into groups with early and late onset has been shown to be of paramount importance.[11] Early onset pneumonia commonly results from aspiration of endogenous community acquired pathogens such as *Staphylococcus aureus*, *Streptococcus pneumoniae*, and *Haemophilus influenzae*, with endotracheal intubation and impaired consciousness being the main risk factors.[12-15] Conversely, late onset pneumonia follows aspiration of oropharyngeal or gastric secretions containing potentially drug resistant nosocomial pathogens. Only late onset VAP is associated with an attributable excess mortality.[9]

The definitions of early and late onset VAP have not been standardised. Firstly, the starting point for early onset pneumonia has varied considerably, including time of hospital admission, of admission to the ICU, or of endotracheal intubation. If the time of admission to the ICU is chosen as the starting point, patients may already have been colonised in hospital and consequently differences between early and late onset pneumonia will no longer be evident.[14 16] In accordance with the American Thoracic Society (ATS) guidelines, we advocate using the time of hospital admission. Secondly, the cut off time separating early and late onset VAP has not been standardised. The ATS suggested using the fifth day after hospital admission.[11] We have shown that colonisation of patients after head injury markedly changed between the third and fourth day in favour of nosocomial pathogens.[13] Whereas the oropharynx, nose, tracheobronchial tree were initially colonized with endogenous community acquired pathogens, this pattern was subsequently changed by an increasing number of typical nosocomial pathogens. Trouillet *et al* have shown that isolation of drug resistant microorganisms can be predicted by the duration of intubation and antimicrobial treatment[17]; the cut off between early and late onset VAP used was 7 days.

Traditionally, nosocomial pneumonia is defined as occurring in patients admitted to hospital (or intubated) for at least 48 hours.[18] However, this definition is no longer adequate at least for VAP because a significant number of cases occur within 48 hours of hospital admission as a consequence of intubation, particularly emergency intubation. In these patients cardiopulmonary resuscitation and continuous sedation were independent risk factors for the development of VAP while antimicrobial treatment was protective.[19]

Key features of the current definitions of nosocomial pneumonia are summarized in box 4.1.

ANTIMICROBIAL TREATMENT

Several investigations have addressed the efficacy of antimicrobial treatment as well as its impact on microbial resistance. Such studies have resolved many of the controversies surrounding the use of antimicrobial agents in the hospital setting (fig 4.1). The immediate administration of treatment

Table 4.1 Differences in nosocomial pneumonia affecting non-ventilated and ventilated patients (ventilator associated pneumonia, VAP)

	Non-ventilated patients	Ventilated patients
Incidence	Relatively low	High
Aetiology	GNEB, *Legionella* spp	Core pathogens; PDRM
Mortality	Probably relatively low	30–50%
Diagnosis	Clinical; TTA; virtually no data on bronchoscopy	Clinical; TBAS; bronchoscopy
Antibiotics	Monotherapy	Early onset: monotherapy. Late onset: combination therapy
Prevention	General measures of infection control	Additionally, measures to reduce risk factors associated with intubation

GNEB = Gram negative enteric bacteria; PDRM = potentially drug resistant microorganisms; TTA = transthoracic aspiration; TBAS = tracheobronchial secretions.

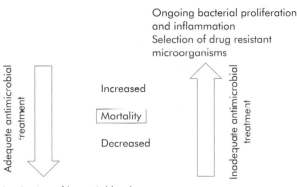

Figure 4.1 Importance of adequate and appropriate antimicrobial treatment.

is crucial and inappropriate treatment is associated with an increased risk of death from pneumonia.[20-22] Moreover, even if the initially inappropriate antimicrobial treatment is corrected according to diagnostic test results, there remains an excess mortality compared with patients treated appropriately from the beginning.[23]

Conversely, antimicrobial treatment is not without risk, particularly prolonged broad spectrum antimicrobial treatment. Rello and coworkers showed that antimicrobial pretreatment was the only adverse prognostic factor in a multivariate model. However, if pneumonia due to high risk organisms (*P aeruginosa*, *A calcoaceticus*, *S marcescens*, *P mirabilis*, and fungi) was included in the model, the presence of these high risk organisms was the only independent predictor and antimicrobial pretreatment dropped out.[20] Thus, antimicrobial pretreatment imposes considerable microbial selection pressure, and is associated with excess mortality due to pneumonia caused by drug resistant microorganisms.

It has become increasingly clear that each antimicrobial treatment policy imposes specific selection pressures, and therefore microbial and resistance patterns in each setting can to some extent be regarded as the footprints of past antimicrobial treatment policies. With this in mind, it is clear that recommendations for initial empirical antimicrobial treatment must be flexible so that they may be modified in accordance with local circumstances.[24-26] Accordingly, changing microbial patterns and increasing rates of microbial resistance must be recognized at the local level so that corresponding changes in general antimicrobial treatment policies may be instituted.[27]

DIAGNOSTIC STRATEGIES

Clinical observations, laboratory results, and chest radiographs are of limited value in diagnosing VAP, and so great effort has been made to establish independent microbiological criteria. In our view these efforts have not yet succeeded. Despite its limitations, clinical assessment is the starting point for diagnosing VAP and alternative strategies must be interpreted with regard to their ability to decrease the rate of false positive clinical judgements (about 10–25%).[28] On the other hand, the 20–40% false negative clinical judgements remain undetected.[29] Moreover, although it is generally recognized that qualitative culture of tracheobronchial secretions is highly sensitive but poorly specific, precluding its use for establishing the diagnosis of VAP in the individual patient, only rarely has it been used for exclusion of VAP and as a tool for local surveillance.[28] Qualitative tracheobronchial aspiration has a high negative predictive value, and a negative culture result in the absence of antimicrobial treatment virtually excludes VAP. Surveillance based on potential pathogens present in patients with suspected VAP is an increasingly

attractive tool to direct local empirical antimicrobial treatment policies. Can quantitative culture overcome the limitations of qualitative tracheobronchial aspirates and allow for an individual diagnostic approach to VAP?

The technique of quantitative culture of bronchoscopically retrieved protected specimen brush (PSB) and bronchoalveolar lavage (BAL) specimens has been evaluated by a variety of approaches. Early animal studies established a relationship between histological pneumonia and bacterial loads, but more recent studies have highlighted limitations of quantitative cultures. In ventilated mini-pigs the severity of bronchial and pulmonary inflammatory lesions and bacterial load were clearly associated. However, there was a large overlap, such that threshold bacterial loads could not differentiate between samples from unaffected pigs, those with bronchitis, and those with pneumonia.[30] Similarly, in a subsequent study evaluating diagnostic tools, none had a satisfactory diagnostic yield.[31]

Studies in healthy non-intubated patients have shown a high specificity for PSB and BAL. In mechanically ventilated patients without suspected VAP the results were less impressive, yielding false positive results in 20–30%, although no strictly independent reference was used.[32-35] In patients with suspected VAP a variety of diagnostic tools have been evaluated with conflicting results.[36-39] These studies provided several general insights, although references and thresholds for the calculation of diagnostic indices varied considerably. Firstly, PSB and BAL had generally comparable diagnostic yields; secondly, tracheobronchial aspirates had comparable yields to PSB and BAL, with a tendency towards a lower specificity; and thirdly, all tools exhibited a rate of false negative and false positive results ranging from 10% to 30%. A study focusing on the variability of PSB showed that the qualitative repeatability was 100%, while in 59% of the patients the quantitative results varied more than tenfold.[40] Based on these studies, several investigations were performed using postmortem histological results or lung culture as an independent reference or gold standard.[41-47] Despite several important methodological limitations, these studies revealed important clues to the relationships between histology, microbiology, and the diagnosis of VAP: (1) limited correlation between histological findings and the bacterial load of lung cultures; (2) the recognition that no single technique would be irrefutable; (3) a surprisingly high rate of false negative and false positive results of 10–50% regardless of the technique used; and (4) a comparable yield from non-invasive and invasive diagnostic tools. Reasons for false negative findings included sampling errors, antimicrobial pretreatment, and the presence of stage specific bacterial loads during the evolution of pneumonia (developing as well as resolving pneumonia). Conversely, false positive results were attributable to contamination of the samples and bronchiolitis or bronchitis, particularly in patients with structural lung disease.

Studies evaluating the influence of diagnostic techniques on outcome have a number of limitations: (1) the usefulness of diagnostic techniques may vary within different populations; (2) this approach ignores the long term effects on microbial resistance; (3) the presence of excess mortality has only been shown for late onset VAP and was low (0–10%) in some studies[4–9]; and (4) outcome measures are most consistently evaluated when antimicrobial treatment is stopped in patients without positive culture results which, in our view, is unethical.[48] Four randomised studies have been published evaluating non-invasive and invasive diagnostic tools, three from Spain and one from France.[49–52] The Spanish studies found no difference in outcome measures such as mortality, cost, duration of hospitalisation, ICU stay, and intubation.[49 51 52] The multicentre French study found a bronchoscopic strategy including quantitative cultures of PSB and/or BAL specimens to be superior to a clinical strategy using qualitative tracheobronchial aspirates in terms of 14 day mortality, morbidity, and use of antimicrobial treatment.[50] Each study had limitations, however, and the results of the French study raise the following concerns: firstly, the clinical strategy did not necessarily reflect routine practice; secondly, it is not clear from the data how the invasive strategy accounted for the better outcome; and, thirdly, the clinical group had a significantly higher rate of inadequate antimicrobial treatment.

In a response to our corresponding critique,[53] the authors indicated that the latter was accounted for by the greater numbers of pathogens detected in tracheobronchial secretions from the clinical group.[54] Although this is plausible, it is contradictory to assume that the higher detection rate of resistant microorganisms in tracheobronchial aspirates was associated with a worse outcome. Thus, it renders even less clear the issue of how the invasive strategy could translate into lower mortality. Moreover, the study does not allow one to draw any conclusion regarding the value of invasive bronchoscopic tools as compared with quantitative tracheobronchial aspirates. In our randomized study evaluating the impact of diagnostic techniques on outcome, we could not find any difference in outcome when quantitative tracheobronchial aspirates were compared with a bronchoscopic strategy.

In view of these data, we draw the following conclusions:

- Quantitative culture cannot confirm a diagnosis of VAP in the individual case.

- Non-invasive and invasive bronchoscopic tools have comparable diagnostic yields and share similar methodological limitations.

- The introduction of microbiological criteria to correct for false positive clinical judgements does not result in more confident diagnoses of VAP ; the microbiological correction of false positive judgements is countered by the misclassification of correctly positive clinical judgements.[29]

STATEMENTS FROM A CONSENSUS CONFERENCE

A consensus conference, sponsored by four societies, on pneumonia acquired in the ICU was held in May 2002, and a summary document was published.[55] Although we do not totally agree with the recommendations, those regarding diagnosis are summarized here.
(1) Microbiological samples must be collected before initiation of antimicrobial agents.
(2) Reliance on qualitative cultures of endotracheal aspirates leads to both over-diagnosis and under-diagnosis of pneumonia.

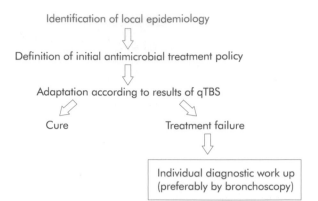

Figure 4.2 Suggested approach to the management of a patient with suspected VAP. qTBS = quantitative tracheobronchial secretions.

(3) The available evidence favours the use of invasive quantitative culture techniques over tracheal aspirates when establishing an indication for antimicrobial therapy.
(4) The available data suggest that the accuracy of non-bronchoscopic techniques for obtaining quantitative cultures of lower respiratory tract samples is comparable to that of bronchoscopic techniques.
(5) The cost effectiveness of invasive as compared with that of non-invasive diagnostic strategies has not been established.

NEW DEVELOPMENTS IN ANTIMICROBIAL TREATMENT

The general limitations of diagnostic criteria for the diagnosis of VAP in the individual patient have fundamental consequences for any antimicrobial treatment strategy. We suggest a change in perspective away from the individual and towards an epidemiological approach, as elaborated in the ATS guidelines.[11] Important components of such an approach include the following.

(1) Initial antimicrobial treatment must always be empirical.

(2) Empirical antimicrobial treatment can be guided by three criteria: severity of pneumonia, time of onset, and specific risk factors. All pneumonias acquired in the ICU are severe by definition in the guidelines.

(3) The selection of antimicrobial agents must be adapted to regional or even local microbial and resistance patterns.

(4) The diagnostic work up may offer additional clues that must be interpreted in the context of the patient's condition. However, it is generally confined to suggesting potential pathogens and their resistance, which may be particularly relevant when there is no response to empirical antibiotics. It is therefore our practice to use quantitative tracheobronchial aspirates regularly, and bronchoscopy with PSB and BAL in patients who are not responding to treatment (fig 4.2).

When can antimicrobial treatment be withheld or stopped? Firstly, patients exhibiting signs of severe sepsis or septic shock must receive empirical treatment. Secondly, patients with clinically suspected VAP, yielding borderline colony counts ($\geqslant 10^2$ but $< 10^3$ cfu/ml in PSB) who were untreated, were found to have an excess mortality if they developed significant colony counts within 72 hours.[48] We therefore argue that stable patients with clinically suspected VAP but without an established pathogen should also receive empirical treatment.

The dilemma of potential overtreatment at the cost of increased microbial selection pressure could be addressed more satisfactorily if our ability to diagnose pneumonia according to clinical criteria improved. This could be achieved, firstly, by improving the clinical criteria for suspected VAP, as those currently in use (a new and persistent

Table 4.2 General framework for empirical initial antimicrobial treatment of VAP

	Class of antimicrobial agents	Examples
Ventilated patients:		
Early onset, no risk factors	Cephalosporin II	• Cefuroxime
	or	
	Cephalosporin III	• Cefotaxime
		• Ceftriaxone
	or	
	Aminopenicillin/β-lacatamase inhibitor	• Amoxicillin/clavulanic acid
	Third or fourth generation quinolone	• Levofloxacin
	or	
	Clindamycin/aztreonam	• Clindamycin
		• Aztreonam
Late onset, no risk factors	Quinolone	• Ciprofloxacin
	or	
	Aminoglycoside	• Gentamicin
		• Tobramycin
		• Amikacin
	plus	
	Antipseudomonal β-lactam/β-lactamase inhibitor	• Piperacillin/tazobactam
	or	
	Ceftazidime	• Ceftazidime
	or	
	Carbapenems	• Imipenem/cilastatin
		• Meropenem
	plus/minus	
	Vancomycin	• Vancomycin
Early or late onset, risk factors	Risk factors for *P aeruginosa*: see late onset	
	Risk factors for MRSA: + vancomycin	• Vancomycin
	Risk factor for legionellosis: macrolide	• Erythromycin
		or
		• Azithromycin
		or
		• Clarithromycin
		or
		• Levofloxacin
		or
		• Moxifloxacin
Non-ventilated patients:		
Early onset, no risk factors	See ventilated patient	
Late onset, no risk factors	See ventilated patient; possibly monotherapy in the absence of severe pneumonia	
Early or late onset, risk factors	See ventilated patient, early or late onset, risk factors	

infiltrate on the chest radiograph plus one to three of the following: fever or hypothermia, leucocytosis or leucopenia, and purulent tracheobronchial secretions) are outdated. In particular, it is inappropriate to ignore changes in oxygenation, and the criteria for severe sepsis and/or septic shock. Pugin *et al*[56] have suggested a scoring system for VAP, including the following six weighted clinical and microbiological variables: temperature, white blood cell count, mean volume and nature of tracheobronchial aspirate, gas exchange ratio, and chest radiograph infiltrates. This score achieved a sensitivity of 72% and a specificity of 85% in a necroscopic study.[45] It is tedious to calculate and includes microbiological criteria, but it indicates that criteria may be developed that significantly improve the predictive value of clinical judgement. A second way in which our ability to diagnose pneumonia could be improved is by developing valid severity criteria. Somewhat surprising is that, in contrast to community acquired pneumonia,[57] severity assessment of VAP has not received much attention. However, it is clear that valid severity criteria may be of great help in determining when antimicrobial treatment may safely be withheld or stopped. Finally, valid markers of the inflammatory response associated with VAP could work as surrogate markers for VAP and thereby be of help in guiding antimcrobial treatment decisions.

In the meantime, our approach is to judge the condition of the patient in view of all available clinical, laboratory, and radiographical information in order to improve our ability to predict the presence or absence of VAP. Culture results are then interpreted within this context and decisions are not made exclusively on the basis of thresholds.

A recent multicenter French study has shown similar clinical efficacy treating VAP with 7 days compared to 14. The confirmation of these findings would be of extreme importance to reduce the amount of antibiotics given in ICUs.[58]

Another approach to reducing the microbial selection pressure imposed by empirical antimicrobial treatment is to reduce exposure by minimising the duration of treatment. The challenge would be to identify low risk groups without drug resistant microorganisms. In an elegant study by Singh *et al*[59] patients with suspected nosocomial pneumonia (58% VAP) with a Pugin score of ≤6 (low clinical probability of pneumonia) received antimicrobial treatment for 10–21 days at the discretion of the attending physician or a 3 day course of ciprofloxacin. After 3 days treatment was stopped in those still considered to have a low clinical probability, whereas those with a higher Pugin score received a full course of standard antibiotics. The length of time in hospital and mortality did not differ but resistance and superinfection rates were higher in the control group (15% *v* 39%). The insight yielded by this important study is that the perspective was shifted away from all conflictive diagnostic issues; instead, a strategy was implemented that allowed reduction in the risk for individual under-treatment and for general over-treatment, with its inherent consequences.

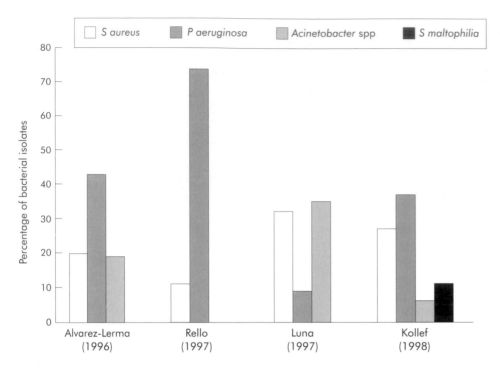

Figure 4.3 Proportion of microorganisms accounting for antimicrobial treatment failures of VAP in four studies.[23 63–65]

In patients with suspected VAP due to Gram negative pathogens, a controlled rotation of one antimicrobial regimen (ceftazidime) to another (ciprofloxacin) was associated with a significant reduction in the incidence of VAP (12% *v* 7%), the incidence of resistant Gram negative pathogens (4% *v* 1%), and the incidence of Gram negative bacteraemia (2% *v* 0.3%).[25] Similarly, controlled rotation of antibiotics including restricted use of ceftazidime and ciprofloxacin over 2 years was associated with a significant reduction in VAP cases from 231 to 161 (70%), of potentially drug resistant microorganisms from 140 to 79 (56%), but with an increase from 40% to 60% of methicillin resistant *Staphylococcus aureus (MRSA)* isolates.[26] It should be stressed that these studies do not practise *rotation* in its strict sense, but simply strategies of controlled antimicrobial treatment. The role of antimicrobial rotation cannot therefore be determined yet, either as a fixed (or blinded) rotation or as a flexible (or controlled) rotation based on local microbial and resistance patterns.[60]

RECOMMENDATIONS FOR EMPIRICAL ANTIMICROBIAL TREATMENT

Based on the ATS guidelines,[11] the following recommendations can be made (table 4.2):

(1) Patients with early onset VAP and no risk factors: core organisms such as community endogenous pathogens (*Staphylococcus aureus*, *Streptococcus pneumoniae*, and *Haemophilus influenzae*) and non-resistant Gram negative enterobacteriaceae (GNEB, including *Escherichia coli*, *Klebsiella pneumoniae*, *Enterobacter* spp, *Serratia* spp, *Proteus* spp) should be appropriately covered. This can be achieved by monotherapy with a second or third generation cephalosporin (cefotaxime or ceftriaxone), or by an aminopenicillin plus a β-lactamase inhibitor. Quinolones or a combination of clindamycin and aztreonam are alternatives.

(2) Patients with late onset VAP and no risk factors: potentially drug resistant microorganisms must also be taken into account. This is particularly true when mechanical ventilation is required for more than 7 days and against a background of broad spectrum antimicrobial treatment.[17] These include multiresistant MRSA, GNEB, and *Pseudomonas aeruginosa*, *Acinetobacter* spp, as well as *Stenotrophomonas maltophilia*. Although not proven by randomized studies, it seems prudent to administer combination treatment, including an antipseudomonal penicillin (plus a β-lactamase inhibitor) or a cephalosporin or a

carbapenem, and a quinolone (ciprofloxacin) or an aminoglycoside. Vancomycin may be added where MRSA is a concern.

(3) Patients with early or late onset VAP and risk factors: treatment is identical to that for late onset VAP without risk factors, except when *Legionella* spp are suspected in which case these pathogens must also be covered.

The guidelines do not make specific recommendations for non-ventilated patients with nosocomial pnuemonia. Instead, patients not meeting severity criteria are treated as early onset VAP with modifications in the presence of additional risk factors. In our view it would be useful to compare this severity based approach with an algorithm that separates pneumonia in the non-intubated and intubated patient, differentiates early and late onset, and considers the presence of risk factors. This is the direction of the recently published German guidelines for the treatment and prevention of nosocomial pneumonia.[61]

This general framework for empirical initial antimicrobial treatment must be modified according to local requirements. Regular updates of data on potential pathogens of VAP indicating trends in microbial and resistance patterns are mandatory.[62] Although data on antimicrobial treatment failures are scarce, we recommend investigating each case. The separate record of these data is particularly useful in detecting patients at risk, as well as microorganisms typically associated with treatment failures. Although few microorganisms are responsible for the vast majority of antimicrobial treatment failures, the distribution of pathogens is widely divergent between centres (fig 4.3).[23 63–65]

CONCLUSION

Much progress has been made in the understanding of nosocomial pneumonia and this has influenced management guidelines. Nevertheless, important issues in diagnosis and treatment remain unresolved. We argue that the controversy over diagnostic tools should be closed. Instead, every effort should be made to increase our ability to make valid clinical predictions about the presence of VAP and to establish criteria to guide restricting empirical antimicrobial treatment without causing harm to patients. At the same time, more emphasis must be put on local infection control measures such as routine surveillance of pathogens, definition of controlled policies of antimicrobial treatment, and effective implementation of strategies of prevention.

REFERENCES

1 **Fagon JY**, Chastre J, Domart Y, et al. Nosocomial pneumonia in patients receiving continuous mechanical ventilation. Prospective analysis of 52 episodes with use of a protected specimen brush and quantitative culture technique. Am Rev Respir Dis 1989;**139**:877–84.

2 **Torres A**, Aznar R, Gatell JM, et al. Incidence, risk, and prognostic factors of nosocomial pneumonia in mechanically ventilated patients. Am Rev Respir Dis 1990;**142**:523–8.

3 **Rello J**, Quintana E, Ausina V, et al. Incidence, etiology, and outcome of nosocomial pneumonia in mechanically ventilated patients. Chest 1991;**100**:439–44.

4 **Fagon JY**, Chastre J, Vuagnat A, et al. Nosocomial pneumonia and mortality among patients in intensive care units. JAMA 1996;**275**:866–9.

5 **Kollef MH**. Ventilator-associated pneumonia. A multivariate analysis. JAMA 1993;**270**:1965–70.

6 **Papazian L**, Bregeon F, Thirion X, et al. Effect of ventilator-associated pneumonia on mortality and morbidity. Am J Respir Crit Care Med 1996;**154**:91–7.

7 **Leu HS**, Kaiser DL, Mori M, et al. Hospital-acquired pneumonia attributable mortality and morbidity. Am J Epidemiol 1989;**129**:1258–67.

8 **Fagon JY**, Chastre J, Hance AJ, et al. Nosocomial pneumonia in ventilated patients: a cohort study evaluating attributable mortality and hospital stay. Am J Med 1993;**94**:281–8.

9 **Kollef M**, Silver P, Murphy DM, et al. The effect of late-onset pneumonia in determining patient mortality. Chest 1995;**108**:1655–62.

10 **Jones RN**, Pfaller MA. Bacterial resistance: a worldwide problem. Diagn Microbiol Infect Dis 1998;**31**:379–88.

11 **American Thoracic Society**. Hospital-acquired pneumonia in adults; diagnosis, assessment, initial severity, and prevention. A consensus statement. Am J Respir Crit Care Med 1996;**153**:1711–25.

12 **Rello J**, Ausina V, Castella J, et al. Nosocomial respiratory tract infections in multiple trauma patients. Influence of level of consciousness with implications for therapy. Chest 1992;**102**:525–9

13 **Ewig S**, Torres A, El-Ebiary M, et al. Bacterial colonization patterns in mechanically ventilated patients with traumatic and medical head injury. Incidence, risk factors, and association with ventilator-associated pneumonia. Am J Respir Crit Care Med 1999;**159**:188–98.

14 **Akca O**, Koltka K, Uzel S, et al. Risk factors for early-onset, ventilator-associated pneumonia in critical care patients: selected multiresistant versus nonresistant bacteria. Anesthesiology 2000;**93**:638–45.

15 **Sirvent JM**, Torres A, Vidaur L, et al. Tracheal colonisation within 24 h of intubation in patients with head trauma: risk factor for developing early-onset ventilator-associated pneumonia. Intensive Care Med 2000;**26**:1369–72.

16 **Ibrahim EH**, Ward S, Sherman G, et al. A comparative analysis of patients with early-onset vs late-onset nosocomial pneumonia in the ICU setting. Chest 2000;**117**:1434–42.

17 **Trouillet JL**, Chastre J, Vugnat A, et al. Ventilator-associated pneumonia caused by potentially drug-resistant bacteria. Am J Respir Crit Care Med 1998;**157**:531–9.

18 **Woodhead M**, Torres A. Definition and classification of community-acquired and nosocomial pneumonias. Eur Respir Mon 1997;**3**:1–12.

19 **Rello J**, Diaz E, Roque M, et al. Risk factors for developing pneumonia within 48 hours of intubation. Am J Respir Crit Care Med 1999;**159**:1742–6.

20 **Rello J**, Ausina V, Ricart M, et al. Impact of previous antimicrobial therapy on the etiology and outcome of ventilator-associated pneumonia. Chest 1993;**104**:1230–5.

21 **Kollef M**. Inadequate antimicrobial treatment: an important determinant of outcome for hospitalized patients. Clin Infect Dis 2000;**31**(Suppl 4):S131–8.

22 **Kollef M**, Ward S, Sherman G, et al. Inadequate treatment of nosocomial infections is associated with certain empiric antibiotic choices. Crit Care Med 2000;**28**:3456–64.

23 **Luna C**, Vujachich P, Niederman MS, et al. Impact of BAL data on the therapy and outcome of ventilator-associated pneumonia. Chest 1997;**111**:676–87.

24 **Rello J**, Sa-Borges M, Correa H, et al. Variations in etiology of ventilator-associated pneumonia across four treatment sites: implications for antimicrobial prescribing practices. Am J Respir Crit Care Med 1999;**160**:608–13.

25 **Kolleff MH**, Vlasnik J, Sharpless L, et al. Scheduled change of antibiotic classes: a strategy to decrease the incidence of ventilator-associated pneumonia. Am J Respir Crit Care Med 1997;**156**:1040–8.

26 **Gruson D**, Hilbert G, Vargas F, et al. Rotation and restricted use of antibiotics in a medical intensive care unit. Impact on the incidence of ventilator-associated pneumonia caused by antibiotic-resistant gram-negative bacteria. Am J Respir Crit Care Med 2000;**162**:8378–43.

27 **Walger P**, Post K, Mayershofer R, et al. Initial antimicrobial policies in the ICU should be based on surveillance rather than on crop rotation. Abstracts of the 40th Interscience Conference on Antimicrobial Agents and Chemotherapy, 401, abstract 89.

28 **Torres A**, Carlet J, and members of the Task Force. ERS task force on ventilator-associated pneumonia. Eur Respir J 2001;**17**:1034–45.

29 **Fabregas N**, Ewig S, Torres A, et al. Clinical diagnosis of ventilator-associated pneumonia revisited: comparative evaluation using immediate postmortem biopsies. Thorax 1999;**54**:867–73.

30 **Marquette CH**, Wallet F, Copin MC, et al. Relationship between microbiologic and histiologic features in bacterial pneumonia. Am J Respir Crit Care Med 1996;**154**:1784–7.

31 **Wermert D**, Marquette CH, Copin MC, et al. Influence of pulmonary bacteriology and histology on the yield of diagnostic procedures in ventilator-acquired pneumonia. Am J Respir Crit Care Med 1998;**158**:139–47.

32 **Wimberley N**, Faling SJ, Bartlett JG. A fiberoptic bronchoscopy technique to obtain uncontaminated lower airway secretion for bacterial culture. Am Rev Respir Dis 1979;**119**:337–43.

33 **Kahn FW**, Jones JM. Diagnosing bacterial respiratory infection by bronchoalveolar lavage. J Infect Dis 1987;**155**:862–9.

34 **Kirkpatrick MB**, Bass JB. Quantitative bacterial cultures of bronchoalveolar lavage fluids and protected brush catheter specimens from normal subjects. Am Rev Respir Dis 1989;**139**:546–8.

35 **Torres A**, Martos A, Puig de la Bellacasa J, et al. Specificity of endotracheal aspiration, protected specimen brush, and bronchoalveolar lavage in mechanically ventilated patients. Am Rev Respir Dis 1993;**147**:952–7.

36 **Fagon JY**, Chastre J, Hance AJ, et al. Detection of nosocomial lung infection in ventilated patients. Use of a protected specimen brush and quantitative culture techniques in 147 patients. Am Rev Respir Dis 1988;**138**:110–6.

37 **Torres A**, De La Bellacasa JP, Xaubet A, et al. Diagnostic value of quantitative cultures of bronchoalveolar lavage and telescoping plugged catheters in mechanically ventilated patients with bacterial pneumonia. Am Rev Respir Dis 1989;**140**:306–10.

38 **El-Ebiary M**, Torres A, Gonzalez J, et al. Quantitative cultures of endotracheal aspirates for the diagnosis of ventilator-associated pneumonia. Am Rev Respir Dis 1993;**148**:1552–7.

39 **Marquette CH**, Georges H, Wallet F, et al. Diagnostic efficency of endotracheal aspirates with quantitative bacterial cultures in intubated patients with suspected pneumonia. Am Rev Respir Dis 1993;**148**:138–44.

40 **Marquette CH**, Herengt F, Mathieu D, et al. Diagnosis of pneumonia in mechanically ventilated patients. Repeatability of the protected specimen brush. Am Rev Respir Dis 1993;**147**:211–4.

41 **Rouby JJ**, Martin De Lassal E, Poete P, et al. Nosocomial bronchopneumonia in the critically ill. Histologic and bacteriologic aspects. Am Rev Respir Dis 1992;**146**:1059–66.

42 **Torres A**, El-Ebiary M, Padró L, et al. Validation of different techniques for the diagnosis of ventilator-associated pneumonia. Am J Respir Crit Care Med 1994;**149**:324–31.

43 **Chastre J**, Fagon JY, Bornet-Lesco M, et al. Evaluation of bronchoscopic techniques for the diagnosis of nosocomial pneumonia. Am J Respir Crit Care Med 1995;**152**:231–40.

44 **Marquette CH**, Copin MC, Wallet F, et al. Diagnostic tests for pneumonia in ventilated patients: prospective evaluation of diagnostic accuracy using histology as a diagnostic gold standard. Am J Respir Crit Care Med 1995;**151**:1878–88.

45 **Papazian L**, Thomas P, Garbe L, et al. Bronchoscopic or blind sampling techniques for the diagnosis of ventilator-associated pneumonia. Am J Respir Crit Care Med 1995;**152**:1982–91.

46 **Fabregas N**, Torres A, El-Ebiary M, et al. Histopathologic and microbiologic aspects of ventilator-associated pneumonia. Anesthesiology 1996;**84**:760–71.

47 **Kirtland SH**, Corley DE, Winterbauer RH, et al. The diagnosis of ventilator-associated pneumonia. A comparison of histologic, microbiologic, and clinical criteria. Chest 1997;**112**:445–57.

48 **Dreyfuss D**, Mier L, Le Bourdelles G, et al. Clinical significance of borderline quantitative protected brush specimen culture results. Am Rev Respir Dis 1993;**147**:946–51.

49 **Sanchez-Nieto JM**, Torres A, Garcia-Cordoba F, et al. Impact of invasive and noninvasive quantitative culture sampling on outcome of ventilator-associated pneumonia: a pilot study. Am J Respir Crit Care Med 1998;**157**:371–6.

50 **Fagon JY**, Chastre J, Wolff M, et al. Invasive and noninvasive strategies for management of suspected ventilator-associated pneumonia. A randomized trial. Ann Intern Med 2000;**132**:621–30.

51 **Ruiz M**, Torres A, Ewig S, et al. Noninvasive versus invasive microbial investigation in ventilator-associated pneumonia: evaluation of outcome. Am J Respir Crit Care Med 2000;**162**:119–25.

52 **Sole Violan J**, Fernandez JA, Benitez AB, et al. Impact of quantitative invasive diagnostic techniques in the management and outcome of mechanically ventilated patients with suspected pneumonia. Crit Care Med 2000;**28**:2737–41.

53 **Ewig S**, Niederman MS, Torres A. Management of suspected ventilator-associated pneumonia. Ann Intern Med 2000;**133**:1008–9.

54 **Fagon JY**, Chastre J. Management of suspected ventilator-associated pneumonia. Ann Intern Med 2000;**133**:1009.

55 **Hubmayr RD**, Burchardi H, Elliot M, et al. Statement of the 4th International Consensus Conference in Critical Care on ICU-Acquired Pneumonia: Chicago, Illinois, May 2002. Intensive Care Med 2002;**28**:1521–36.

56 **Pugin J**, Auckenthaler R, Mili N, et al. Diagnosis of ventilator-associated pneumonia by bacteriologic analysis of bronchoscopic and nonbronchoscopic "blind" bronchoalveolar lavage fluid. Am Rev Respir Dis 1991;**143**:1121–9.

57 **Ewig S**, Schäfer H, Torres A. Severity assessment in community-acquired pneumonia. Eur Respir J 2000;**16**:1193–201.

58 **Chastre J**, Wolff M, Fagon JY, et al. Comparisons of two durations of antibiotic therapy to treat ventilator-associated pneumonia. Am J Respir Crit Care Med 2003;**167**:(Suppl) A21.

59 **Singh N**, Rogers P, Atwood CW, *et al*. Short-course empiric antibiotic therapy for patients with pulmonary infiltrates in the intensive care unit. A proposed solution for indiscriminate antibiotic prescription. *Am J Respir Crit Care Med* 200; **162**:505–11.

60 **Niederman MS**. Is "crop rotation" of antibiotics the solution to a "resistant" problem in the ICU? *Am J Respir Crit Care Med* 1997;**156**:1029–31.

61 **Ewig S**, Dalhoff K, Lorenz J, *et al*. Deutsche Geselschaft für Pneumologie: Empfehlungen zur Therapie und Prävention der nosokomilaen Pneumonie. *Pneumologie* 2000;**54**:525–38.

62 **Niederman MS**. An approach to empiric therapy of nosocomial pneumonia. *Med Clin North Am* 1994;**78**:1123–41.

63 **Alvarez-Lerma F**. Modification of empiric antibiotic treatment in patients with pneumonia acquired in the intensive care unit. ICU-Acquired Pneumonia Study Group. *Intensive Care Med* 1996;**22**:387–94.

64 **Rello J**, Gallego M, Mariscal D, *et al*. The value of routine microbial investigation in ventilator-associated pneumonia. *Am J Respir Crit Care Med* 1997;**156**:196–200.

65 **Kollef MH**, Ward S. The influence of mini-BAL cultures on patient outcomes: implications for the antibiotic management of ventilator-associated pneumonia. *Chest* 1998;**113**:412–20.

5 Acute lung injury and the acute respiratory distress syndrome: definitions and epidemiology

K Atabai, M A Matthay

The acute respiratory distress syndrome (ARDS) is a common clinical disorder characterised by injury to the alveolar epithelial and endothelial barriers of the lung, acute inflammation, and protein rich pulmonary oedema leading to acute respiratory failure. Since its first description by Ashbaugh et al,[1] a considerable volume of both basic and clinical research has led to a more sophisticated appreciation of the pathogenesis and pathophysiology of the syndrome.[2] However, our understanding of the epidemiology and effects of treatments have been hampered by the lack of uniform definitions. Several attempts have been made to provide workable definitions that would be useful in both clinical management and research. This chapter reviews the definitions and epidemiology of ARDS, with particular attention to how changes in defining the syndrome have affected our understanding of the natural history and treatment options.

DEFINITIONS
Basic definition
In 1967 Ashbaugh and colleagues described a clinical syndrome of tachypnoea, hypoxaemia resistant to supplemental oxygen, diffuse alveolar infiltrates, and decreased pulmonary compliance in 12 patients who required positive pressure mechanical ventilation. The onset of the syndrome was acute, typically within hours of the inciting clinical disorder. The majority of patients did not have a history of pulmonary disease. Adequate oxygenation required the use of continuous positive pressure with end expiratory pressures (PEEP) of 5–10 cm H_2O. The earliest radiographic findings were patchy infiltrates indistinguishable from cardiogenic pulmonary oedema that usually became confluent with progressive clinical deterioration. Lung compliance was substantially decreased. Gross lung specimens resembled hepatic tissue with large airways being free from obstruction. Histological examination revealed hyaline membranes in the alveoli with microscopic atelectasis and intra-alveolar haemorrhage similar to the infant respiratory distress syndrome.[1]

In a subsequent paper Petty and Ashbaugh refined and elaborated on what they coined the "*adult* respiratory distress syndrome".[3] In a review of 40 cases the mechanism of lung injury was either direct (chest trauma, aspiration) or indirect (pancreatitis, sepsis) and, in some cases, was attributed to mechanical ventilation. Despite the heterogeneity of inciting events, the physiological and pathological response of the lung was uniform. The use of PEEP was critical in maintaining acceptable oxygen saturation by reducing the right to left intrapulmonary shunt and increasing the functional residual capacity. Recovery from lung injury could be rapid and complete or could progress to interstitial fibrosis and progressive respiratory failure. Fatalities were primarily due to septic complications.[3]

Expanded definition
Over the next two decades the basic definition was thought by many experts to be a hindrance to understanding the syndrome. The definition was not sufficiently specific, was open to varying interpretations, and did not require the clinical aetiology of the syndrome to be specified. Investigators used different criteria to enrol patients in clinical studies making comparison of results across trials difficult. In 1988 Murray and colleagues proposed an expanded definition of ARDS intended to describe whether the syndrome was in an acute or chronic phase, the physiological severity of pulmonary injury, and the primary clinical disorder associated with the development of lung injury (table 5.1).[4] The first part of the definition addressed the clinical course separating acute from chronic cases; patients with a prolonged course (chronic) were presumably more likely to develop pulmonary fibrosis and to have poor outcomes. The second part, the lung injury score (LIS), quantified the severity of lung injury from the degree of arterial hypoxaemia, the level of PEEP, the respiratory compliance, and the radiographic abnormalities (table 5.2). Finally, the cause or associated medical condition was to be specified.[4] This proposal was accompanied by an editorial by Petty endorsing the new definition.

The expanded definition had several advantages. By describing whether patients had an acute course with rapid resolution or a more chronic course, the definition differentiated between the rapidly resolving course typical of ARDS secondary to drug overdoses or pulmonary contusion and the complicated and protracted course of many patients with severe pneumonia or sepsis syndrome. The LIS quantified the severity of lung injury separating patients with severe lung injury (LIS >2.5) from those with mild lung injury (LIS <2.5->0.1). Most importantly, the identification of the cause or associated medical condition addressed the aetiology of lung injury. As the authors argued, grouping all causes of ARDS under an umbrella classification potentially prevented the discovery of beneficial treatments aimed at a particular cause.[4]

Abbreviations: ALI, acute lung injury; ARDS, acute respiratory distress syndrome; PEEP, positive end expiratory pressure; Pao_2, arterial oxygen tension; Fio_2, fractional inspired oxygen; Pao_2, alveolar oxygen tension; LIS, lung injury score; PAOP, pulmonary artery occlusion pressure.

Table 5.1 Three part expanded definition of clinical acute lung injury (ALI) and the acute respiratory distress syndrome (ARDS) proposed by Murray and colleagues[4]

Part 1	Acute or chronic, depending on course
Part 2	Severity of physiological lung injury as determined by the lung injury score (see table 5.2)
Part 3	Lung injury caused by or associated with known risk factor for ARDS such as sepsis, pneumonia, aspiration, or major trauma

Table 5.3 1994 consensus conference definition of acute lung injury (ALI) and the acute respiratory distress syndrome (ARDS)

Onset	● Acute and persistent
Oxygenation criteria	● Pao_2/Fio_2 ≤300 for ALI
	● Pao_2/Fio_2 ≤200 for ARDS
Exclusion criteria	● PAOP ≥18 mm Hg
	● Clinical evidence of left atrial hypertension
Radiographic criteria	● Bilateral opacities consistent with pulmonary oedema

Table 5.2 Calculation of the lung injury score[4]

	Score
Chest radiograph	
No alveolar consolidation	0
Alveolar consolidation confined to 1 quadrant	1
Alveolar consolidation confined to 2 quadrants	2
Alveolar consolidation confined to 3 quadrants	3
Alveolar consolidation confined to 4 quadrants	4
Hypoxaemia score	
Pao_2/Fio_2 ≥300	0
Pao_2/Fio_2 225–299	1
Pao_2/Fio_2 175–224	2
Pao_2/Fio_2 100–174	3
Pao_2/Fio_2 <100	4
PEEP score (when mechanically ventilated)	
≤5 cm H_2O	0
6–8 cm H_2O	1
9–11 cm H_2O	2
12–14 cm H_2O	3
≥15 cm H_2O	4
Respiratory system compliance score (when available)	
≥80 ml/cm H_2O	0
60–79 ml/cm H_2O	1
40–59 ml/cm H_2O	2
20–39 ml/cm H_2O	3
≤19 ml/cm H_2O	4
The score is calculated by adding the sum of each component and dividing by the number of components used.	
No lung injury	0
Mild to moderate lung injury	0.1–2.5
Severe lung injury (ARDS)	>2.5

NAECC definition

In 1994 the North American-European Consensus Conference (NAECC) on ARDS proposed a revised definition for acute lung injury (ALI) and ARDS (table 5.3).[5] The panel recognised that accurate estimates of the incidence and outcomes of ARDS were hindered by the lack of a simple uniform definition, especially one that could be used to enrol patients in clinical studies. The panel changed "adult" back to "acute respiratory distress syndrome", recognising that the syndrome was not limited to adults (the original Ashbaugh report included one 11 year old patient). Mechanical ventilation was not a requirement, although it was anticipated that most clinical trials would only enrol intubated patients. In order to exclude chronic lung disease, the definition required an acute onset of respiratory failure.

The physiological severity of lung injury was addressed by using the term ALI to refer to patients with a Pao_2/Fio_2 ratio of <300 and ARDS in those with a Pao_2/Fio_2 ratio of <200. Although this was an arbitrary separation of the clinical spectrum of lung injury, previous studies had suggested that these cut off values were reasonable.[6] The more liberal oxygenation criteria might allow clinical trials to capture patients with lung injury earlier in their course and perhaps facilitate identification of risk factors important in predicting outcomes.[6] In contrast to the definition of Murray et al, the NAECC definition

did not incorporate the level of PEEP. There was considerable debate on this issue but it was decided that, for the sake of simplicity, the level of PEEP should not be used to make the diagnosis of ALI or ARDS.

The NAECC definition included exclusion criteria for patients with cardiogenic pulmonary oedema. The pulmonary artery occlusion pressure (PAOP), if measured, should be <18 mm Hg and there should be no clinical evidence of left atrial hypertension, although left atrial hypertension might occasionally coexist with ARDS. In each case it would be up to the clinician to assess whether the clinical, radiographic, or physiological abnormalities could be explained primarily by left atrial hypertension. The radiographic criteria for the diagnosis of ALI/ARDS were simplified to the presence of bilateral opacities consistent with pulmonary oedema. There was no quantification of the radiological abnormalities nor was there an effort to separate ALI from ARDS by radiographic findings.

The NAECC definition, as with previous attempts, had limitations (table 5.4). The definition was descriptive and did not address the cause of lung injury. Although it stipulated an acute onset, it did not provide guidelines on how to define acute. Most importantly, the radiological criteria were not sufficiently specific. In a recent study 21 critical care specialists, including seven members of the ARDS Network group of investigators, were asked to evaluate 28 chest radiographs of patients with a Pao_2/Fio_2 ratio of <300 and to decide if they would qualify for the 1994 definition of ALI.[7] The inter-observer statistical agreement was moderate, with substantially worse agreement when analysis was limited to digital radiographs. A similar study showed excellent agreement between one intensive care specialist and a radiologist in diagnosing ALI only after the two had undergone a period of training during which diagnostic discrepancies were discussed and guidelines for interpreting ambiguous radiographs were established.[8]

The NAECC definition does not account for the level of PEEP used, which affects the Pao_2/Fio_2 ratio. However, there is no simple solution to this issue because the level of PEEP, as well as other ventilator settings, would have to be stipulated in advance before the diagnosis could be made.

Relationship between definitions

Several studies have examined the relationship between the definition of ARDS proposed by Murray et al and that of the NAECC. A prospective trial using strict diagnostic criteria for ARDS as the gold standard evaluated the diagnostic accuracy of the LIS, the NAECC definition, and a modified LIS in identifying patients with ARDS.[9] The modified LIS consisted of two components: a Pao_2/Fio_2 of ≤174 (corresponding to grade 3 or higher LIS (table 5.2)) and bilateral infiltrates on a chest radiograph. The following diagnostic criteria for ARDS served as the gold standard: concomitant presence of respiratory failure requiring mechanical ventilation; bilateral pulmonary infiltrates; Pao_2/Pao_2 <0.2; PAOP <18 mm Hg; and static respiratory system compliance <50 ml/cm H_2O. One hundred and twenty three patients with at least one of seven "at risk"

Table 5.4 Strengths and limitations of the different definitions of ARDS

Definition	Strengths	Limitations
Petty and Ashbaugh (1971)[3]	• Detailed clinical description of the hallmarks of ARDS which remains relevant today	• No formal criteria for identification of patients
Murray et al (1988)[4]	• Three part definition evaluates chronicity, severity, and cause of lung injury	• Lung injury score has not been predictive of mortality • No formal criteria to exclude cardiogenic pulmonary oedema
North American-European Consensus Conference (1994)[5]	• Simple criteria which are easy to apply in the clinical setting • Disease spectrum recognised by separation of ARDS from ALI	• Cause of lung injury not required • Radiographic criteria not sufficiently specific

diagnoses were followed prospectively for the development of ARDS. The diagnostic accuracy in the "at risk" population (true positive + true negative/total number of patients) was 90% for the LIS definition and 97% for both the modified LIS and the NAECC definitions (p=0.03). The authors concluded that the three scoring systems identified similar populations when applied to patients with clearly defined at risk diagnoses.

A more recent study assessed the agreement between the definitions of Murray et al and the NAECC in diagnosing ARDS in a prospective trial of 118 patients comparing ventilation strategies.[10] The incidence using the LIS was 62% while that using the NAECC definition was 55%. Statistical agreement between the two definitions was moderate and improved when analysis was limited to patients who had undergone compliance measurements (65%). A more liberal Pao_2/Fio_2 ratio decreased agreement, as did increasing the LIS threshold diagnostic of ARDS to 3 or decreasing it to 2. Omitting data on oxygenation, chest radiography, PAOP, PEEP, or respiratory compliance either decreased agreement or left it unchanged. While agreement between the definitions was only moderate, there was no difference in mortality between the two groups of patients identified. The authors concluded that, for investigative purposes, the two criteria could be used interchangeably.

Significance of definitions in clinical trials

The NAECC updated its recommendations in 1998.[11 12] Although no formal changes were made, the Committee emphasised the importance of addressing epidemiological and aetiological differences between patients when designing clinical trials. Several prospective studies had identified risk factors present at the onset of lung injury that predicted poorer outcomes[13–16]; clinical trial organisers would need to ensure an equal distribution of these risk factors in their experimental and control arms. They also encouraged further research focused on identifying markers predictive of progression to or poor outcomes from lung injury.[11] Previous definitions had relied on abnormalities of lung physiology to grade injury[1 3–5]; however, neither the initial LIS nor the initial Pao_2/Fio_2 ratio was predictive of mortality in clinical trials.[13 14 16 17] Some biological markers, on the other hand, had already been proved to be useful in identifying patients at risk for poor outcomes. For example, raised levels of procollagen III peptide in early bronchoalveolar lavage and pulmonary oedema fluid samples predicted a protracted clinical course with progression to pulmonary fibrosis in patients with ALI/ARDS,[18 19] and increased levels of von Willebrand factor antigen in plasma predicted the development of lung injury in patients with non-pulmonary sepsis syndrome.[20] Also, a recent study reported that higher levels of von Willebrand factor antigens in the plasma of ALI/ARDS patients independently predicted mortality early in the clinical course.[21]

The importance of standard definitions and a mechanistic approach to enrolling patients in clinical trials are apparent in the results of two recent randomised multicentre trials. The first, conducted by the ARDS Network, evaluated the benefits of a low tidal volume strategy of mechanical ventilation and found an absolute reduction in the primary outcome of death prior to hospital discharge of 9% using lower tidal volumes (22% relative reduction in mortality).[22] Patients were enrolled using the 1994 definition and the benefit of a protective ventilation strategy was maintained in all subsets of patients with ALI/ARDS.[23] This was the first large trial to show the benefit of any intervention in ALI/ARDS.[2 24]

The importance of identifying the mechanism of lung injury is borne out by a recent trial of recombinant human activated protein C in severe sepsis.[25] A 96 hour infusion of protein C resulted in an absolute reduction in mortality of 6.1% (20% relative reduction) in a large international multicentre trial; 54% of the 1690 patients had a pulmonary source of sepsis and 75% required mechanical ventilation on entry into the study. Although the study did not report the number of patients who met the criteria for ALI/ARDS, it is likely that most did since ARDS is the most common cause of respiratory failure in sepsis and sepsis is the most common predisposing factor for the development of ARDS.[2 26] Based on this study, it is likely that a trial of protein C in patients with lung injury due to sepsis will show a treatment benefit while the same trial in patients with ARDS due to trauma or fat emboli may not. As more is learned about the epidemiology and pathophysiology of ARDS, identifying the cause of injury in designing treatment trials will become increasingly critical.

EPIDEMIOLOGY
Incidence

The incidence of ALI and ARDS has been difficult to establish. Most studies were conducted before the NAECC definition was proposed and used different criteria to enrol patients. Defining the population at risk in a given study has been equally problematic. Accurate measurement of disease incidence requires knowledge of the number of people with the disease within a defined population at risk for developing it. Prospective trials must account for the catchment area of the hospitals studied; each hospital's catchment area may overlap with that of several other hospitals.

In 1972 the National Heart and Lung Institute (NHLI) task force estimated an incidence of 75 cases of ARDS per 100 000 population per year.[27] Several subsequent studies have estimated a much lower annual incidence of 1.5–13.5 cases per 100 000 population (table 5.5).[28–32] There are several reasons why the number of cases may have been overestimated. The task force predated the widespread acceptance of the definition of ARDS and used a broad definition of lung injury that included conditions such as renal failure and volume overload. In addition, the population at risk was not clearly

Table 5.5 Annual incidence of the acute respiratory distress syndrome (ARDS) and acute lung injury (ALI) in different clinical studies

Study	Criteria used to diagnose ALI/ARDS	Incidence (cases/100 000 population/year)	Study limitations
NHLI task force[27]		75	• Broad definition of respiratory distress syndrome including patients with volume overload
Canary Islands[31]	Pao_2/Fio_2 <110 Pao_2/Fio_2 <150	1.5 3.5	• Mean age of study population was 32 • Non-urban setting
Utah[30]	Pao_2/Fio_2 <110	4.8–8.3	• Incomplete sampling of hospitals • Use of ICD-9 codes to diagnose ARDS
Berlin[28]	Lung injury score >2.5 Lung injury score >1.75–<2.5	3.0 17.1	• 2 month study may miss seasonal variation in incidence of ALI/ARDS • No correction for migration in and out of study population
Scandinavia[29]	Pao_2/Fio_2 <300 Pao_2/Fio_2 <200 Lung injury score >2.5	17.9 13.5 7.6	• 2 month study may miss seasonal variation in incidence of ALI/ARDS • No correction for migration in and out of study population

defined.[33] [34] A three year study conducted in the Canary Islands was unique in that all patients requiring mechanical ventilation were cared for at one hospital.[29] Using a Pao_2/Fio_2 ratio of <110 to define ARDS, the population incidence was 1.5 cases per 100 000 population. A Pao_2/Fio_2 cut off of <150 resulted in an incidence of 3.5 cases per 100 000 population. Although the study strictly defined the population at risk, extrapolation of incidence data from this young population (average age 32) to an urban setting is questionable. A prospective three year study in Utah using a Pao_2/Pao_2 ratio of <0.2 (corresponding to a Pao_2/Fio_2 ratio of <110) to define ARDS estimated an annual incidence of 4.8–8.3 cases per 100 000 population. The authors recorded all cases of ARDS in six Utah hospitals and estimated the number of cases in the remaining 34 acute care hospitals using ICD-9 codes.[30] Although the investigators made corrections for the population migrating in and out of Utah as well as for visitors developing ARDS, the incomplete sampling of hospitals and the use of ICD-9 codes weakened the study. Also, the incidence of alcohol and tobacco use is probably much less in Utah than in other states. A 2 month prospective study in Berlin found an annual incidence of 3 cases per 100 000 population using the expanded definition proposed by Murray *et al.*[28] The population of Berlin was the study population and 97% of all intensive care units were surveyed. No corrections were made for migration in and out of the catchment area. Finally, a prospective 2 month study in Sweden, Denmark, and Iceland using the NAECC definition found an annual incidence of ARDS and of ALI of 13.5 per 100 000 and 17.9 cases per 100 000, respectively.[29] The annual incidence of ARDS using the LIS was 7.6 cases per 100 000 population. Interestingly, only 71 of 110 patients who met the criteria for ARDS using the LIS also met the criteria using a Pao_2/Fio_2 ratio of <200.

The true incidence of ALI/ARDS is currently unknown, but may not be as high as the 1972 NHLI estimate nor as low as estimates made in the Canary Islands or Berlin. A definitive study using the NAECC definition has been completed at the University of Washington and preliminary results suggest that the original NHLI estimate may have been reasonable.[33]

Incidence of ARDS in patients with known risk factors

Lung injury can be caused by direct or indirect mechanisms (table 5.6). Identifying risk factors for the development of ALI/ARDS is particularly important in evaluating treatments that may prevent progression to lung injury in high risk populations. Three prospective studies from the early 1980s evaluated the incidence of ARDS in patients with known risk factors.[35–37] In each study investigators followed patients with

Table 5.6 Clinical disorders associated with the development of ALI/ARDS

Direct	Indirect
Common • Aspiration pneumonia • Pneumonia	Common • Sepsis • Severe trauma with prolonged hypotension and/or multiple fractures • Multiple transfusions of blood products
Less common • Inhalation injury • Pulmonary contusion • Fat emboli • Near drowning • Reperfusion injury	Less common • Acute pancreatitis • Cardiopulmonary bypass • Drug overdose • Disseminated intravascular coagulation • Burns • Head injury

respiratory failure and clinical conditions thought to predispose to ARDS for the development of the syndrome. All three used stricter Pao_2/Fio_2 ratios to diagnose ARDS than the NAECC definition.

In the first of two studies from Seattle, 136 patients with one or more risk factors were followed for the development of ARDS defined by a Pao_2/Fio_2 ratio of <150.[37] The risk factors were sepsis syndrome, aspiration of gastric contents, pulmonary contusion, multiple transfusions, near drowning, pancreatitis, multiple major fractures, and prolonged hypotension not due to sepsis or cardiogenic shock. Multiple major fractures were defined as either fractures of two or more major long bones, an unstable pelvic fracture, or one major long bone fracture and a major pelvic fracture. Multiple transfusions were defined as infusion of 10 or more units of packed red blood cells or whole blood within a 12 hour period. Although 34% of the patients identified developed ARDS, the majority of patients who developed ARDS during the study time frame were missed. Of the patients captured by the study, those with sepsis and aspiration pneumonia had the highest risk of developing ARDS (38% and 30% risk, respectively), followed by patients receiving multiple blood transfusions and pulmonary contusions (24% and 17% risk, respectively). Patients with more than one risk factor were at increased risk for developing the syndrome. Of the patients who developed ARDS, 76% had done so within 2–24 hours of the inciting event and 93% by 72 hours.

The second study from Seattle defined ARDS as a PaO_2/FiO_2 ratio of <150 or <200 in patients on PEEP and captured 80% of patients who developed ARDS during the study.[36] Sepsis syndrome was again associated with the highest incidence of ARDS (41%), followed by multiple transfusions (36%), aspiration pneumonia (22%), and pulmonary contusion (22%). Interestingly, massive transfusions were equally likely to cause ARDS in medical patients as in patients with trauma.

A study from Denver identified risk factors as cardiopulmonary bypass, burn, bacteraemia, hypertransfusion, fracture, pneumonia requiring care in the intensive care unit (ICU), aspiration, and disseminated intravascular coagulation (DIC).[35] ARDS was diagnosed in patients with a PaO_2/PAO_2 ratio of <0.2, PAOP <12 mm Hg, and a static pulmonary compliance of <50 ml/cm H_2O. Aspiration pneumonia was associated with a 35% incidence of developing ARDS, followed by DIC (22%), and pneumonia requiring ICU care (12%). The study missed 22% of patients who developed ARDS, most of whom had presumed sepsis. Bacteraemia, defined as two positive blood cultures, was associated with a 3.8% risk of ARDS.

The data from these prospective and other studies[6] identify sepsis as the most common risk factor for developing ARDS, followed by aspiration pneumonia, pneumonia, trauma, and multiple transfusions. The relative incidence of ALI/ARDS with each risk factor will depend on the exact definitions used; for example, if patients with pneumonia and sepsis syndrome are classified as pneumonia, then the incidence with pneumonia will be greater. Overall, approximately 20–40% of patients with well established risk factors and respiratory failure develop ARDS,[9 15 35 36] and the more risk factors in any individual, the greater the likelihood of developing the syndrome.[15 35 36 38] As with most of the epidemiological data currently available, these numbers may change as newer studies use the NAECC criteria to define ALI/ARDS.

In addition to the risk factors discussed above, recent reports have identified additional conditions that influence the susceptibility of individuals to developing lung injury. In a prospective study of 351 patients the incidence of ARDS with one of seven known "at risk" diagnoses was compared in patients with and without a history of chronic alcohol abuse.[15] Experimental data demonstrating the activating effect of alcohol on neutrophil adherence, chemotaxis, and phagocytosis[39] led investigators to speculate that patients who chronically abuse alcohol would be at a higher risk for developing ARDS. The incidence of ARDS was 43% in patients with a history of chronic alcohol abuse compared with 22% in the control group. Patients with higher APACHE II scores at the time of the "at risk" diagnosis also had a significantly higher incidence of ARDS. Both the history of chronic alcohol abuse and the APACHE II score remained significant with multivariate analysis.

The same investigators hypothesised that patients with diabetes mellitus may be protected from ARDS due to the impaired neutrophil function associated with hyperglycaemia. In a study of 113 patients with septic shock, the incidence of ARDS was 25% in diabetic and 47% in non-diabetic patients.[40] After multivariate analysis adjusting for age, a history of cirrhosis, and source of infection, the difference in incidence remained significant. Mortality was not significantly different in the two groups. This was the first study to identify a risk factor that decreased the risk of developing ARDS.[41]

Clinical risk factors predictive of a poor outcome
Several prospective trials using the NAECC definition have identified risk factors that are independent predictors of mortality (table 5.7).[13 14 16 29 45] Each study enrolled a slightly different study population which may contribute to differences in risk factors identified. In a prospective trial of 123 medical and surgical (not trauma) patients with lung injury, liver dysfunction, sepsis and non-pulmonary organ system dysfunction

Table 5.7 Risk factors predictive of increased mortality in multivariate analysis of patients with ALI/ARDS

Risk factor	Study
Liver dysfunction/cirrhosis	Doyle et al[13]
	Zilberberg et al[16]
	Monchi et al[14]
	Luhr et al[29]
	Roupie et al[45]
Sepsis	Doyle et al[13]
	Zilberberg et al[16]
	Monchi et al[14]
Non-pulmonary organ dysfunction	Doyle et al[13]
	Monchi et al[14]
Age	Zilberberg et al[16]
	Luhr et al[29]
Organ transplantation	Zilberberg et al[16]
HIV infection	Zilberberg et al[16]
Active malignancy	Zilberberg et al[16]
Length of mechanical ventilation prior to ARDS	Monchi et al[14]
Oxygenation index (mean airway pressure × FiO_2 × $100/PaO_2$)	Monchi et al[14]
Mechanism of lung injury	Monchi et al[14]
Right ventricular dysfunction	Monchi et al[14]
PaO_2/FiO_2 <100	Luhr et al[29]
Chronic alcoholism	Moss et al[15]

during the period between hospitalisation and admission to the ICU were associated with significantly increased mortality.[13] A study of 107 medical intensive care patients with lung injury found sepsis, cirrhosis, organ transplantation, HIV infection, active cancer, and age above 65 years to be independent predictors of mortality.[16] A French study of 259 patients with ARDS in a medical ICU found cirrhosis, sepsis, the duration of mechanical ventilation prior to ARDS, oxygenation index (mean airway pressure × FiO_2 × $100/PaO_2$), the mechanism of lung injury, and the occurrence of right ventricular dysfunction to be independent predictors of death.[14] A Scandinavian study of 132 intensive care patients in three countries (including medical, surgical and neurological patients) found chronic liver disease, a PaO_2/FiO_2 ratio of <100, and age to be independent predictors of death.[29]

In most studies the initial oxygenation abnormality defined by the PaO_2/FiO_2 ratio did not predict mortality unless it was grossly abnormal.[6 13 14 16 17 29 42] Similarly, the initial severity of lung injury defined by the LIS has not predicted mortality,[13 16] although in one study the LIS measured after 4 days predicted a complicated clinical course.[43]

Although identification of independent predictors of mortality using multivariate analysis in any single study depends on which risk factors are evaluated, cumulative data convincingly show that patients with ALI/ARDS and sepsis, liver disease, non-pulmonary organ dysfunction, or advanced age have higher mortality rates.[6 13 14 16 29 43–7] Equal distribution of these risk factors among experimental and control groups is essential when enrolling patients in clinical trials.

CONCLUSION
The understanding of ARDS and its definition continues to evolve as we learn more about its epidemiology and pathophysiology. The first two decades of research after Ashbaugh and Petty's classic articles describing ARDS were hampered by the lack of uniform definitions. The expanded definition of ARDS proposed by Murray and colleagues in 1988 incorporating the chronicity, severity, and cause of lung

injury represented a turning point towards a more quantitative approach. The NAECC 1994 definition simplified the diagnostic criteria proposed by Murray and colleagues by eliminating the level of PEEP from the oxygenation criteria and the measurement of respiratory compliance, and reducing the chest radiographic inclusion criteria to the presence of bilateral opacities consistent with pulmonary oedema. As with the definition of Murray *et al*, the NAECC definition graded lung injury by defining different oxygenation criteria for ALI and ARDS. In the past decade the application of these two definitions has led to substantial progress in the understanding of the natural history of lung injury. Although the two criteria define overlapping populations with a similar prognosis, it is not clear whether conclusions generated using one definition can be extrapolated to populations defined by the other. It is hoped that future trials will use the NAECC definition exclusively.

Several aspects of the definition of ALI/ARDS need further refinement. Although initial oxygenation indices have little prognostic value, the more liberal oxygenation criteria describing ALI appear to identify patients with similar baseline characteristics and prognosis at an earlier stage of the illness. If there is no prognostic or epidemiological difference between ALI and ARDS patients, then the two categories should be combined. On the other hand, in certain subsets such as trauma, patients with ALI may have better a prognosis than those with ARDS. While the radiographic criteria of the NAECC definition are easy to apply, recent data suggest that there is significant interobserver variability. Although a more standardised approach is desirable, complex schemas quantifying the severity of infiltrates in different quadrants have no prognostic value. It therefore appears that an approach that combines the simplicity of the NAECC definition with more standardised and specific criteria would be ideal.

The risk of an individual developing lung injury and its prognosis will be more predictable as more accurate physiological markers are identified. Interestingly, a recent large prospective clinical study of 179 patients has found that a markedly raised dead space fraction (0.58) occurs early in the course of ARDS and is independently associated with mortality.[48] As the pathogenesis and epidemiology of lung injury are elucidated, treatment may be individualised around the mechanism of injury and the clinical characteristics of each patient.

REFERENCES

1 **Ashbaugh DG**, Bigelow DB, Petty TL, *et al*. Acute respiratory distress in adults. *Lancet* 1967;**ii**:319–23.
2 **Ware LB**, Matthay MA. The acute respiratory distress syndrome. *N Engl J Med* 2000;**342**:1334–49.
3 **Petty TL**, Ashbaugh DG. The adult respiratory distress syndrome. Clinical features, factors influencing prognosis and principles of management. *Chest* 1971;**60**:233–9.
4 **Murray JF**, Matthay MA, Luce JM, *et al*. An expanded definition of the adult respiratory distress syndrome. *Am Rev Respir Dis* 1988;**138**:720–3; erratum 1989;**139**:1065.
5 **Bernard GR**, Artigas A, Brigham KL, *et al*. The American-European Consensus Conference on ARDS. Definitions, mechanisms, relevant outcomes, and clinical trial coordination. *Am J Respir Crit Care Med* 1994;**149**:818–24.
6 **Sloane PJ**, Gee MH, Gottlieb JE, *et al*. A multicenter registry of patients with acute respiratory distress syndrome. Physiology and outcome. *Am Rev Respir Dis* 1992;**146**:419–26.
7 **Rubenfeld GD**, Caldwell E, Granton J, *et al*. Interobserver variability in applying a radiographic definition for ARDS. *Chest* 1999;**116**:1347–53.
8 **Meade MO**, Cook RJ, Guyatt GH, *et al*. Interobserver variation in interpreting chest radiographs for the diagnosis of acute respiratory distress syndrome. *Am J Respir Crit Care Med* 2000;**161**:85–90.
9 **Moss M**, Goodman PL, Heinig M, *et al*. Establishing the relative accuracy of three new definitions of the adult respiratory distress syndrome. *Crit Care Med* 1995;**23**:1629–37.
10 **Meade MO**, Guyatt GH, Cook RJ, *et al*. Agreement between alternative classification of acute respiratory distress syndrome. *Am J Respir Crit Care Med* 2001;**163**:490–3.
11 **Abraham E**, Matthay MA, Dinarello CA, *et al*. Consensus conference definitions for sepsis, septic shock, acute lung injury, and acute respiratory distress syndrome: time for a reevaluation. *Crit Care Med* 2000;**28**:232–5.
12 **Artigas A**, Bernard GR, Carlet J, *et al*. The American-European Consensus Conference on ARDS, Part 2. Ventilatory, pharmacologic, supportive therapy, study design strategies and issues related to recovery and remodeling. *Intensive Care Med* 1998;**24**:378–98.
13 **Doyle RL**, Szaflarski N, Modin GW, *et al*. Identification of patients with acute lung injury. Predictors of mortality. *Am J Respir Crit Care Med* 1995;**152**:1818–24.
14 **Monchi M**, Bellenfant F, Cariou A, *et al*. Early predictive factors of survival in the acute respiratory distress syndrome. A multivariate analysis. *Am J Respir Crit Care Med* 1998;**158**:1076–81.
15 **Moss M**, Bucher B, Moore FA, *et al*. The role of chronic alcohol abuse in the development of acute respiratory distress syndrome in adults. *JAMA* 1996;**275**:50–4.
16 **Zilberberg MD**, Epstein SK. Acute lung injury in the medical ICU: comorbid conditions, age, etiology, and hospital outcome. *Am J Respir Crit Care Med* 1998;**157**:1159–64.
17 **Krafft P**, Fridrich P, Pernerstorfer T, *et al*. The acute respiratory distress syndrome: definitions, severity and clinical outcome. An analysis of 101 clinical investigations. *Intensive Care Med* 1996;**22**:519–29.
18 **Chesnutt AN**, Matthay MA, Tibayan FA, *et al*. Early detection of type III procollagen peptide in acute lung injury. Pathogenetic and prognostic significance. *Am J Respir Crit Care Med* 1997;**156**:840–5.
19 **Clark JG**, Milberg JA, Steinberg KP, *et al*. Type III procollagen peptide in the adult respiratory distress syndrome. Association of increased peptide levels in bronchoalveolar lavage fluid with increased risk for death. *Ann Intern Med* 1995;**122**:17–23.
20 **Rubin DB**, Wiener-Kronish JP, Murray JF, *et al*. Elevated von Willebrand factor antigen is an early plasma predictor of acute lung injury in nonpulmonary sepsis syndrome. *J Clin Invest* 1990;**86**:474–80.
20 **Pugin J**, Verghese G, Widmer MC, *et al*. The alveolar space is the site of intense inflammatory and profibrotic reactions in the early phase of acute respiratory distress syndrome. *Crit Care Med* 1999;**27**:304–12.
21 **Ware LB**, Conner ER, Matthay MA. Von Willebrand factor antigen is an independent marker of poor outcome in patients with early acute lung injury. *Crit Care Med* 2001;**29**:2325–31.
22 **ARDS Network**. Ventilation with lower tidal volumes as compared with traditional tidal volumes for acute lung injury and the acute respiratory distress syndrome. The Acute Respiratory Distress Syndrome Network. *N Engl J Med* 2000;**342**:1301–8.
23 **Eisner MD**, Thompson T, Hudson LD, *et al*. Efficacy of low tidal volume ventilation in patients with different clinical risk factors for acute lung injury and the acute respiratory distress syndrome. *Am J Respir Crit Care Med* 2001 (in press).
24 **McIntyre RC Jr**, Pulido EJ, Bensard DD, *et al*. Thirty years of clinical trials in acute respiratory distress syndrome. *Crit Care Med* 2000;**28**:3314–31.
25 **Bernard GR**, Vincent J, Laterre P, *et al*. Efficacy and safety of recombinant human activated protein C for severe sepsis. *N Engl J Med* 2001;**344**:699–709.
26 **Matthay MA**. Severe sepsis: a new treatment with both anticoagulant and antiinflammatory properties. *N Engl J Med* 2001;**344**:759–61.
27 **National Heart and Lung Institute**. *Task force on problems, research approaches, needs: the lung program*. Washington, DC: Department of Health, Education, and Welfare, 1972: 165–80.
28 **Lewandowski K**, Metz J, Deutschmann C, *et al*. Incidence, severity, and mortality of acute respiratory failure in Berlin, Germany. *Am J Respir Crit Care Med* 1995;**151**:1121–5.
29 **Luhr OR**, Antonsen K, Karlsson M, *et al*. Incidence and mortality after acute respiratory failure and acute respiratory distress syndrome in Sweden, Denmark, and Iceland. The ARF Study Group. *Am J Respir Crit Care Med* 1999;**159**:1849–61.
30 **Thomsen GE**, Morris AH. Incidence of the adult respiratory distress syndrome in the state of Utah. *Am J Respir Crit Care Med* 1995;**152**:965–71.
31 **Villar J**, Slutsky AS. The incidence of the adult respiratory distress syndrome. *Am Rev Respir Dis* 1989;**140**:814–6.
32 **Webster NR**, Cohen AT, Nunn JF. Adult respiratory distress syndrome: how many cases in the UK? *Anaesthesia* 1988;**43**:923–6.
33 **Hudson LD**, Steinberg KP. Epidemiology of acute lung injury and ARDS. *Chest* 1999;**116**:74–82S.
34 **Steinberg KP**, Hudson LD. Acute lung injury and acute respiratory syndrome. *Clin Chest Med* 2000;**21**:401–17.
35 **Fowler AA**, Hamman RF, Good JT, *et al*. Adult respiratory distress syndrome: risk with common predispositions. *Ann Intern Med* 1983;**98**:593–7.
36 **Hudson LD**, Milberg JA, Anardi D, *et al*. Clinical risks for development of the acute respiratory distress syndrome. *Am J Respir Crit Care Med* 1995;**151**:293–301.
37 **Pepe PE**, Potkin RT, Reus DH, *et al*. Clinical predictors of the adult respiratory distress syndrome. *Am J Surg* 1982;**144**:124–30.
38 **Hyers TM**. Prediction of survival and mortality in patients with adult respiratory distress syndrome. *New Horiz* 1993;**1**:466–70.
39 **Hallengren B**, Forsgren A. Effect of alcohol on chemotaxis, adherence and phagocytosis of human polymorphonuclear leucocytes. *Acta Med Scand* 1978;**204**:43–8.
40 **Moss M**, Guidot DM, Steinberg KP, *et al*. Diabetic patients have a decreased incidence of acute respiratory distress syndrome. *Crit Care Med* 2000;**28**:2187–92.

41 **Frank JA**, Nuckton TJ, Matthay MA. Diabetes mellitus: a negative predictor for the development of acute respiratory distress syndrome from septic shock. *Crit Care Med* 2000;**28**:2645–6.

42 **Bell RC**, Coalson JJ, Smith JD, *et al*. Multiple organ system failure and infection in adult respiratory distress syndrome. *Ann Intern Med* 1983;**99**:293–8.

43 **Heffner JE**, Brown LK, Barbieri CA, *et al*. Prospective validation of an acute respiratory distress syndrome predictive score. *Am J Respir Crit Care Med* 1995;**152**:1518–26.

44 **Ferring M**, Vincent JL. Is outcome from ARDS related to the severity of respiratory failure? *Eur Respir J* 1997;**10**:1297–300.

45 **Roupie E**, Lepage E, Wysocki M, *et al*. Prevalence, etiologies and outcome of the acute respiratory distress syndrome among hypoxemic ventilated patients. SRLF Collaborative Group on Mechanical Ventilation. Société de Réanimation de Langue Française. *Intensive Care Med* 1999;**25**:920–9.

46 **Suchyta MR**, Clemmer TP, Elliott CG, *et al*. The adult respiratory distress syndrome. A report of survival and modifying factors. *Chest* 1992;**101**:1074–9.

47 **Ely WE**, Wheeler AP, Thompson BT, *et al*. Recovery rate and prognosis in older persons who develop lung injury and the acute respiratory distress syndrome. *Ann Intern Med* 2002;**136**:25–36.

48 **Nuckton TJ**, Alonso J, Kallet RH, *et al*. Pulmonary dead space fraction as a risk factor for mortality in the acute respiratory distress syndrome. *N Engl J Med* 2002;**346**:1281–6.

6 The pathogenesis of acute lung injury/acute respiratory distress syndrome

G J Bellingan

Lung injury is the term used to describe the pulmonary response to a broad range of injuries occurring either directly to the lung or as the consequence of injury or inflammation at other sites in the body. Acute respiratory distress syndrome (ARDS) represents the more severe end of the spectrum of this condition in which there are widespread inflammatory changes throughout the lung, usually accompanied by aggressive fibrosis.[1-5] The pathogenesis of lung injury is not well understood.[1 5] We do not know why some people progress to ARDS while others who sustain indistinguishable injuries remain relatively unaffected.[6] ARDS is unique among pulmonary fibrotic conditions in that the fibrosis resolves almost completely in many cases; once again the mechanisms for this are not understood.[7] It is now well recognised that some of the damage is created and exacerbated by mechanical ventilation.[8] However, mortality from ARDS has improved in certain centres over the last 10 years,[9 10] predating major changes in ventilatory practice; the reasons for this improvement in mortality are thus also not clear.

ARDS often occurs as part of a wider picture of multiorgan dysfunction syndrome (MODS).[11] Central to the pathogenesis are an explosive inflammatory process and the reparative responses invoked in an attempt to heal this. This chapter will outline the pathological processes which occur during ARDS and their evolution as our understanding of the inflammatory, immune, and fibroproliferative responses has grown. It will describe the underlying cellular and molecular processes, correlate these with the clinical picture, and highlight how such insights can lead to novel therapeutic approaches.

DEFINITIONS

Lung injury (acute lung injury (ALI) and ARDS) is currently defined clinically by gas exchange and chest radiographic abnormalities which occur shortly after a known predisposing injury and in the absence of heart failure.[1] The definition and range of predisposing conditions are discussed in chapter 5.

The pathophysiology of ARDS is driven by an aggressive inflammatory reaction. Indirect injury occurs as part of a systemic inflammatory response syndrome (SIRS), which can be due to infective or non-infective causes such as pancreatitis or trauma; when SIRS is caused by infection it is called sepsis. SIRS with organ dysfunction is called severe sepsis and, in the presence of significant hypotension, septic shock.[12] ARDS can thus occur in conjunction with failure of other organs, the multiorgan dysfunction syndrome (MODS). A number of endogenous anti-inflammatory mechanisms are also initiated to counterbalance the effects of such an aggressive

inflammatory response and this is termed the compensatory anti-inflammatory response syndrome (CARS), although these responses too may be excessive and contribute to a state of immunoparesis.[13 14]

PATHOLOGY

Lung injury is an evolving condition and the pathological features of ARDS are typically described as passing through three overlapping phases (table 6.1)—an inflammatory or exudative phase, a proliferative phase and, lastly, a fibrotic phase.[2-5] These phases are complicated by other variables—for example, episodes of nosocomial pneumonia and the deleterious effects of ventilator induced lung injury. Moreover, the initiating insults themselves may influence the pathophysiological picture. Radiographic differences have been identified between patients with ARDS arising from direct pulmonary injuries compared with those from indirect injuries.[15] Likewise, a small study has suggested greater areas of alveolar collapse and oedema in patients dying with ARDS from direct rather than indirect injuries.[16] Although these differences may translate into differences in outcome, no clear mechanistic differences between these groups have been identified.[17] A recent study has suggested, however, that lung cyclo-oxygenase-2 (COX-2) gene expression (a gene implicated in the early proinflammatory response) is only induced by indirect mechanisms related to the systemic response to endotoxin rather than directly in response to inhaled endotoxin.[18]

Exudative phase

Typically, this lasts for the first week after the onset of symptoms. The histological changes are termed diffuse alveolar damage.[5] At necroscopic examination the lungs are heavy, rigid and, when sectioned, do not exude fluid because of its high protein content. Bachofen and Wiebel were among the first to study the histopathological changes in detail in patients who died with ARDS.[19] An acute stage commencing within the first 24 hours of symptoms was marked by significant proteinaceous and often markedly haemorrhagic interstitial and alveolar oedema with hyaline membranes. The hyaline membranes are eosinophilic containing fibrin, immunoglobulin, and complement. The microvascular and alveolar barriers have focal areas of damage and the alveolar wall is oedematous with areas of necrosis within the epithelial lining, although the basal lamina is intact initially. The early endothelial lesions are more subtle, containing areas of necrosis and denuded spaces usually filled with fibrin clot. Neutrophils are found increasingly during the initial phases in capillaries, interstitial tissue, and progressively within airspaces.[20]

Table 6.1 Summary of some histopathological changes in ARDS

	Exudative phase	Proliferative phase	Fibrotic phase
Macroscopic	• Heavy, rigid, dark	• Heavy, grey	• Cobblestoned
Microscopic	• Hyaline membranes • Oedema • Neutrophils • Epithelial>endothelial damage	• Barrier disruption • Oedema • Alveolar type II cell proliferation • Myofibroblast infiltration • Neutrophils • Alveolar collapse • Alveoli filled with cells and organising matrix • Epithelial apoptosis • Fibroproliferation	• Fibrosis • Macrophages • Lymphocytes • Matrix organisation • Deranged acinar architecture • Patchy emphysematous change
Vasculature	• Local thrombus	• Loss of capillaries • Pulmonary hypertension	• Myointimal thickening • Tortuous vessels

Proliferative phase

Typically occupying the second 2 weeks after the onset of respiratory failure, the proliferative phase is characterised by organisation of the exudates and by fibrosis.[2-5] [19] [21] The lung remains heavy and solid, and microscopically the integrity of the lung architecture becomes steadily more deranged. The capillary network is damaged and there is a progressive decline in the profile of capillaries in tissue sections; later, intimal proliferation is evident in many small vessels further reducing the luminal area. The interstitial space becomes grossly dilated, necrosis of type I pneumocytes exposes areas of epithelial basement membrane, and the alveolar lumen fills with leucocytes, red cells, fibrin, and cell debris. Alveolar type II cells proliferate in an attempt to cover the denuded epithelial surfaces and differentiate into type I cells.[22] Fibroblasts become apparent in the interstitial space and later in the alveolar lumen.[23] These processes result in extreme narrowing or even obliteration of the airspaces. Fibrin and cell debris are progressively replaced by collagen fibrils. The main site of fibrosis is the intra-alveolar space, but it also occurs within the interstitium.

Fibrotic phase

This can begin from day 10 after initiating injury. Macroscopically, the lungs have a cobblestoned character due to scarring.[2-5] The vasculature is grossly deranged with vessels narrowed by myointimal thickening and mural fibrosis. The microscopic events occurring in the repair phase are not well documented, mainly because of a paucity of histological data as patients recover. Some insights have been obtained from bronchoalveolar lavage (BAL), radiology, and from animal models.[21] BAL confirms a marked decline in neutrophils and a relative accumulation of lymphocytes and macrophages. The most dramatic, although unpredictable, changes are those of lung collagen.[25] Total lung collagen content may double within the first 2 weeks,[26] but this burden can be eliminated and many, albeit small, studies show that survivors can return to relatively normal lung function.[27] Interestingly, although the severity of pathological changes in the first few weeks (hyaline membrane, airspace organisation, or cellularity) do not seem to correlate with late functional recovery, the degree of fibrosis is a key predictor of outcome.[28] [29] High levels of procollagen peptides detected early in ARDS have been repeatedly shown to predict a poor outcome.[30] [31] Moreover, established fibrosis reduces lung compliance thereby increasing the work of breathing, decreasing the tidal volume, and resulting in CO_2 retention. Also, because of the alveolar obliteration and inter-

stitial thickening, gas exchange is reduced which contributes to hypoxia and ventilator dependence. Although late deaths from ARDS have been ascribed mainly to sepsis rather than progressive hypoxia, sepsis is a common complication in these patients. It is usually the consequence of ventilator associated pneumonia or other nosocomial infections related to their ventilator dependence.[32] [33]

Recent evidence suggests that there is a much greater overlap of the inflammatory and fibroproliferative phases than previously thought,[7] and many mediators are common to both processes.[24] The fibroproliferative response begins remarkably early with N-terminal procollagen III peptide levels, a marker for collagen turnover, being raised in BAL fluid within 24 hours of ventilation for ARDS.[30] Myofibroblast cells also show an early increase in the alveolar walls, and BAL fluid from ARDS patients within 48 hours of diagnosis is intensely mitogenic for fibroblasts.[31] This all suggests that the fibrosis characteristic of ARDS may not be a late event but is switched on at a very early stage. This is particularly important as the inflammatory and fibrotic processes, although closely overlapping, appear to be separately regulated, thus offering the possibility for early directed treatments against fibrosis independent of the effects on inflammation.[34]

PATHOGENESIS

Lung injury is initiated by a specific insult but can be exacerbated by inappropriate mechanical ventilatory strategies (reviewed in chapter 8). Briefly, alveolar overdistension can generate a proinflammatory response which is exacerbated by repetitive opening and closing of alveoli as occurs through the use of inappropriately low levels of positive end expiratory pressure (PEEP).[8] Indeed, overdistension or recurrent opening/closing of alveoli can also induce structural damage to the lung.[35] [36] The effect of high inspired concentrations of oxygen on the disease process is uncertain, particularly in humans. However, prolonged exposure to 100% oxygen is fatal in most animal models, producing neutrophil influx and alveolar oedema that can be blocked in rodents using anti-inflammatory strategies such as inhaled low dose carbon monoxide.[37] [38]

The main players in the inflammatory process are neutrophils and multiple mediator cascades.[39-41] The fibroblast is key in the fibroproliferative response and is the target of regulators of matrix deposition.[42] A complex interplay of regulatory cytokines counteracts the inflammatory mediators; similarly, matrix deposition is balanced by the actions of the metalloproteases. There is no uniform response to injury: some patients develop ARDS, some ALI, and some do not develop pulmonary symptoms at all. The reasons for this are not clear but may be partly genetic. There is evidence for a genetic susceptibility to sepsis and, recently, to ARDS itself.[43-45]

Because of the difficulties in obtaining histological samples in humans, studies have been undertaken in animals and have provided a valuable understanding of the mechanisms driving lung injury.[46] It is important to be aware of the limitations of these models as animals differ in their sensitivity to the initiating insult (especially endotoxin) and in their pulmonary responses. The timing and severity of the insults and, especially, the degree of subsequent resuscitation also do not mirror the clinical condition. Models include direct challenge to the lung such as bleomycin, endotoxin or acid aspiration, surfactant washout and oxygen toxicity, or intravenous challenges including endotoxin, complement or microemboli: all have features in common with the human counterpart including inflammatory cell influx and endothelial damage.[38 47 48] Animals challenged with endotoxin develop endothelial and epithelial barrier dysfunction although the endothelium appears to be more sensitive than the epithelium, whereas in humans it is the epithelium that shows greater damage.[49] Animal models have also been used to examine the later stages of ARDS. The best are studies in primates exposed to high concentrations of oxygen which showed enlarged airspaces, thickened alveolar walls and interstitial fibrosis, and in the survivors there was decreased alveolarisation and bronchopulmonary dysplasia.[38]

INFLAMMATION

With initiation of inflammation there is increased leucocyte production and rapid recruitment to the inflamed site. There is also activation of mediator cascades including the production of cytokines, chemokines, acute phase proteins, free radicals, complement, coagulation pathway components, and focal upregulation of adhesion molecule expression. The "anti-inflammatory" response includes the glucocorticoids, cytokines (interleukin (IL)-4, IL-10 and IL-1 receptor antagonist (IL-1ra)) and other mechanisms such as shedding of adhesion molecules.[39-41]

The neutrophil

This is the dominant leucocyte found both in BAL fluid and in histological specimens from patients with ARDS.[20] In many animal models the degree of lung injury is reduced dramatically if neutrophil influx is ablated, although this is not a universal finding.[50 51] However, ARDS can develop in neutropenic patients, hence neutrophils are believed to be an important but not essential component of the injurious response.[52] Neutrophils cause cell damage though the production of free radicals, inflammatory mediators, and proteases. Excessive quantities of neutrophil products including elastase, collagenase, reactive oxygen species, and cytokines such as tumour necrosis factor α (TNF-α) have been found in patients with ARDS.[20 41 53-56] Recent studies with mice deficient in neutrophil elastase suggest that this enzyme may be an important mediator of damage to the alveolar epithelium and the progression to fibrosis.[57]

Adhesion molecules, notably β_2 integrins, mediate neutrophil binding to the pulmonary endothelium. This process is believed to promote leucocyte induced lung injury although some investigators suggest that adhesion molecules have a diminished role in the pulmonary compared with the systemic circulation.[58 59] Adhesion molecules also modulate activation and mediator release by neutrophils. In a landmark study Folkesson and Matthay induced pulmonary injury in the presence of β_2 integrin blocking antibodies and demonstrated that, while neutrophil migration still occurred, a number of indices of inflammation were reduced.[60] Neutrophil activation leads to cytoskeletal changes that reduce cell deformability

and slow their transit time through the lung capillary bed, providing an integrin independent mechanism whereby neutrophil contact with the pulmonary endothelium is increased.[61] Other inflammatory cells including macrophages and, later, lymphocytes are involved, while platelets may exacerbate the vascular injury and endothelial cells themselves are capable of producing many damaging mediators of inflammation.

Inflammatory mediators

The inflammatory process is driven in part by cytokines including TNF-α and IL-1β, IL-6, and IL-8. All have been found in BAL fluid and plasma of patients with ARDS.[56 62 63] TNF-α and IL-1β can both produce an ARDS-like condition when administered to rodents. They are produced by inflammatory cells and can promote neutrophil-endothelial adhesion, microvascular leakage, and amplify other proinflammatory responses. Despite their profile in the septic response, the importance of these cytokines in the pathogenesis of ARDS is unclear. Levels of TNF-α are not uniformly increased in patients with lung injury and anti-TNF-α and IL-1 therapies have been disappointing. The increase in TNF-α levels occurs very early in the clinical course and may be missed by the time of presentation, although anti-TNF-α therapies can still be of benefit in some cases of sepsis.[64] The huge redundancy in the proinflammatory mediator systems suggests that the search for a "common pathway" susceptible to inhibition may be too simplistic.[39] Many proinflammatory mediators including endotoxin, proinflammatory cytokines, vascular endothelial growth factor (VEGF), high mobility group-1 protein, and thrombin are implicated in the increased vascular permeability that contributes to oedema in lung injury.[65] The balance of "anti-inflammatory" cytokines and mediators must also be considered. There is now good experimental evidence that mediators such as IL-1ra, soluble TNF receptors (sTNF-R), IL-4, IL-10, and even other molecules such as carbon monoxide at very low concentrations are powerful downregulators of the inflammatory response.[37 64]

The intense neutrophilic infiltrate has led to a search for the chemotactic factors responsible. Early studies implicated complement; however, more recently, the focus has been on chemokines. IL-8 levels are raised in the BAL fluid of patients at risk who ultimately develop ARDS.[63] It is a powerful neutrophil chemoattractant derived from alveolar macrophages and other cells that is regulated by hypoxia/hyperoxia.[66] Another neutrophil chemoattractant, ENA-78, may account for IL-8 independent neutrophil adhesion in ARDS. MIF, a neuropeptide, is increased in ARDS but its role is unclear.

Animal model work suggests that free radicals are fundamental to the tissue damage resulting from proinflammatory stimuli and that antioxidants, including glutathione and superoxide dismutase, are important protective mechanisms. Similarly, in humans oxidant stress is increased and plasma antioxidant levels are reduced in patients with ARDS.[55 67] Nitric oxide may play a role in septic lung injury as nitrotyrosine, a product derived from peroxynitrite, is found in increased amounts in patients with ARDS.[68] The lipid mediator platelet activating factor (PAF) can activate both neutrophils and platelets and administration can mimic many features of lung injury. Other mechanisms for the generation of barrier dysfunction during the inflammatory phase include pathological changes in the regulation of apoptosis. In this regard soluble Fas ligand (sFasL) has been shown to drive alveolar epithelial cell apoptosis in vitro, and to cause lung injury with increased airway cell apoptosis in vivo, to be released in the airspaces of and be localised to the lung epithelial cells in patients with ARDS.[69] In addition to excess apoptosis in the parenchymal cells, delayed apoptosis in the infiltrating neutrophils may contribute to the proinflammatory load.[70]

Mediators of pulmonary hypertension

Mild pulmonary arterial hypertension is frequently seen in patients with ARDS, and loss of normal control over pulmonary vasomotor tone is an important mechanism underlying refractory hypoxaemia. Hypoxic pulmonary vasoconstriction is lost in sepsis induced lung injury as inhalation of 100% oxygen before and during endotoxin challenge does not prevent pulmonary hypertension and hypoxic vasoconstriction is inhibited for several hours after endotoxin challenge.[71] Studies with knockout mice have demonstrated a central role for nitric oxide (NO) in the normal modulation of pulmonary vascular tone. The mechanisms whereby this regulation is lost in lung injury are not clear, but it is known that endotoxin induces COX-2 and inducible nitric oxide synthase (iNOS) expression in the pulmonary vasculature.[72] The situation is complicated, however, as endotoxin contributes to an early marked pulmonary hypertension despite the induction of iNOS and irrespective of the pulmonary artery occlusion pressure or cardiac output.[73] Increased expression of the powerful vasoconstrictor endothelin-1 is associated with pulmonary hypertension in sepsis and ARDS.[74] Thromboxane B$_2$, another pulmonary vasoconstrictor, may also be an important mediator of pulmonary hypertension in ARDS as COX inhibitors reduce the early pulmonary hypertension induced by endotoxin. Other pulmonary vasoconstrictors may also be released in ARDS and other mechanisms of pulmonary hypertension such as microthromboembolism probably contribute. Inflammation leads to a procoagulant state and disseminated intravascular coagulation which is well recognised in ARDS and sepsis. Thrombin can also potentiate inflammation and lead to endothelial barrier dysfunction, in addition to its profibrotic effects (see below).

Surfactant dysfunction

Inflammation leads to surfactant dysfunction in ARDS.[75] Surfactant is secreted mainly by alveolar type II cells and consists of phospholipids (predominantly phosphatidylcholine) and surfactant specific proteins, SP-A, SP-B, SP-C and SP-D.[76] The ability of surfactant to lower surface tension is critically dependent on both the phospholipid and the protein components, especially the hydrophobic proteins SP-B and SP-C. The phospholipids are stored in the lamellar bodies of type II cells and interact with surfactant proteins upon release from the cells, forming large aggregates called tubular myelin. During the normal cycle of breathing these functional large surfactant aggregates become dissipated, reducing to smaller aggregates which do not have the same surface tension lowering properties. Type II cells take up these small aggregates and recycle them into new surfactant. The hydrophilic surfactant protein SP-A, quantitatively the major surfactant protein, plays a key role in this process. The other hydrophilic surfactant protein is SP-D, which may also have a function in phospholipid recycling. SP-A and SP-D are members of the collectin family and form part of the innate immune system in the lung; interestingly, both have significant antibacterial activity and inhibit neutrophil apoptosis.[77]

Surfactant levels are dramatically decreased in the infant respiratory distress syndrome due to immaturity of the type II cells. By contrast, in ARDS surfactant deficiency is not a primary causal event; rather, the inflammatory processes lead to surfactant dysfunction as a secondary factor. Damage and loss of type II cells leads to decreased synthesis and recirculation of surfactant. This defect in turnover can lead to accumulation of small aggregates, while overall surfactant performance follows a reduction in the functional large surfactant aggregates and damage to surfactant proteins.[78] In addition, the protein rich oedema in ARDS "contaminates" surfactant, further reducing its functional capacity. Furthermore, in lung injury the ratio of minor phospholipids to phosphatidylcholine increases, possibly indicating damage and release of cell membrane lipids. The degree to which surfactant dysfunction contributes to the pathogenesis of ARDS is currently not clear.

THE FIBROPROLIFERATIVE RESPONSE

Fibroproliferation is a stereotypical part of the normal repair process which, if not closely regulated, can have serious consequences. The fibrotic response is fuelled by mediators that stimulate local fibroblasts to migrate, replicate, and produce excessive connective tissue.[7 24 42] Animal models have suggested a number of potential profibrotic factors. For example, the expression of TNF-α in the lung, using an SP-C promoter for tissue specificity, led to the development of a T lymphocyte predominant alveolitis which progressed steadily to a histological picture resembling idiopathic pulmonary fibrosis.[79] These data suggest that TNF-α and other proinflammatory mediators, including IL-1β, play important roles in the development of pulmonary fibrosis. Similarly, expression of transforming growth factor α (TGF-α) in the distal pulmonary epithelium induced pulmonary fibrosis, the extent of which is related to the level of gene expression.[46] The Th2 cytokines have been implicated in fibroproliferative disorders and both IL-4 and IL-13 are increased in a bleomycin model of fibrosis; interestingly, inhibition of IL-13 significantly abrogated this fibrotic response.[80] Although many mediators regulate collagen metabolism in pulmonary fibrosis, studies of these in ARDS are very limited. There is evidence that the levels of TGF-α and a platelet derived growth factor (PDGF)-like factor are increased in BAL fluid from patients with ARDS.[81 82] A number of products of the coagulation cascade—particularly fibrin, thrombin, and factor Xa—are important mediators of the pulmonary profibrotic response and are increased in patients with ARDS.[24]

The archetypal profibrotic cytokine is TGF-β, of which there are three closely related isoforms (TGF-β1, 2 and 3) that exert nearly identical effects as modulators of inflammation, inhibitors of growth and differentiation, and regulators of extracellular matrix production.[83] Studies in animals and in humans strongly suggest that TGF-β is important in the pathogenesis of pulmonary fibrosis.[84] It has been shown be mitogenic and chemotactic for fibroblasts, to increase the synthesis of extracellular matrix proteins, and to inhibit the production of matrix degrading enzymes.[24] TGF-β1 should not be simply viewed as a profibrotic cytokine, however, as it has multiple other actions—it is anti-inflammatory, decreases epithelial proliferation, and can be pro-apoptotic for many cell types. It is also a powerful chemotactic agent for monocytes and macrophages, essential cells in the process of wound healing. In the normal repair process the secretion of TGF-β1 is thus a powerful effector for resolution and it is only when its expression is persistent or excessive that it leads to pathological fibrosis. TGF-β1 is produced as a latent precursor that is converted into the mature bioactive form after cleavage of the N-terminal portion, termed the latency associated peptide (LAP). In animal models the transfection of active (but not latent) TGF-β1 results in severe fibrosis.[85] More recently it has been shown that the integrin αvβ6, an adhesion molecule that binds matrix and anchors cells, can bind LAP and activate TGF-β1.[86] The expression of this integrin is very low or absent on most normal adult epithelial cells but is upregulated dramatically after injury.[46] Failure to express this adhesion molecule confers almost complete protection against bleomycin induced lung injury and fibrosis in mice. This highlights the role of the alveolar epithelium, integrins, and TGF-β1 in the regulation of the inflammatory and repair processes.

RESOLUTION OF ARDS

Liquid is gradually cleared from airspaces by ion pumps that transport sodium with osmotically driven water movement across the alveolar epithelium via membrane water channels.[87] Catecholamines may increase this while propranolol or amiloride inhibit sodium transport and impede clearance of alveolar fluid. Repair of the injured lung requires an intact epithelial basal lamina which facilitates restoration of the epithelial barrier and may thus further promote clearance of oedema.[88] Lung lymph flow, a much ignored subject, may also contribute to the clearance of pulmonary oedema.

Histologically, the resolution phase of ARDS has been the least clearly documented. Apoptosis is essential to the clearance of neutrophils and has been clearly demonstrated in the lung in patients with ARDS.[70 89] Apoptosis is also responsible for removing surplus alveolar type II cells while survivors differentiate into a type I phenotype. BAL fluid recovered from patients with ALI during the repair phase can induce fibroblast and endothelial cell death. This provides a mechanism to clear excess cells while retaining underlying normal lung structure. Resolution of ARDS requires more than the clearance of leucocytes; for successful healing the fibroproliferative response must be terminated and excess mesenchymal cells cleared. As the inflammatory and fibroproliferative processes are intimately linked and many mediators such as thrombin and IL-1 are central to both, it is likely that the resolution of inflammation makes a major contribution to the resolution of fibroproliferation.[34] Other mediators will be produced that promote resolution—for example, interferon (IFN)γ produced by activated T cells downregulates the transcription of the TGF-β1 gene. The generation of pulmonary fibrosis involves a complex interplay between collagen deposition and degradation, with the early balance shifted dramatically towards deposition. In ARDS type III collagen is initially deposited which is more flexible and susceptible to breakdown; later this is remodelled to the thicker and more resistant type I collagen.[26] The mechanisms involved in the clearance of the fibrotic matrix are not well established but are likely to involve matrix metalloproteases (MMPs) and gelatinases that digest collagens. At least two of these—MMP-2 and MMP-9—are increased in the lungs of patients with ARDS.[90] The MMPs are further regulated by tissue inhibitors of metalloproteases (TIMPs), although the relative balance of these systems during ARDS is unknown.

The pulmonary fibrosis in ARDS does not necessarily completely resolve and can lead to persisting pulmonary problems both during weaning and after patients leave the intensive care unit. Recovery of lung function can be slow, with some patients taking up to 12 months to return to baseline while others have persisting abnormalities. In the majority, however, lung mechanics fully recover suggesting that the pulmonary fibrosis in ARDS is reversible.[2 27]

PATHOPHYSIOLOGY RELATED TO PATHOLOGY

Refractory hypoxaemia may be multifactorial, but intrapulmonary shunting with ventilation-perfusion mismatching is believed to be the primary cause. Studies on patients with ARDS have shown that the degree of intrapulmonary shunting is sufficient to account for the entire alveolar-arterial oxygen gradient, suggesting that a decrease in transfer factor may be of secondary importance.[2] Microscopic studies have shown that the alveolar airspaces are filled with oedema, debris, hyaline membranes, and matrix or lost through alveolar collapse, creating a huge physiological deadspace. The effects of this on gas exchange are maximised by loss of hypoxic pulmonary vasoconstriction and by the widespread patchy vascular defects so common in ARDS. Pulmonary oedema will also lead to a significant diffusion block. The causes of pulmonary oedema are multiple and include mediator induced vascular permeability, increased pulmonary pressures, and alterations to the oncotic pressure as suggested in the seminal studies by Guyton in 1959.[91]

- There is much greater overlap of the inflammatory and fibroproliferative phases of ARDS than previously imagined, with the fibroproliferative response beginning within 24 hours and its severity being directly related to the outcome.
- An exaggerated inflammatory response underlies the pathogenesis of ARDS. The neutrophil is the dominant leucocyte, while many proinflammatory agents including endotoxin, proinflammatory and chemotactic cytokines, vascular endothelial growth factor, high mobility group-1 protein and thrombin, together with oxidant stress, are all implicated in vascular leakage and lung damage.
- Surfactant deficiency is not a primary causal event in ARDS; rather, the inflammatory processes lead to surfactant dysfunction as a secondary factor.
- Alveolar type II cell proliferation and enhanced fibroproliferation are key steps in attempts at repair in the lung; both offer potential targets for future therapies.

Lung compliance is markedly decreased in ARDS. This will be related initially to flooding of the alveoli and the interstitial spaces with fluid inflammatory cells and debris. Progressively, this inflammatory response is organised and replaced by matrix that further reduces compliance. The effects of this on the pressure-volume curve and on mechanical ventilation will be reviewed in greater detail in chapter 9.

CONCLUSIONS

Understanding the pathogenesis of ARDS is essential both to choosing effective management strategies and to looking for novel treatments. We have seen that mechanical ventilation can induce inflammation if applied inappropriately or reduce mortality if correctly used, and that this has a clear pathophysiological rationale. Similar concepts have led to ongoing studies of prone ventilation and to the investigation of other ventilatory strategies such as high frequency ventilation and lung rest with extracorporeal membrane oxygenation.

This chapter has outlined the key mediators involved in both the inflammatory and fibroproliferative responses and highlighted some of the important mechanisms through which these responses are regulated. Many of these mediators will be examined in more detail in other chapters in this book that deal with treatment options.

Funded by the Medical Research Council (MRC) UK.

REFERENCES

1 **Bernard GR**, Artigas A, Brigham KL, et al. The American-European Consensus Conference on ARDS. Definitions, mechanisms, relevant outcomes, and clinical trial co-ordination. Am J Respir Crit Care Med 1994;**149**:818–24.
2 **Griffiths MJD**, Evans TW. Adult respiratory distress syndrome. In: Brewis RAL, Corrin B, Geddes DM, Gibson GJ, eds. Respiratory medicine. 2nd ed. Philadelphia: WB Saunders, 1995: 605–29.
3 **Luce JM**. Acute lung injury and the acute respiratory distress syndrome. Crit Care Med 1998;**26**:369–76.
4 **Deby-Dupont G**, Lamy M. Pathophysiology of acute respiratory distress syndrome and acute lung injury. In: Webb A, Shapiro MJ, Singer M, Suter PM, eds. Oxford textbook of critical care. Oxford: Oxford University Press, 1999: 55–9.
5 **Tomashefski JF Jr**. Pulmonary pathology of the adult respiratory distress syndrome. Clin Chest Med 1990;**11**:593–619.
6 **Hudson LD**, Milberg JA, Anardi D, et al. Clinical risks for development of the acute respiratory distress syndrome. Am J Respir Crit Care Med 1995;**151**:293–301.
7 **Marshall R**, Bellingan G, Laurent G. The acute respiratory distress syndrome: fibrosis in the fast lane. Thorax 1998;**53**:815–7.
8 **Ranieri VM**, Suter PM, Tortorella C, et al. Effect of mechanical ventilation on inflammatory mediators in patients with acute respiratory distress syndrome: a randomised controlled trial. JAMA 1999;**282**:54–61.
9 **Milberg JA**, Davis DR, Steinberg KP, et al. Improved survival of patients with acute respiratory distress syndrome (ARDS):1983–1993. JAMA 1995;**273**:306–9.
10 **Abel SJ**, Finney SJ, Brett SJ, et al. Reduced mortality in association with the acute respiratory distress syndrome (ARDS). Thorax 1998;**53**:292–4.

11 **Bion J**. Pathophysiology of acute respiratory distress syndrome and acute lung injury. In: Webb A, Shapiro MJ, Singer M, Suter PM, eds. *Oxford textbook of critical care.* Oxford: Oxford University Press, 1999: 923–6.

12 **Bone RC**, Balk RA, Cerra FB, et al. Definitions for sepsis and organ failure and guidelines for the use of innovative therapies in sepsis. The American College of Chest Physicians/Society of Critical Care Medicine (ACCP/SCCM) Consensus Conference Committee. *Chest* 1992;**101**:1644–55.

13 **Bone RC**. Sir Isaac Newton, sepsis, SIRS, and CARS. *Crit Care Med* 1996;**24**:1125–8.

14 **Docke WD**, Randow F, Syrbe U, et al. Monocyte deactivation in septic patients: restoration by IFN-gamma treatment. *Nature Med* 1997;**3**:678–81.

15 **Desai SR**, Wells AU, Suntharalingam G, et al. Acute respiratory distress syndrome caused by pulmonary and extrapulmonary injury: a comparative CT study. *Radiology* 2001;**218**:689–93.

16 **Hoelz C**, Negri EM, Lichtenfels AJ, et al. Morphometric differences of pulmonary lesions in primary and secondary ARDS: a preliminary study in autopsies. *Am J Respir Crit Care Med* 2001;**163**:450.

17 **Finney SJ**, Robb JD, Suntharalingam G, et al. ARDS due to direct and indirect pulmonary injuries: ICU survival, broncho-alveolar lavage neutrophil counts and oxygenation. *Am J Respir Crit Care Med* 2001;**163**:139.

18 **Sadikot RT**, Hao C, Jansen D, et al. Bioluminescent measurement of multiorgan Cox-2 gene expression in transgenic mice treated with LPS. *Am J Respir Crit Care Med* 2001;**163**:208.

19 **Bachofen M**, Wiebel ER. Structural alteration of lung parenchyma in the adult respiratory distress syndrome. *Clin Chest Med* 1982;**3**:35–6.

20 **Weiland JE**, Davis WB, Holter JF, et al. Lung neutrophils in the adult respiratory distress syndrome. Clinical and pathophysiologic significance. *Am Rev Respir Dis* 1986;**133**:218–25.

21 **Matsubara O**, Tamura A, Ohdama S, et al. Alveolar basement membrane breaks down in diffuse alveolar damage: an immunohistochemical study. *Pathol Int* 1995;**45**:473–82.

22 **Anderson WR**, Thielen K. Correlative study of adult respiratory distress syndrome by light, scanning and transmission electron microscopy. *Ultrastruct Pathol* 1992;**16**:615–28.

23 **Snyder LS**, Hertz MI, Peterson MS, et al. Acute lung injury. Pathogenesis of intraalveolar fibrosis. *J Clin Invest* 1991;**88**:663–73.

24 **Marshall RP**, Bellingan GJ, Laurent GJ. The fibroproliferative response to acute lung injury. In: Bellingan GJ, Laurent GJ, eds. *Acute lung injury: from inflammation to repair.* Amsterdam: IOS Press, 2000: 104–14.

25 **Zapol WM**, Trelstad R, Coffey JW, et al. Pulmonary fibrosis in severe acute respiratory failure. *Am J Respir Crit Care Med* 1979;**119**:547–54.

26 **Raghu G**, Striker LJ, Hudson LD, et al. Extracellular matrix in normal and fibrotic human lungs. *Am Rev Respir Dis* 1985;**131**:281–9.

27 **McHugh LG**, Milberg JA, Whitcomb ME, et al. Recovery of function in survivors of the acute respiratory distress syndrome. *Am J Respir Crit Care Med* 1994;**150**:90–4.

28 **Suchyta MR**, Elliott CG, Colby T, et al. Open lung biopsy does not correlate with pulmonary function after the adult respiratory distress syndrome. *Chest* 1991;**99**:1232–7.

29 **Martin C**, Papazian L, Payan MJ, et al. Pulmonary fibrosis correlates with outcome in adult respiratory distress syndrome. A study in mechanically ventilated patients. *Chest* 1995;**107**:196–200.

30 **Chesnutt AN**, Matthay MA, Tibayan FA, et al. Early detection of type III procollagen peptide in acute lung injury. Pathogenic and prognostic significance. *Am J Respir Crit Care Med* 1997;**156**:840–5.

31 **Marshall RP**, Bellingan GJ, Gunn S, et al. Fibroproliferation occurs early in the acute respiratory distress syndrome and impacts on outcome. *Am J Respir Crit Care Med* 2000;**162**:1783–8.

32 **Montgomery AB**, Stager MA, Carrico CJ, et al. Causes of mortality in patients with the adult respiratory distress syndrome. *Am Rev Respir Dis* 1985;**132**:485–9.

33 **Bell RC**, Coalson JJ, Smith JD, et al. Multiple organ system failure and infection in adult respiratory distress syndrome. *Ann Intern Med* 1983;**99**:293–8.

34 **Bellingan GJ**, Marshall RP, Laurent GJ. Fibrosis in ARDS: how close is the link between inflammation and fibroproliferation? In: Vincent JL, ed. *Yearbook of intensive care and emergency medicine.* Berlin: Springer, 2000: 217–24.

35 **Acute Respiratory Distress Syndrome Network**. Ventilation with lower tidal volumes as compared with traditional tidal volumes for acute lung injury and the acute respiratory distress syndrome. *N Engl J Med* 2000;**342**:1301–8.

36 **Rouby JJ**, Lherm T, Martin de Lassale E, et al. Histologic aspects of pulmonary barotrauma in critically ill patients with acute respiratory failure. *Intensive Care Med* 1993;**19**:383–9.

37 **Otterbein LE**, Mantell LL, Choi AM. Carbon monoxide provides protection against hyperoxic lung injury. *Am J Physiol* 1999;**276**:L688–94.

38 **Kapanci Y**, Wiebel ER, Kaplan HP, et al. Pathogenesis and reversibility of the pulmonary lesions of oxygen toxicity in monkeys. 2. Ultrastructural and morphometric studies. *Lab Invest* 1969;**20**:101–8.

39 **Bellingan G**. Inflammatory cell activation in Sepsis. In: Evans TW, Bennett D Bion JF, et al, eds. *Intensive care medicine. Br Med Bull* 1999;**55**:12–29.

40 **Bellingan GJ**. Leukocyte: friend or foe? *Intensive Care Med* 2000;**26**:111–8.

41 **Chollet-Martin S**, Jourdain B, Gibert C, et al. Interactions between neutrophils and cytokines in blood and alveolar spaces during ARDS. *Am J Respir Crit Care Med* 1996;**154**:594–601.

42 **Coker RK**, Laurent GJ. Pulmonary fibrosis: cytokines in the balance. *Eur Respir J* 1998;**11**:1218–21.

43 **Wax RS**, Angus DC. The molecular genetics of sepsis. In: Vincent JL, ed. *Yearbook of intensive care and emergency medicine.* Berlin: Springer, 2000: 3–17.

44 **Marshall RP**, Webb S, Bellingan GJ, et al. Angiotensin converting enzyme I/D polymorphism in the acute respiratory distress syndrome. *Am J Respir Crit Care Med* 2000;**161**:209.

45 **Marshall RP**, Webb S, Brull D, et al. Interleukin-6 (-174G>C) polymorphism predicts outcome in acute respiratory failure. *Am J Respir Crit Care Med* 2000;**163**:305.

46 **Griffiths M**. Transgenic and knockout mouse models of pulmonary inflammatory diseases. In: Bellingan GJ, Laurent GJ, eds. *Acute lung injury: from inflammation to repair.* Amsterdam: IOS Press, 2000: 93–104.

47 **Meyrick B**, Brigham KL. Acute effects of *Escherichia coli* endotoxin on the pulmonary microcirculation of anaesthetised sheep structure:function relationships. *Lab Invest* 1983;**48**:458–70.

48 **Adler KB**, Callahan LM, Evans JN. Cellular alterations in the alveolar wall in bleomycin-induced pulmonary fibrosis in rats. An ultrastructural morphometric study. *Am Rev Respir Dis* 1986;**133**:1043–8.

49 **Wiener-Kronish JP**, Albertine KH, Matthay MA. Differential responses of the endothelial and epithelial barriers of the lung in sheep to *Esherichia coli* endotoxin. *J Clin Invest* 1991;**88**:864–75.

50 **Heflin AC**, Brigham KL. Prevention by granulocyte depletion of increased lung vascular permeability of sheep following endotoxaemia. *J Clin Invest* 1981;**68**:1253–60.

51 **Winn R**, Maunder R, Chi E, et al. Neutrophil depletion does not prevent lung edema after endotoxin infusion in goats. *J Appl Physiol* 1987;**62**:116–21.

52 **Braude S**, Apperley J, Krausz T, et al. Adult respiratory distress syndrome after allogenic bone-marrow transplantation; evidence for a neutrophil-independent mechanism. *Lancet* 1985;i:1239–42.

53 **Lee CT**, Fein AM, Lippmann M, et al. Elastolytic activity in pulmonary lavage fluid from patients with adult respiratory-distress syndrome. *N Engl J Med* 1981;**304**:192–6.

54 **Ward PA**, Till GO, Kunkel R, et al. Evidence for the role of hydroxyl radical in complement and neutrophil dependent tissue injury. *J Clin Invest* 1983;**72**:789–801.

55 **Zhang H**, Slutsky AS, Vincent JL. Oxygen free radicals in ARDS, septic shock and organ dysfunction. *Intensive Care Med* 2000;**26**:474–6.

56 **Armstrong L**, Millar AB. Relative production of tumour necrosis factor alpha and interleukin 10 in adult respiratory distress syndrome. *Thorax* 1997;**52**:442–6.

57 **Chua F**, Dunsmore SE, Mutsaers SE, et al. Characterisation of the response to mice deficient in neutrophil elastase or cathepsin G to bleomycin. *Am J Respir Crit Care Med* 2001;**163**:231.

58 **Donnelly SC**, Haslett C, Dransfield I, et al. Role of selectins in development of adult respiratory distress syndrome. *Lancet* 1994;**344**:215–9.

59 **Doershuk CM**, Winn RK, Coxson HO, et al. CD18 dependent and independent mechanisms of neutrophil emigration in pulmonary and systemic microcirculation in rabbits. *J Immunol* 1990;**144**:2327–33.

60 **Folkesson HG**, Matthay MA. Inhibition of CD18 or CD11b attenuates acute lung injury after acid instillation in rabbits. *J Appl Physiol* 1997;**82**:1743–50.

61 **Worthen GS**, Schwab B III, Elson EL, et al. Mechanics of stimulated neutrophils: cell stiffening induces retention in capillaries. *Science* 1989;**245**:183–6.

62 **Pugin J**, Ricou B, Steinberg KP, et al. Pro-inflammatory activity in bronchoalveolar lavage fluids from patients with ARDS, a prominent role for interleukin-1. *Am J Respir Crit Care Med* 1996;**153**:1850–6.

63 **Donnelly SC**, Strieter RM, Kunkel SL, et al. Interleukin-8 and development of adult respiratory distress syndrome in at-risk patient groups. *Lancet* 1993;**341**:643–7.

64 **Panacek EA**. Results of the "MONARCS" phase III clinical trial of an anti-TNF-α antibody (afelimomab) in sepsis. *Am J Respir Crit Care Med* 2000;**161**:318.

65 **Albertine KH**. Histopathology of pulmonary oedema and the acute respiratory distress syndrome. In: Matthay MA, Ingbar DH, eds. *Pulmonary edema. Lung Biology in Health and Disease. Volume 116.* New York: Marcel Dekker, 1998: 37–84.

66 **Hirani N**, Clay, M, Sri-Pathmanathan, R, et al. A role for acute hypoxia/hyperoxia in the pathogenesis of the acute respiratory distress syndrome – an in vivo model. *Thorax* 1999;**54**(Suppl 3):A13.

67 **Metnitz PG**, Bartens C, Fischer M, et al. Antioxidant status in patients with acute respiratory distress syndrome. *Intensive Care Med* 1999;**25**:180–5.

68 **Haddad IY**, Pataki G, Hu P, et al. Quantitation of nitrotyrosine levels in lung sections of patients and animals with acute lung injury. *J Clin Invest* 1994;**94**:2407–13.

69 **Matute-Bello G**, Winn RK, Jonas M, et al. Fas (CD95) induces alveolar epithelial cell apoptosis in vivo: implications for acute pulmonary inflammation. *Am J Pathol* 2001;**158**:153–61

70 **Matute-Bello G**, Liles WC, Radella F, et al. Neutrophil apoptosis in the acute respiratory distress syndrome. *Am J Respir Crit Care Med* 1997;**156**:1969–77.

71 **Robbins IM**, Newman JH, Brigham KL. Increased-permeability pulmonary edema from sepsis/endotoxaemia. In: Matthay MA, Ingbar DH, eds. *Pulmonary edema. Lung Biology in Health and Disease. Volume 116.* New York: Marcel Dekker, 1998: 203–46.

72 **Griffiths MJ**, Curzen NP, Mitchell JA, et al. In vivo treatment with endotoxin increases rat pulmonary vascular contractility despite NOS induction. *Am J Respir Crit Care Med* 1997;**156**:654–8.

73 **Sibbald WJ**, Paterson NA, Holliday RL, *et al.* Pulmonary hypertension in sepsis: measurement by the pulmonary artery diastolic wedge pressure gradient and the influence of passive and active factors. *Chest* 1978;**73**:583–91.

74 **Druml W**, Steltzer H, Waldhausl W, *et al.* Endothelin-1 in adult respiratory distress syndrome. *Am Rev Respir Dis* 1993;**148**:1169–73.

75 **Baudouin SV**. Surfactant medication for acute respiratory distress syndrome. *Thorax* 1997;**52**:S9–15.

76 **Rooney SA**, Young SL, Mendelson CR. Molecular and cellular processing of lung surfactant. *FASEB J* 1994;**8**:957–67.

77 **Greene KE**, Gardai S, Henson PM. SP-A and SP-D inhibit spontaneous neutrophil apoptosis via activation of the PI-3 kinase/AKT. *Am J Respir Crit Care Med* 2001;**163**:23.

78 **Baker CS**, Evans TW, Randle BJ, *et al.* Damage to surfactant-specific protein in acute respiratory distress syndrome. *Lancet* 1999;**353**:1232–7.

79 **Miyazaki Y**, Araki K, Vesin C, *et al.* Expression of a tumor necrosis factor-alpha transgene in murine lung causes lymphocytic and fibrosing alveolitis. A mouse model of progressive pulmonary fibrosis. *J Clin Invest* 1995;**96**:250–9.

80 **Keane MP Belperio JA**, Burdick MD, *et al.* IL-13 is an important cytokine in the pathogenesis of pulmonary fibrosis. *Am J Respir Crit Care Med* 2001;**163**:43.

81 **Madtes DK**, Rubenfeld G, Klima LD, *et al.* Elevated transforming growth factor-alpha levels in bronchoalveolar lavage fluid of patients with acute respiratory distress syndrome. *Am J Respir Crit Care Med* 1998;**158**:424–30.

82 **Henke C**, Marineili W, Jessurun J, *et al.* Macrophage production of basic fibroblast growth factor in the fibroproliferative disorder of alveolar fibrosis after lung injury. *Am J Pathol* 1993;**143**:1189–99.

83 **Clark DA**, Coker R. Transforming growth factor-beta (TGF-beta). *Int J Biochem Cell Biol* 1998;**30**:293–8.

84 **Khalil N**, Greenberg AH. The role of TGF-beta in pulmonary fibrosis. *Ciba Found Symp* 1991;**157**:194–207

85 **Sime PJ**, Xing Z, Graham FL, *et al.* Adenovector-mediated gene transfer of active transforming growth factor-beta1 induces prolonged severe fibrosis in rat lung. *J Clin Invest* 1997;**100**:768–76.

86 **Munger JS**, Huang X, Kawakatsu H, *et al.* The integrin alpha v beta 6 binds and activates latent TGF beta 1: a mechanism for regulating pulmonary inflammation and fibrosis. *Cell* 1999;**96**:319–28.

87 **Folkesson HG**, Matthay MA, Hasegawa H, *et al.* Transcellular water transport in lung alveolar epithelium through mercury sensitive water channels *Proc Natl Acad Sci USA* 1994;**91**:4970–4.

89 **Matthay MA**, Wiener-Kronish JP. Intact epithelial barrier function is critical for the resolution of alveolar oedema in humans. *Am Rev Respir Dis* 1990;**142**:1250–7.

89 **Haslett C**. Granulocyte apoptosis and its role in the resolution and control of lung inflammation. *Am J Respir Crit Care Med* 1999;**160**:S5–11.

90 **Ricou B**, Nicod L, Lacraz S, *et al.* Matrix metalloproteinases and TIMP in acute respiratory distress syndrome. *Am J Respir Crit Care Med* 1996;**154**:346–52.

91 **Guyton AC**, Lindsey AW. Effect of elevated left atrial pressure and decreased plasma protein concentration on the development of pulmonary oedema. *Circ Res* 1959;**VII**:649–57.

7 Critical care management of severe acute respiratory syndrome

J T Granton, S E Lapinsky

Severe acute respiratory syndrome (SARS) is a viral illness characterised by a syndrome of fever and respiratory symptoms that can progress to respiratory failure and death. Initial reports of a highly contagious atypical pneumonia originated from the Guangdong province of the People's Republic of China in November 2002. The condition remained isolated to China until February 2003 when an infected physician travelled to Hong Kong. Since that time the disease has spread, with 8437 probable cases in 32 countries and 813 deaths providing a case fatality rate of 9.6% (WHO website http://www.who.int/csr/sars/en/).[1] The largest outbreaks have been in China, Toronto (Canada), and Singapore. This review describes the current state of knowledge of SARS, with particular reference to the management of the critically ill patient and the safety and protection of the staff in intensive care units (ICU). The recommendations are based on the published data available at the time of writing, collaborations between physicians in many affected centres, recommendations from the WHO and Centres for Disease Control (CDC), and local experience. Given the novelty of this illness, it is inevitable that treatments will evolve. The reader should therefore refer to more current sources to guide patient management.

AETIOLOGICAL AGENT

The worldwide cooperative effort to identify the aetiological agent for SARS has been summarised elsewhere.[1] The speed at which the aetiological agent was identified is a testimony to the progress in advances in molecular biology, the automation of molecular methods, and the power of genomic information available in databases accessible on the Internet. Initial efforts focused on several potential viruses—most notably, metapneumoviruses and paramyxovirus. On 21 March 2003 an agent isolated from patients meeting the case definition for SARS was found to be capable of producing cytopathic changes in a Vero and a murine cell line from a laboratory in Germany, and in rhesus monkey renal cell lines in a laboratory in Hong Kong. Using electron microscopy, coronavirus-like particles were identified (fig 7.1). Subsequent sequencing using reverse transcription-polymerase chain reaction (RT-PCR) of the isolated product identified the virus as a novel coronavirus.[2 3] Further study of this agent and sequencing its 29 751 base genomic structure supported the notion that this virus is not merely a mutation of an existing strain, but that it represents a novel infectious agent.[4]

The SARS coronavirus (SARS-CoV) is an RNA virus belonging to the family Coronaviridae. The genome sequence revealed that SARS-CoV was not significantly related to other coronaviruses, including two human coronaviruses (HCoV-OC43 and HCoV 229E). Marra and coworkers reported that the virus did not closely resemble any of the three previously known groups of coronaviruses.[4] Coronaviridae are capable of producing both enteric and respiratory disease in a variety of hosts. Indeed, their cellular tropism has been exploited to develop models of gastroenteritis and hepatitis (G Levy, personal communication). A glycoprotein projection on the surface of the virus (S protein; in effect, a cellular anchor) is thought to provide the virus with its cellular and host preferences. Interestingly (and of some concern), two distinct genotypes of the SARS-CoV have been described.[5] The different genotypes were partitioned between two epidemiologically distinct epidemics. Disturbingly, they also reported that there was a common variant with an amino acid substitution in the sequence coding for the S protein of the SARS coronavirus. They suggested that this substitution may have resulted from immunological pressure mounted by the host. Given the purported role of the S protein, changes in its structure have the potential both to affect the cellular tropism and, in turn, the clinical features of the illness, and further to complicate future vaccine development. Until changes in the structure of the virus divert its attention to other mammalian hosts, SARS is likely to remain a global health concern to humans.

CLINICAL FEATURES

In the absence of a rapid early diagnostic assay, case definitions of SARS are based on the presence of epidemiological risk factors (close contact with SARS cases or travel to SARS "affected" areas) with a combination of fever and respiratory symptoms, with or without hypoxia and chest radiographic changes. However, as the SARS epidemic spread, the ability to distinguish it from other community acquired pneumonias based on such epidemiological clues became increasingly tenuous. Although more recent definitions have incorporated serological assays or identification of viral RNA to confirm cases (see below), at this time SARS must be considered in the differential diagnosis of any community acquired or nosocomial pneumonia. The sensitivity of the WHO definition of a SARS case has been shown to be limited when applied as a screening method for individuals at risk of infection. Using clinical criteria and progression of the disease in the face of conventional therapy as a gold standard, the current WHO definition of SARS had a specificity of 96% and negative predictive value of 86%.[6] These findings were attributed to the absence of respiratory symptoms in many cases at presentation and because radiographic features were not used in the WHO definition of a case. However, their results are not surprising as the WHO definition was not intended as a screening

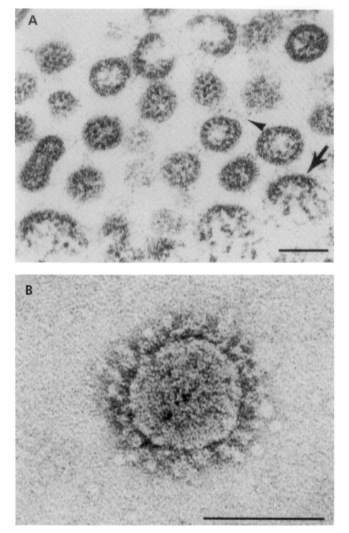

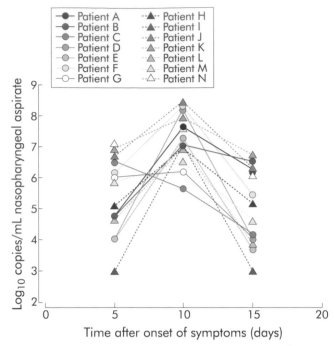

Figure 7.2 Sequential quantitative reverse transcription polymerase chain reaction (RT-PCR) for SARS coronavirus in the nasopharyngeal secretions of 14 patients reported by Peiris and coworkers. A peak in the viral loads was seen on the 10th day of sampling. Reproduced with permission from Ksiazek *et al*.[2] **[AQ:3]**

Figure 7.1 Electron micrographs of the SARS coronavirus. (A) Thin section electron micrograph of viral nucleocapsids aligned along the membrane of the rough endoplasmic reticulum (arrow) as particles bud into the cisternae. (B) A methylamine tungstate penetrated coronavirus particle with an internal helical nucleocapsid-like structure and club shaped surface projections surrounding the periphery of the particle. Reproduced with permission from Ksiazek *et al*.[2]

tool. Screening methods should incorporate questions surrounding potential exposure, travel history, and an evaluation of the presence of fever, both respiratory and non-respiratory complaints such as malaise, headache, fatigue, and abdominal symptoms. The importance of proper screening, a rational and aggressive local health policy, sweeping quarantines, and infection control measures in the management of the epidemic cannot be overemphasised.[7–10] It is through these efforts that affected regions have been able to contain the spread of this disease. In the absence of specific treatment for SARS, such measures are (and will remain) the cornerstone of global therapy. The current case definitions can be found at the websites for the Centre for Disease Control (http://www.cdc.gov/ncidod/sars/) and WHO (http://www.who.int/csr/sars/en/).

DIAGNOSTIC TESTING

At present, specific testing for SARS-CoV infection has limitations that prohibit definitive early confirmation of disease. Diagnostic tests for the SARS virus include (a) detection of antibodies produced in response to SARS infection; (b) molecular tests—for example, PCR to detect genetic material of the SARS-CoV in blood, stool or respiratory secretions; and (c) cell culture techniques which allow the identification of live virus. Immunofluorescence assays become positive later in the illness, but may be useful to confirm undifferentiated cases or to assist with epidemiological studies. IgG seroconversion occurs in most patients by day 20.[11] Positive antibody test results, seroconversion, or a fourfold rise in titre indicate previous infection with the SARS virus. A negative antibody test result more than 21 days after the onset of illness is likely to exclude infection with SARS-CoV. At the time of writing, antibody testing is unsuitable during the acute illness. Clearly there is a need to develop an assay that will allow the earlier detection of infected individuals to facilitate infection control.

PCR based assays have been developed by different groups around the world and, although such assays are available commercially, results of these tests should still not be used to exclude the diagnosis of SARS. Studies evaluating viral loads in respiratory secretions using quantitative PCR describe an "inverted V" pattern with peak viral load occurring near day 10 (fig 7.2).[11] The presence of the infectious virus can be confirmed by inoculating suitable cell cultures (such as Vero cells) with respiratory secretions, blood or stool, and propagating the virus in vitro. Once isolated, the virus must be identified as SARS-CoV using further tests performed under biosafety precautions that are not routinely available.

Initial diagnostic testing should also include a search for other respiratory pathogens including blood cultures, sputum Gram stain and culture, and serological tests. Bronchoscopy is valuable to exclude other diagnoses but is not recommended in patients with a typical clinical picture and clear epidemiological link because of the high risk of transmitting the infection. In patients who are immunosuppressed and in whom concerns regarding other diagnoses are high, the risk of bronchoscopy may be acceptable. Clinicians should save any available clinical specimens (respiratory, blood, and serum) for additional testing with RT-PCR.

Lymphopenia commonly complicates SARS. Additional laboratory findings in patients with SARS include thrombocytopenia, leucocytosis, and raised levels of creatine kinase, lactate dehydrogenase (LDH), bilirubin, and transaminases.[12–14] A high peak LDH level and an increased white cell count at presentation may carry a poor prognosis. Anaemia has been reported in up to 60% of patients[14] and may be secondary to ribavirin mediated haemolysis.[12] Haemolysis may also contribute to the hyperbilirubinaemia and high LDH levels seen in some patients.

NATURAL HISTORY

The reported incubation period of SARS varies from 2 to 7 days (http://www.cdc.gov/mmwr). However, based on the infectious characteristics of other members of the Coronaviridae, there is concern that the incubation period may be up to 21 days. Indeed, in a recent case in Toronto a medical student developed symptoms beyond the 10 day quarantine period. The mean duration of symptoms to time of admission to hospital is 3–5 days and in one study was observed to shorten throughout the epidemic.[9] The viral load may play a role in both the transmission and severity of subsequent disease. The notion of "super spreaders" has been suggested to describe the occasional patient who is associated with spread to large numbers of contacts. At present it is unknown if asymptomatic individuals are capable of spreading the disease. The mode of transmission is thought to be droplet spread. Consequently, protective measures have focused on barrier methods, the intensity of which varies with the risk of aerosolisation of secretions.

To date, several studies have provided valuable information regarding the natural progression of the disease.[9 11 15 16] The Hong Kong group has provided an excellent summary of their prospective evaluation of the temporal progression of the disease in a cohort of individuals who were infected following exposure to sewage in a local housing complex, Amoy Gardens.[11] A three phase illness was described.

The first stage was characterised by influenza-like symptoms such as fever, myalgia and headache. Our current understanding is that fever eventually occurs in all patients and is often the presenting symptom. However, we also recognise that fever may occasionally be absent on presentation in the elderly.[17] Patients often have mild respiratory symptoms at the onset, and gastrointestinal manifestations are relatively uncommon initial features. Patients may deffervesce at the end of this phase. Peiris et al correlated this first phase with an increase in viral load and ascribed the symptoms to direct viral infection and cytolysis.[11] The chest radiograph is abnormal at presentation in up to 70% of patients,[18 19] featuring patchy or focal airspace disease with a predilection for the periphery and bases of the lungs (fig 7.3). Half of the opacities are initially unilateral. In addition to a progression of the focal opacities during the course of the illness, the opacities are also often migratory (fig 7.3). Spontaneous pneumomediastinum has been reported in some patients.[11 19] The studies that have included CT evaluation reveal a pattern that shares remarkable similarities with cryptogenic organising pneumonia or bronchiolitis obliterans organising pneumonia (COP/BOOP).[18 20 21] CT changes may be present in the absence of detectable abnormalities on chest radiographs (fig 7.4). Ground glass opacification and the peripheral distribution of the opacities on the CT scan are characteristic.[21] Pleural effusions are notably absent.

Recurrence of fever occurs in up to 85% of patients after 5–7 days and heralds the onset of the second phase. During this phase respiratory symptoms are often intensified with worsening breathlessness and dry cough.[11] In one cohort 73% of patients developed diarrhoea a week into their illness. Diarrhoea may pose special risks for healthcare providers as the virus can probably spread by the faecal-oral route. The observed decrease in viral load during this phase supports the notion that this phase may be related to the immunological response by the host. In some cases these symptoms are followed by hypoxaemia and progression in the severity and distribution of the pulmonary infiltrates.

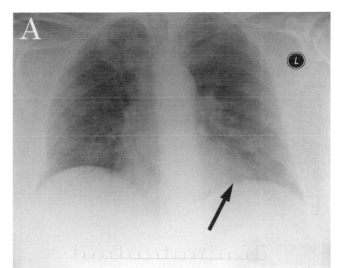

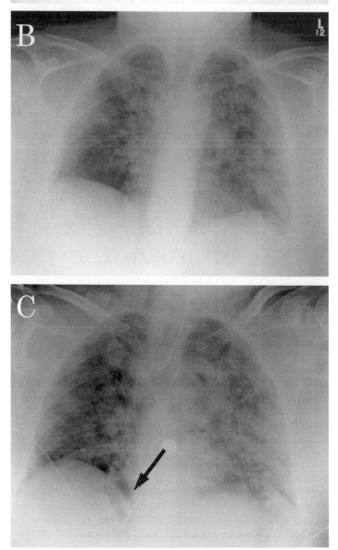

Figure 7.3 Progression in appearances on the chest radiograph of a patient with SARS. (A) Radiograph taken on presentation to the emergency department with fever and cough. Ill defined airspace filling disease is seen in the left base (arrow). (B) 48 hours after admission the patient developed progressive hypoxaemia and worsening of the chest radiograph with involvement of both lungs. (C) 72 hours after admission the patient was mechanically ventilated via an endotracheal tube. This chest radiograph taken 96 hours after admission demonstrates bilateral patchy airspace disease consistent with the acute respiratory distress syndrome (ARDS). Evidence of extrapulmonary air is also seen (arrow).

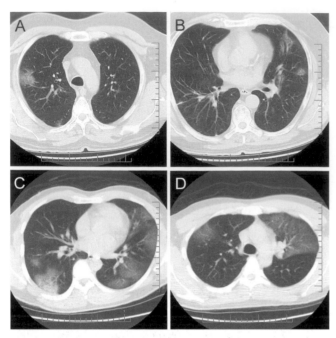

Figure 7.4 Computed tomographic images of two patients with SARS. The first images (A and B) were taken of the patient described in fig 7.3 on the same day as the first chest radiograph (fig 7.3A). Peripheral ground glass opacities (arrow) were seen on multiple sections affecting both lung fields. The second patient (C and D) also shows the peripheral opacities and ground glass pattern that characterise SARS.

Respiratory failure

About 20–25% of patients with SARS become critically ill and require ICU admission.[22 23] The mean duration from the onset of illness to ICU admission is 5–10 days and respiratory failure is the usual indication. A recent report from the Singapore group found that 45 of 199 infected patients eventually fulfilled the criteria for the diagnosis of acute lung injury (Pao_2/Fio_2 <300) or ARDS (Pao_2/Fio_2 <200).[22] In 10–15% of patients lung injury may progress to the point where mechanical ventilatory support is required. Advanced age, male sex, chronic hepatitis B carriage, raised creatinine levels, and recurrence of fever were associated with the development of ARDS in one study.[11] However, after multivariate analysis, only advanced age and chronic hepatitis C infection correlated with the development of ARDS, although the importance of coexisting hepatitis C infection will probably be less relevant in areas where hepatitis C is less prevalent. Classic histological features of ARDS, including hyaline membranes, have been observed in post mortem samples from patients with SARS (fig 7.5).[24 25] Loss of cilia, bronchial wall denudation, and squamous bronchial metaplasia have also been described. The presence of giant cells and macrophages in the alveolar space early in the disease has been claimed to be a diagnostic pathological characteristic of SARS related ARDS. However, in our view the specificity of these findings for SARS infection is not clear; for example, both multinucleated type II pneumocytes and macrophages are seen in other forms of ARDS. The histological appearances change with the duration of the illness, with cases of less than 10 days' duration having acute phase diffuse alveolar damage, airspace oedema, and bronchiolar fibrin deposition. Specimens from patients after 10 days of respiratory failure had features of the organising phase of diffuse alveolar damage, type II pneumocyte hyperplasia, squamous metaplasia, multinucleated giant cells, and acute bronchopneumonia.[26] It is unclear how the differences in histological appearance relate to prognosis.

Following a period of clinical improvement, some patients experience new chest infiltrates or sudden progression of respiratory failure. This third phase appears to be associated with the development of IgG seroconversion,[11] although nosoco-

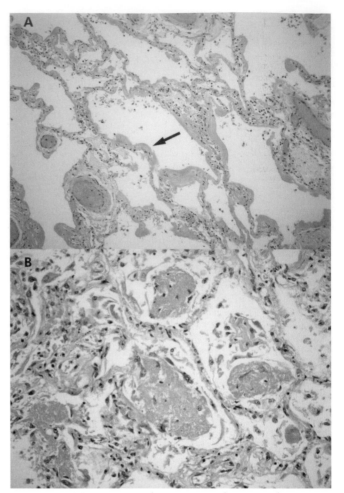

Figure 7.5 (A) Necroscopic lung specimen showing early ("exudative phase") diffuse alveolar damage with vascular congestion and airspaces (alveoli/alveolar ducts) lined by fibrinous fluid exudate ("hyaline membranes", arrow). These changes are non-specific with respect to the cause of injury (H&E; original magnification ×200). (B) Necroscopic lung specimen showing more advanced and more severe acute lung injury reflected by fibrinous exudates in alveoli undergoing early organisation with ingrowth of mesenchymal cells. This pattern of acute lung injury has been called "acute fibrinous and organising pneumonia"(AFOP).[27] This is non-specific with respect to cause and implies that the process will evolve into a more classical picture of organising pneumonia (formerly called BOOP: H&E; original magnification ×200). Photograph courtesy of Dr Dean Chamberlain.

mial superinfection may account for this deterioration in some of the patients. Haemophagocytosis in the lung biopsy specimens from these patients lends support to the hypothesis that SARS may cause cytokine dysregulation and indirect organ injury through host mediated mechanisms.

TREATMENT

If the diagnosis is uncertain, empirical treatment for community acquired pneumonia should be started. In most series of SARS treatment has included broad spectrum antibiotics including a fluoroquinolone or macrolide. The antiviral agent ribavirin has been used in the majority of patients treated in Hong Kong and in the first SARS outbreak in Toronto, without evidence of efficacy or even a strong anecdotal suggestion that patients benefit. The adverse effects of ribavirin are significant, particularly haemolytic anaemia and electrolyte disturbances such as hypokalaemia and hypomagnesaemia. The drug is also teratogenic. These features have led to the use of ribavirin falling out of favour. Similarly, the use of antiretroviral agents remains speculative. In a presentation at the international WHO SARS conference, the use of Lopinavir (an inhibitor of the HIV protease) in 34 patients with SARS was reported. Early in the

Table 7.1 High risk procedures for transmission of SARS in the ICU

Procedure	Concern	Possible solution
Nasopharyngeal swabs	Coughing	Use nasal swabs
Bag-valve-mask ventilation	Difficult to seal at face	Limit as much as possible
Tracheal intubation	Coughing, agitation	Sedation and neuromuscular blockade, PAPR hoods
Bronchoscopy	Coughing, aerosolisation	Limit use of PAPR hoods, neuromuscular blockade
Suctioning	Coughing, aerosolisation	Minimise, in-line suction
Non-invasive ventilation	Unfiltered aerosolised exhalation	Prohibited
High frequency oscillation	Unfiltered exhalation, uncontrolled secretions	Avoid at present until an in-line filter is developed

PAPR=powered air purification respirators.

disease there was a significantly lower rate of mortality (0 *v* 10.4%, p=0.04) and mechanical ventilation (0 *v* 12.2%, p=0.03) in the group treated with Lopinavir compared with historical controls (n=690; http://www.who.int/csr/sars/conference/june_2003/). Lopinavir may also have had benefit as rescue therapy when used with pulsed corticosteroids.

Anecdotal evidence suggests that corticosteroids show some benefit, particularly in patients with progressive pulmonary infiltrates and hypoxaemia. Various methylprednisolone regimens have been used at different centres with doses ranging from 40 mg twice daily (similar to treatment of *Pneumocystis* pneumonia) to 2 mg/kg/day (similar to treatment of late phase ARDS), to pulsed doses of 500 mg IV daily.[28 29] Physicians must search for other causes for fever and infection as secondary nosocomial infections may be responsible for the clinical progression seen in some critically ill patients later in their illness. Indeed, early reports in coronaviral models of hepatitis suggest that the use of corticosteroids may worsen outcome.[30 31] The use and correct timing of steroids in patients with SARS may be important and needs to be prospectively evaluated.

More recently the use of interferon beta has been advocated. The rationale for its use stems from the concern that the later phases of the illness are driven by the host's immune response. Anecdotal reports on the use of interferon appear promising and a clinical study is currently underway. Plasmapheresis as rescue therapy has also been used in some centres with uncertain benefit (http://www.who.int/csr/sars/conference/june_2003/).

SURVIVAL

The case fatality rate varies from 3% to 12%, depending on whether the denominator includes suspected and probable cases (3%) or probable cases alone (12%).[11 12 15 16 32] Older patients or those with pre-existing disease (diabetes, cardiac disease) have a higher mortality rate.[1 12–13 16 22 23 33] In one study the mortality rate of patients over 60 years was 43% compared with 13.2% in their younger counterparts.[9] While the mortality rate is higher in older patients, particularly those with pre-existing co-morbidity, young previously healthy people succumb to SARS, possibly because of higher viral loads or their vigorous host response. In multivariate analysis age, LDH level, and an increased neutrophil count at presentation were associated with a higher odds ratio for a poor outcome (death or ICU admission). Children appear to have a much less severe course than adults.[32] For patients admitted to the ICU, the mortality rates at 28 days have been reported to be 34–37%. In the series reported by Fowler and coworkers,[23] ICU outcome was worse in patients over 65 years, in diabetics, and in those with a higher heart rate and creatine kinase level on admission. Lew and colleagues[22] correlated a delayed recovery (requiring ventilation beyond 14 days) or death with both the APACHE II score (odds ratio for each 1 unit increase of 0.87, CI 0.78 to 0.97) and Pao_2/Fio_2 ratio (odds ratio for each 1 unit increase of 1.02, CI 1.0 to 1.04) on admission to the ICU. The

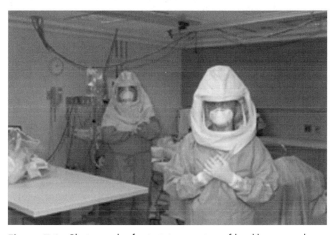

Figure 7.6 Photograph of a training session of healthcare workers performing an intubation on a patient simulator system. Photograph courtesy of Dr Randy Wax.

majority of deaths (75%) occurred late in the course of the ICU admission from ARDS, multisystem organ failure, thrombosis, or septic shock.

MANAGEMENT OF RESPIRATORY FAILURE

The risk of droplet spread is increased by various procedures (table 7.1). Efforts to avoid viral spread include the avoidance of nebulisers for drug administration and limitation or avoidance of the use of non-invasive ventilation. Nebulised humidification for oxygen therapy may carry similar risks, and our practice is to provide non-humidified oxygen using nasal prongs or a Venturi mask. A non-rebreather mask with expiratory port allowing for gas filtration is available and may be of value. During bag-mask-valve ventilation a filter should be used on the expiratory port.

Tracheal intubation poses a special risk to healthcare providers. Indeed, several of the outbreaks among healthcare workers in Toronto occurred following intubation of patients with SARS. As a result, strict guidelines for intubation and the management of cardiac arrest have been developed.[34] Recommendations for general anaesthesia have also been published.[35] In all instances, when a patient with known or suspected SARS requires tracheal intubation, perfect execution of infection control measures and donning of protective equipment is required (fig 7.6). In Toronto mock cardiac arrests and patient simulators with relevant clinical scenarios have been used. Intubation should be performed by the most skilled person available using the method with which they are most comfortable. Awake intubation may be associated with agitation and coughing which can severely compromise infection control precautions. We therefore recommend rapid sequence induction to facilitate airway stabilisation. A powered air purification respirator (PAPR) such as 3M Airmate can be used for these procedures.

Designated mechanical ventilators should have two filters (for example, Conserve 50 PALL filters) placed to eliminate the exhalation of viral particles into the environment and to protect the inside of the ventilator from contamination. One filter should be interposed between the distal end of the expiratory tubing and the ventilator itself, and the second should be placed on the exhalation outlet of the ventilator. Ideally, the exhalation port should then be connected to a central scavenging system that would eliminate release of viral particles into the ICU. High frequency oscillation may be associated with increased risk of droplet spread and exposure to respiratory secretions, and our practice is to avoid this intervention in patients with SARS. High frequency jet ventilation for those failing conventional ventilation may be used safely (owing to the ability to place in-line filters).

If a ventilated patient desaturates requiring manual bag-valve-mask ventilation, it is important to turn the ventilator to standby before disconnection to avoid droplet spray. In fact, in an intubated patient with SARS we recommend avoiding this intervention unless there is an obvious mechanical ventilator failure, even in the event of a cardiac arrest. Similarly, tracheobronchial suctioning of patients should be minimised and an in-line suction catheter system should be used. Because of the effect of infection control measures on bedside care, the use of kinetic beds may be considered for patients who are unable to move without assistance.

The severity of ARDS complicating SARS has been singularly impressive. Aside from the advanced infection control measures, the ventilatory management of these patients is no different from others with ARDS. We therefore use a low tidal volume strategy to minimise the risk of ventilator associated lung injury and adopt an open lung approach using recruitment manoeuvres and higher levels of PEEP to maintain alveolar patency. The use of routine recruitment manoeuvres is offset by the desire to minimise exposure to respiratory therapists and nurses. Little experience exists with the use of interventions such as prone positioning or inhaled nitric oxide in patients with SARS. In the report by Lew et al[22] three of seven patients had a significant improvement in oxygenation with prone positioning. Anecdotally, the experience in Toronto and Singapore has been that nitric oxide offers little benefit.

The development of air leaks appears to be high in patients with SARS related ARDS, ranging between 20% and 34%. Eleven episodes of venous thromboembolism and seven episodes of proven or suspected pulmonary embolism were reported by Lew and colleagues,[22] although the mode of prophylaxis was not stated.

INFECTION CONTROL PRECAUTIONS

Initial unfamiliarity and, later in the SARS outbreak, the failure to adhere to infection control procedures resulted in the spread of SARS to many healthcare personnel.[23] The organism appears to be transmitted by droplet spread, although surface contamination and possibly airborne spread may play a role. Recent data suggest that the virus may remain viable for considerable periods (up to 24 hours) on a dry surface.[36] As a result, staff education and continued vigilance are essential. Infection of healthcare workers involved in high risk procedures is a very real threat. Despite the use of infection control precautions, nine healthcare workers developed SARS following a prolonged intubation procedure, eight of whom required hospitalisation.[36] Droplet aerosolisation also occurs during bronchoscopy and similar precautions should be employed, including sedation and paralysis to prevent coughing.

Some recommendations for ICU staff have been published and are shown in box 7.1.[34] To avoid repeatedly breaking the negative pressure barrier, individual rooms should be stocked with basic supplies and modified cardiac arrest carts containing emergency drugs should be available in the room. Staff

---

Box 7.1 Infection control precautions in the ICU

Staff education

- High risk procedures, alternatives and precautions.
- Ways of minimising exposure and effective use of time when in the room.
- Instructions to staff on how to "undress" and "re-dress" without contamination.
- Importance of vigilance and adherence to all infection control precautions.
- Importance of monitoring own health.
- Information on SARS as it evolves.

Dress precautions

- Airborne precautions using an N-95 mask or equivalent.
- Contact precautions.
- Eye protection with a non-reusable goggles or face shield.
- Pens, paper, other personal items should not be allowed into or removed from the room.
- Powered air purification respirator (PAPR) hoods should be used during high risk procedures.

Environment/equipment

- Negative pressure isolation rooms with antechambers, and doors closed at all times.
- Individual isolation rooms stocked with basic supplies and emergency drugs.
- Alcohol based hand and equipment disinfectants.
- Gloves, gowns, masks and disposal units readily available.
- Use of video camera equipment or windows to monitor patients.
- Careful and frequent cleaning of surfaces with disposable clothes and alcohol based detergents.
- No equipment should be shared.

Transport

- Avoid patient transport where possible.
- Reflect on need for investigations and whether the benefits justify the transportation risks.
- Intubated patients should have a filter (Conserve PALL 50) inserted between the bag-valve and the swivel connector.
- Infection control should be alerted.

---

should remain outside the negative pressure rooms as much as possible. This means timing venesection and administration of treatment to minimise entries and the use of video camera equipment or windows to monitor patients without exposing staff. An antechamber (preferably with a sink) helps to maintain strict infection control precautions. Pens, paper, and other personal items should not be allowed into or removed from the room. Airborne precautions using a N-95 mask or equivalent should be taken; it is important that manufacturers' specifications are adhered to—for example, some N-95 masks maintain protection for 8 hours and some only for 4 hours. Touching the mask or lifting it to wipe the face or nose should be avoided. It is crucial to maintain a close seal to the skin and to ensure a proper fit. Sessions to determine optimum fit and mask type should be provided to all personnel. In addition, contact precautions—including the use of double gowns (at least one of which is waterproof) and double gloves, hats and shoe covers—should be used. Gowns, gloves, hats, boots, masks, and goggles should be changed after seeing each patient. Eye protection with non-reusable goggles or a face shield is required and staff should change into hospital scrubs upon arrival and change into their own clothing at the end of the day to avoid formite spread. Scrubs should not leave the hospital and should be sterilised after each use. The importance of proper removal of protective equipment cannot be overemphasised as contact with droplets on the surface of masks and gowns may occur.

Transportation of a patient with SARS is an infection control challenge that should be avoided whenever possible. SARS patients should never be transported while being supported by bag-valve-mask ventilation and should preferably be intubated. If bag ventilation is used, a filter should be placed between the bag and the endotracheal tube. The infection control department should be consulted for advice on proper precautions.

An important component of infection control is the limitation of personnel and visitors having contact with the patient. It is crucial that staff do not work if they are ill, even if the diagnosis is not clear. After unprotected contact with a SARS patient, staff are subject to a compulsory 10 day quarantine period. Visitors were restricted in Toronto hospitals during the outbreak. Indeed, several of the restrictions remain in place and will continue to do so for an indefinite period. All visitors are screened for symptoms of SARS and adhere to the same precautions as hospital staff. Visits with SARS patients are prohibited even on compassionate grounds.

CONCLUSIONS

SARS has resulted in significant challenges for critical care medicine. The ability of this disease to incapacitate staff has resulted in staff safety becoming a priority to maintain adequate critical care services. Indeed, the impact of this infection on the healthcare system and regional economy cannot be understated. Resources of individual hospitals were rapidly outstripped as scores of administrative and front line care providers were quarantined or became ill. In Toronto 18% of the critically ill patients were healthcare workers. The ability of this infection to spread is singularly impressive and devastating. Our understanding of the virus, its diagnosis, and treatment continues to evolve. Infection control measures remain the mainstay of regional and global health. The concept of "universal precautions" has expanded beyond policies regarding blood borne infections and now includes strict respiratory and contact precautions. The effect of these stringent policies on patients without SARS was devastating. As a result of the outbreak, hospitals were closed and advanced surgical and medical care programmes such as transplantation and organ donation were shut down. In one instance 35 critical care beds were closed (representing 38% of our tertiary ICU beds) because of an inadvertent exposure of ICU staff to a patient with SARS. The secondary morbidity and mortality from this disease on patients who were placed on hold or whose surgery was delayed remains to be determined. The guidelines and recommendations discussed here will change as our knowledge grows. No doubt information technology played an important role in allowing collaboration and rapid transfer of information throughout the SARS pandemic. Indeed, through such collaboration we can hope to improve the mortality and morbidity of our patients and, indeed, ourselves.

REFERENCES

1 **Anon.** Update: severe acute respiratory syndrome—United States, June 18, 2003. *MMWR* 2003;**52**:570.
2 **Ksiazek TG**, Erdman D, Goldsmith CS, *et al.* A novel coronavirus associated with severe acute respiratory syndrome. *N Engl J Med* 2003;**348**:1953–66.
3 **Drosten C**, Gunther S, Preiser W, *et al.* Identification of a novel coronavirus in patients with severe acute respiratory syndrome. *N Engl J Med* 2003;**348**:1967–76.
4 **Marra MA**, Jones SJ, Astell CR, *et al.* The genome sequence of the SARS-associated coronavirus. *Science* 2003;**300**:1399–404.
5 **Ruan YJ**, Wei CL, Ee AL, *et al.* Comparative full-length genome sequence analysis of 14 SARS coronavirus isolates and common mutations associated with putative origins of infection. *Lancet* 2003;**361**:1779–85.
6 **Rainer TH**, Cameron PA, Smit D, *et al.* Evaluation of WHO criteria for identifying patients with severe acute respiratory syndrome out of hospital: prospective observational study. *BMJ* 2003;**326**:1354–8.
7 **Yang W.** Severe acute respiratory syndrome (SARS): infection control. *Lancet* 2003;**361**:1386–7.
8 **Zhong NS**, Zeng GQ. Our Strategies for fighting severe acute respiratory syndrome (SARS). *Am J Respir Crit Care Med* 2003;**168**:7–9.
9 **Donnelly CA**, Ghani AC, Leung GM, *et al.* Epidemiological determinants of spread of causal agent of severe acute respiratory syndrome in Hong Kong. *Lancet* 2003;**361**:1761–6.
10 **Pearson H**, Clarke T, Abbott A, *et al.* SARS: what have we learned? *Nature* 2003;**424**:121–6.
11 **Peiris JS**, Chu CM, Cheng VC, *et al.* Clinical progression and viral load in a community outbreak of coronavirus-associated SARS pneumonia: a prospective study. *Lancet* 2003;**361**:1767–72.
12 **Booth CM**, Matukas LM, Tomlinson GA, *et al.* Clinical features and short-term outcomes of 144 patients with SARS in the greater Toronto area. *JAMA* 2003;**289**:2801–9.
13 **Tan YM**, Chow PK, Soo KC. Severe acute respiratory syndrome: clinical outcome after inpatient outbreak of SARS in Singapore. *BMJ* 2003;**326**:1394.
14 **Wong RS**, Wu A, To KF, *et al.* Haematological manifestations in patients with severe acute respiratory syndrome: retrospective analysis. *BMJ* 2003;**326**:1358–62.
15 **Avendano M**, Derkach P, Swan S. Clinical course and management of SARS in health care workers in Toronto: a case series. *Can Med Assoc J* 2003;**168**:1649–60.
16 **Lee N**, Hui D, Wu A, *et al.* A major outbreak of severe acute respiratory syndrome in Hong Kong. *N Engl J Med* 2003;**348**:1986–94.
17 **Fisher DA**, Lim TK, Lim YT, *et al.* Atypical presentations of SARS. *Lancet* 2003;**361**:1740.
18 **Grinblat L**, Shulman H, Glickman A, *et al.* Severe acute respiratory syndrome: radiographic review of 40 probable cases in Toronto, Canada. *Radiology* 2003;**228**:802–9.
19 **Wong KT**, Antonio GE, Hui DS, *et al.* Severe acute respiratory syndrome: radiographic appearances and pattern of progression in 138 patients. *Radiology* 2003;**228**:401–6.
20 **Wong KT**, Antonio GE, Hui DS, *et al.* Thin-section CT of severe acute respiratory syndrome: evaluation of 74 patients exposed to or with the disease. *Radiology* 2003;**228**:395–400.
21 **Muller NL**, Ooi GC, Khong PL, *et al.* Severe acute respiratory syndrome: radiographic and CT findings. *AJR* 2003;**181**:3–8.
22 **Lew TW**, Kwek TK, Tai D, *et al.* Acute respiratory distress syndrome in critically ill patients with severe acute respiratory syndrome. *JAMA* 2003;**290**:374–80.
23 **Fowler RA**, Lapinsky SE, Hallett D, *et al.* Critically ill patients with severe acute respiratory syndrome. *JAMA* 2003;**290**:367–73.
24 **Nicholls JM**, Poon LL, Lee KC, *et al.* Lung pathology of fatal severe acute respiratory syndrome. *Lancet* 2003;**361**:1773–8.
25 **Ding Y**, Wang H, Shen H, *et al.* The clinical pathology of severe acute respiratory syndrome (SARS): a report from China. *J Pathol* 2003;**200**:282–9.
26 **Franks TJ**, Chong PY, Chui P, *et al.* Lung pathology of severe acute respiratory syndrome (SARS): a study of 8 autopsy cases from Singapore. *Hum Pathol* 2003;**34**:729.
27 **Beasley MB**, Franks TJ, Galvin JR, *et al.* Acute fibrinous and organizing pneumonia: a histological pattern of lung injury and possible variant of diffuse alveolar damage. *Arch Pathol Lab Med* 2002;**126**:1064–70.
28 **Gagnon S**, Boota AM, Fischl MA, *et al.* Corticosteroids as adjunctive therapy for severe Pneumocystis carinii pneumonia in the acquired immunodeficiency syndrome. A double-blind, placebo-controlled trial. *N Engl J Med* 1990;**323**:1444–50.
29 **Meduri GU**, Headley AS, Golden E, *et al.* Effect of prolonged methylprednisolone therapy in unresolving acute respiratory distress syndrome: a randomized controlled trial. *JAMA* 1998;**280**:159–65.
30 **Fingerote RJ**, Leibowitz JL, Rao YS, *et al.* Treatment of resistant A/J mice with methylprednisolone (MP) results in loss of resistance to murine hepatitis strain 3 (MHV-3) and induction of macrophage procoagulant activity (PCA). *Adv Exp Med Biol* 1995;**380**:89–94.
31 **Fingerote RJ**, Abecassis M, Phillips MJ, *et al.* Loss of resistance to murine hepatitis virus strain 3 infection after treatment with corticosteroids is associated with induction of macrophage procoagulant activity. *J Virol* 1996;**70**:4275–82.
32 **Hon KL**, Leung CW, Cheng WT, *et al.* Clinical presentations and outcome of severe acute respiratory syndrome in children. *Lancet* 2003;**361**:1701–3.
33 **Chan JW**, Ng CK, Chan YH, *et al.* Short term outcome and risk factors for adverse clinical outcomes in adults with severe acute respiratory syndrome (SARS). *Thorax* 2003;**58**:686–9.
34 **Lapinsky SE**, Hawryluck L. ICU management of severe acute respiratory syndrome. *Intensive Care Med* 2003;**29**:870–5.
35 **Kamming D**, Gardam M, Chung F. Anaesthesia and SARS. *Br J Anaesth* 2003;**90**:715–8.
36 **Anon.** Cluster of severe acute respiratory syndrome cases among protected health-care workers—Toronto, Canada, April 2003. *MMWR* 2003;**52**:433–6.

8 Ventilator induced lung injury

T Whitehead, A S Slutsky

Mechanical ventilation has become an indispensable tool, facilitating general anaesthesia and supporting life in the critically ill. However, its application has adverse effects including an increased risk of pneumonia, impaired cardiac performance, and neuromuscular problems relating to sedation and muscle relaxants. Moreover, it has become clear that applying pressure—whether positive or negative—to the lung can cause damage known as ventilator induced lung injury (VILI). This concept is not new. In his treatise on resuscitation of the apparently dead, John Fothergill in 1745 suggested that mouth to mouth inflation of the victim's lungs might be preferable to using a pair of bellows as "the lungs of one man may bear, without injury, as great a force as another man can exert; which by the bellows cannot always be determin'd".[1] Although not specifically addressed, Forthergill's admonition against the use of the bellows probably related to gross air leaks produced by large pressures. This type of injury is now called barotrauma and was the first widely recognised manifestation of VILI. The clinical and radiological manifestations of barotrauma include pneumothorax, pneumomediastinum, and surgical emphysema.

Later, evidence accumulated to suggest that ventilation causes more subtle morphological and functional changes and can excite an inflammatory response within the lung. This type of injury was not recognised for many years as the pattern of damage is often indistinguishable from that seen in other forms of lung injury such as the acute respiratory distress syndrome (ARDS), for which mechanical ventilation is an indispensable treatment. Studies using animal models were necessary to define key aspects of VILI. Based on these, many clinicians in the 1990s began to adopt ventilatory strategies designed to minimise lung injury, although the clinical importance of VILI has only recently been established.[2]

In this chapter we summarise the main risk factors for VILI, its possible mechanisms, and its clinical relevance. Specific ventilation techniques for ARDS are addressed in chapter 9, and will only be alluded to here for the purpose of illustrating general principles.

MAJOR DETERMINANTS OF VILI

Most research into VILI is based on positive pressure ventilation delivered via an endotracheal tube, although the principles are equally relevant to non-invasive or negative pressure ventilation. It has become clear that the degree of VILI is determined by the interaction of the ventilator settings and patient related factors, particularly the condition of the ventilated lung.

Ventilator determinants of VILI
Airway pressure and lung distension
Conceptually, it seems obvious that inflation of the lung will cause damage if airway pressures are high enough. The important issues for the clinician have been (1) what levels of airway pressure are dangerous and (2) can they be avoided in the mechanical ventilation of patients with stiff lungs, as in ARDS?

The association between high airway pressure and air leaks has long been recognised.[3 4] However, this relationship does not necessarily imply causality as damaged, stiff lungs that require high airway pressures for ventilation may be intrinsically more prone to air leaks. Recent large studies in patients with ARDS have, in fact, shown a poor correlation between airway pressure (or tidal volume) and the occurrence of air leaks, which occurred in 8–14% of the patients.[2 5–7] However, these data should not be interpreted as demonstrating that the degree of lung distension is unimportant in the development of barotrauma. In these studies airway pressures and tidal volumes were lower than those used in the past when barotrauma rates as high as 39% were reported in patients ventilated for acute respiratory failure.[8]

More subtle lung damage was first unequivocally shown by Webb and Tierney who ventilated rats for 1 hour using different airway pressures with and without positive end expiratory pressure (PEEP).[9] Animals ventilated with a peak airway pressure of 14 cm H_2O had no histological changes in the lung, while those ventilated with a pressure of 30 cm H_2O had mild perivascular oedema. In contrast, all rats ventilated at 45 cm H_2O (without PEEP) developed severe hypoxia and died before the end of the hour. Their lungs had marked perivascular and alveolar oedema. Similar findings have been observed in other species, although there is considerable variation in the susceptibility to VILI. Whereas in rats ventilation at high peak inspiratory pressure for just 2 minutes is sufficient to induce pulmonary oedema, larger animals such as rabbits and sheep require much longer periods of ventilation for changes to be evident.[10–12] This is clearly important when extrapolating data from animal studies to humans.

Pressure or volume?
Although the term *barotrauma* is commonly used when discussing VILI, the evidence indicates that the degree of lung inflation is a more important determinant of lung injury than airway pressure per se. This may be inferred from the observation that trumpet players commonly achieve airway pressures of 150 cm H_2O without developing repetitive episodes of gross air leakage.[13] The relative contribution of pressure and volume to lung injury was first studied by ventilating rats whose tidal excursion was limited by strapping the chest and abdomen.[14] High airway pressure without a high tidal volume did not produce lung injury. By contrast, animals ventilated without thoracic restriction using high tidal volumes, achieved either with high positive inspiratory pressure or

negative pressure in an iron lung, developed severe injury. These results have been confirmed in other species.[15 16]

The term *volutrauma* is therefore more accurate than *barotrauma*, although in practice the two are closely related. The degree of alveolar distension is determined by the pressure gradient across the alveoli, approximated by the transpulmonary pressure, the difference between the static airway pressure (estimated clinically by the plateau airway pressure) and the pleural pressure. Peak airway pressure is not necessarily a reflection of alveolar pressure and is greatly influenced by the resistance to flow in the airways. Recent guidelines have therefore emphasised the importance of limiting plateau pressures and of being aware of factors that increase (or decrease) the degree of alveolar distension for a given alveolar pressure.[17] For example, conditions associated with increased chest wall compliance such as immaturity increase lung distension, and hence damage, for a given alveolar pressure. Conversely, chest wall compliance is commonly reduced by abdominal distension,[18] which can result in lower alveolar inflation, derecruitment, and hypoxaemia if the plateau pressure is inappropriately low.

Lung injury at low lung volumes

There is evidence that lung damage may also be caused by ventilation at low lung volume (meaning low *absolute* lung volume rather than low tidal volume). This has been well defined in animal models, but the relevance to humans is not firmly established. Several studies have shown that the injurious effects of mechanical ventilation can be attenuated by the application of PEEP.[9 14 19 20] Ventilation with high tidal volume and low or zero PEEP appears to be more damaging than low tidal volume and high PEEP, even though both strategies result in similar high levels of end inspiratory pressure and alveolar distension. Ventilation of isolated lavaged rat lungs with small tidal volumes (5–6 ml/kg) and low or zero PEEP caused lung injury that could be reduced by the application of higher levels of PEEP.[21]

A number of mechanisms may explain lung injury associated with ventilation at low absolute lung volumes. Cyclic opening and closing (recruitment-derecruitment) of small airways/lung units may lead to increased local shear stress—so called *atelectrauma*. PEEP effectively splints open the distal airways, maintaining recruitment throughout the ventilatory cycle. The static pressure-volume curve (fig 8.1) is often used to illustrate the balance between overdistension and recruitment. As airway pressure is increased from functional residual capacity (FRC), an abrupt change in the lung compliance is often evident, particularly in injured or surfactant deficient lungs. This lower inflection point (LIP) may represent the approximate pressure (volume) at which lung units are recruited. The upper inflection point (UIP) at which lung compliance decreases at higher airway pressure was thought to reflect the point at which alveoli are becoming overdistended, and therefore potentially damaged.[23] Based on these concepts, an ideal ventilatory strategy would be one in which all the tidal ventilation would take place on the "steep" portion of the pressure-volume curve where the lung is most compliant. The value of PEEP would be sufficient to prevent derecruitment but not so great as to lead to overdistension. High frequency oscillatory ventilation (HFOV) potentially offers the ideal combination of minimum tidal volume while maintaining maximal recruitment (the "open lung"), provided sufficient end expiratory lung volume is maintained.[24 25]

Although theoretically sound, the explanation of VILI according to the pressure-volume curve is certainly a gross oversimplification. Recruitment is not complete at the LIP and continues at higher inflating pressures.[26 27] Similarly, the UIP does not necessarily reflect the onset of overdistension. Instead, it may represent the point at which recruitment is complete and therefore compliance decreases. Furthermore,

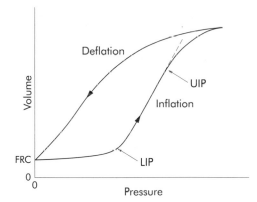

Figure 8.1 Pressure-volume curve derived from a patient with ARDS. FRC=functional residual capacity; LIP=lower inflection point; UIP=upper inflection point. Adapted from Matamis *et al*[22] with permission.

inflation may be expanding alveoli without necessarily overdistending them.[27] In addition, it is difficult to show that recruitment-derecruitment actually occurs,[28] and dynamic ventilation may not follow the pattern of the static pressure-volume curve. Indeed, a recent study using saline lavaged rabbits suggested that ventilation follows the deflation limb of the pressure-volume curve, provided an adequate recruitment manoeuvre is performed.[29] Thus, theoretically, a lung could be maintained in a recruited state at lower airway pressures than the inflation limb of the pressure-volume curve would indicate and, conversely, pressures applied on the basis of the inflation limb would cause overdistension. Finally, but of perhaps greatest importance, the damaged lung in the clinical setting is not homogeneously affected, as detailed below. Applied airway pressure that may be ideal to recruit and ventilate some lung units may be inadequate to open the most densely atelectatic regions, and yet simultaneously cause overdistension in the most compliant areas.[30 31]

Other ventilator parameters

Few studies have addressed the effect of ventilator parameters other than tidal volume, airway pressure, and PEEP in VILI. Increased respiratory frequency may augment lung injury through greater stress cycling, a phenomenon well described in engineering, or through the deactivation of surfactant. Isolated perfused rabbit lungs ventilated with a frequency of 20 breaths/min show greater oedema and perivascular haemorrhage than those ventilated at 3 breaths/min.[32] The relevance of these findings to clinical practice is unclear.

Inspired oxygen fraction

Oxidant stress is believed to be an important mechanism in mediating lung injury in a variety of lung diseases including ARDS, and exposure of animals or humans to a high inspired oxygen fraction (FIO_2) leads to lung damage, probably through the increased generation of reactive oxygen species.[33 34] Current practice in ARDS is to use the lowest FIO_2 giving an oxygen saturation of around 90%.

Carbon dioxide

Arterial carbon dioxide tensions ($PaCO_2$) reflect minute ventilation. The advent of protective ventilatory strategies in ARDS, with lower tidal volumes and minute ventilation, was accompanied by the acceptance of higher levels of $PaCO_2$ (permissive hypercapnia) and mild respiratory acidosis.[35] Rather than being harmful, some animal studies suggest that hypercapnia exerts a protective effect in lung injury, although to date there is no clear evidence from clinical studies.[36]

Patient determinants of VILI

The condition of the ventilated lung is of considerable importance in determining susceptibility to VILI. At one extreme,

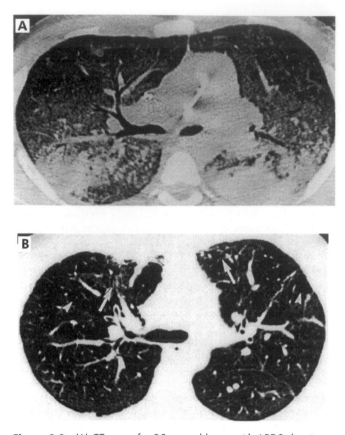

Figure 8.2 (A) CT scan of a 25 year old man with ARDS showing the typically heterogeneous distribution of opacification within the lungs, mostly in the posterior dependent regions. (B) CT scan of the same patient 8 months later showing remarkably little abnormality in the posterior regions but with reticular changes anteriorly (large arrows). Reproduced with permission from Desai *et al.*[44]

VILI does not appear to be a clinical problem in patients with normal lungs who can undergo prolonged periods of mechanical ventilation without detrimental effect.[37] In these instances the pressures and flows within the lung closely resemble the physiological situation. At the other extreme, the grossly abnormal lungs of patients with ARDS are highly susceptible to VILI, and it may be that in some patients no mechanical ventilation strategy is entirely devoid of detrimental effects.

Ventilating the injured lung

Animal studies using isolated lungs and intact animals have indicated that injured lungs are more susceptible to VILI.[38–40] An important factor underlying this predisposition to VILI is the uneven distribution of disease and inflation seen in injured lungs. Based on the diffuse relatively homogeneous distribution of shadowing on a plain chest radiograph, it was thought that the lung was uniformly affected in ARDS. However, CT scanning showed that the posterior dependent

portions of the lung are more severely affected (fig 8.2A), a distribution determined largely by gravity. The greater compliance of less affected areas means that they receive a much greater proportion of the delivered tidal volume.[41] This may result in substantial regional overdistension and hence injury.

In a recent study, piglets with multifocal pneumonia were ventilated using a tidal volume of 15 ml/kg for 43 hours.[42] Approximately 75% of the lung volume was consolidated, so the residual 25% of normally ventilated lung may have received a tidal volume equivalent to 40–50 ml/kg. Histological examination showed emphysema-like lesions in these areas, whereas in consolidated areas the alveoli were "protected" against overdistension, but the bronchioles that remained patent were injured through overdistension and by the forces generated through interdependence and recruitment-derecruitment (fig 8.3). Lesions similar to those described above have been reported in a necropsy series of patients with ARDS[43]; furthermore, CT scans of ARDS survivors have shown greatest residual abnormality in the anterior parts of the lung, even though the posterior areas had been most abnormal in the acute phase (fig 8.2B).[44] These changes may be due to injury caused by overdistension.

Other factors that may promote VILI in already injured lungs are surfactant abnormalities and the presence of an activated inflammatory infiltrate which may be further stimulated by mechanical ventilation.

Lung immaturity

The immature lung may be particularly susceptible to VILI.[45] The volume of the lung relative to body weight and the number of alveoli are lower in premature infants, making a tidal volume based on weight potentially more injurious. The resilience of the lung tissue is lower, due to less well developed collagen and elastin elements, and surfactant deficiency leads to alveolar instability and favours airway closure. At delivery the fluid filled, surfactant deficient airways of the preterm neonate require high inflation pressures to establish patency, with potential generation of high shear stress. Preterm lambs show evidence of lung injury after only six high volume insufflations.[46]

MANIFESTATION OF VILI
Pulmonary oedema

Pulmonary oedema is a prominent feature of experimental models of VILI, particularly those using small animals.[9 12 47] The high protein content of the oedema fluid suggests that it is, at least in part, due to increased permeability, and experimental studies have implicated changes at both the epithelial and microvascular endothelial barriers. Increased static inflation of fluid filled lung lobes in sheep led to the passage of larger solutes across the epithelium, a finding observed in other models.[48 49] Increased microvascular permeability has been shown by the redistribution of ^{125}I-labelled albumin into the extravascular space in mechanically ventilated rats,[50] with

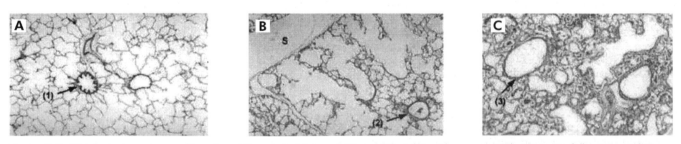

Figure 8.3 Histological specimens of lung from (A) control piglets and (B) and (C) piglets with experimental pneumonia following ventilation for 2 days. (A) shows normal lung architecture and bronchioles (arrow 1). In piglets with pneumonia there are emphysematous changes in the ventilated regions (B), but bronchioles are of normal size (arrow 2). In consolidated areas (C) there is bronchiolar dilatation (arrow 3). Reproduced with permission from Goldstein *et al.*[42]

parallel findings in other species.[16][51] In contrast to the clear evidence for increased permeability, relatively little is known about the contribution of hydrostatic pressures to the development of pulmonary oedema in mechanical ventilation. This stems largely from the great difficulty in assessing transmural pressures at the microvascular level. Studies in lambs have indicated that high tidal volume ventilation causes a relatively modest increase in transmural pulmonary vascular pressures.[16] Hydrostatic forces may still be important. Firstly, regional differences in lung perfusion and atelectasis may generate far greater filtration forces in some areas[52] and, secondly, in the injured lung even small increases in transmural pressure may greatly increase oedema formation.

Morphological changes

The acute structural changes of "injurious" mechanical ventilation have been best defined using small animal models. Under the light microscope the development of oedema is first evident as perivascular cuffing which progresses to florid interstitial oedema and alveolar flooding with continued ventilation at high pressure.[9][50] Changes in the endothelium are detectable by electron microscopy within only a few minutes of high airway pressure ventilation of rats, and appear to precede alterations in the epithelium. Some endothelial cells become focally separated from their basement membrane forming intracapillary blebs. Eventually, diffuse alveolar damage is evident; the epithelial surface becomes grossly disrupted in some areas with destruction of type I but sparing of type II cells.[14][47]

Larger animals have been used to study the longer term effects of mechanical ventilation. In piglets with experimental pneumonia, alveolar damage is seen in the ventilated regions after 2–3 days, with bronchiolar dilatation in the consolidated regions (fig 8.3).[42] An inflammatory reaction also becomes prominent. Ventilation of piglets with high peak airway pressures leads to neutrophil recruitment within 24 hours and fibroproliferative changes after 3–6 days.[53] Similarly, conventional ventilation (tidal volume 12 ml/kg) of saline lavaged rabbits led to accumulation of neutrophils in the lungs, as well as severe epithelial damage and hyaline membrane formation. By contrast, animals ventilated with HFOV had minimal injury.[54][55]

Increased vascular permeability, diffuse alveolar damage, inflammatory cell infiltrates, and later fibroproliferative changes are not specific to VILI. ARDS and other forms of lung injury are associated with identical pathological appearances. The pertinent question for the clinician is the degree to which the changes classically ascribed to ARDS are in fact attributable to VILI?

MECHANISMS OF VILI

The mechanical forces applied through ventilation may have deleterious effects in at least two ways: (1) through physical disruption of the tissues and cells, which depends not only on the magnitude and pattern of the applied stress but also on the resilience of the lung tissue, and (2) through the aberrant activation of cellular mechanisms leading to inappropriate and harmful responses. Both certainly occur, although it is not clear which is more important clinically.

Physical disruption (stress failure)
How forces are generated within the lung
Macklin and Macklin proposed that air leaks are caused by a momentary high pressure gradient between the alveolus and the bronchovascular sheath.[3] Air ruptures across the epithelial surface and tracks along the bronchovascular sheath. It may then pass into the interstitium causing pulmonary interstitial emphysema, into the pleural space causing pneumothorax, into the pericardial cavity leading to pneumopericardium, and so on. The endothelium, in close apposition to the epithelial surface, is subject to stress failure due to forces derived both from transpulmonary and intravascular pressures. The extremely thin blood gas barrier (0.2–0.4 μM) permits free gas exchange by diffusion but exposes the capillary to high wall stress, determined by the ratio of the wall tension to thickness.[56] In rabbits stress failure occurs at capillary transmural pressures of 52.5 cm H_2O (~40 mm Hg) or greater and the microscopic lesions of endothelial and epithelial disruption are similar to those caused by high volume ventilation.[56][58] Importantly, the blood-gas barrier is more prone to stress failure at higher lung volumes, probably due to increased longitudinal forces acting on the blood vessel.[59] The forces generated by mechanical ventilation may therefore interact with those due to pulmonary vascular perfusion to magnify lung injury. Isolated rabbit lungs ventilated with a peak static pressure of 30 cm H_2O exhibit greater oedema and haemorrhage when perfused with high flow rates corresponding to higher pulmonary artery pressures.[60]

Interdependence
Adjacent alveoli and terminal bronchioles share common walls so that forces acting on one lung unit are transmitted to those around it. This phenomenon, known as interdependence, is believed to be important in maintaining uniformity of alveolar size and surfactant function.[61] Under conditions of uniform expansion all lung units will be subject to a similar transalveolar pressure, approximately equal to the alveolar minus the pleural pressure. However, if the lung is unevenly expanded, such forces may vary considerably. When an alveolus collapses the traction forces exerted on its walls by adjacent expanded lung units increase and these are applied to a smaller area. These forces will promote re-expansion at the expense of greatly increased and potentially harmful stress at the interface between collapsed and expanded lung units. At a transpulmonary pressure of 30 cm H_2O it has been calculated that re-expansion pressures could reach 140 cm H_2O.[61][62] In a necroscopic study of patients who had died with ARDS, expanded cavities and pseudocysts were found particularly around atelectatic areas, suggesting that these forces do indeed play a role in VILI.[43]

Recruitment-derecruitment
Theoretically, small airways may become occluded by exudate or apposition of their walls.[63][64] In either event, the airway pressure required to restore patency greatly exceeds that in an unoccluded passage. The resulting shear stress may damage the airways, particularly if the cycle is repeated with each breath (~20 000 times per day). The pressure required to reopen an occluded airway is inversely proportional to its diameter,[65] which is consistent with the observation that small airway damage in isolated lungs ventilated at zero PEEP occurs more distally as PEEP is applied.[21]

Airway collapse is favoured by surfactant deficiency or conditions in which the interstitial support of the airways is weakened or underdeveloped.[65][66] Conversely, recruitment-derecruitment may not occur at all in normal lungs, which tolerate periods of negative end expiratory pressure without evident harm.[67]

Importance of surfactant
Surfactant plays a role in VILI in two related ways; firstly, surfactant dysfunction or deficiency appears to amplify the injurious effects of mechanical ventilation and, secondly, ventilation itself can impair surfactant function thereby favouring further lung damage.

Abnormalities of the surfactant system may contribute to injury in the mature lung as in preterm infants. Surfactant isolated from patients with ARDS and experimental models of pneumonia is functionally impaired.[68][69] This is associated with a decrease in the functionally active large aggregate (LA) component of the surfactant pool relative to the less active small aggregate (SA) component. Although stretch of type 2 cells in vitro and a modest degree of hyperventilation stimulate surfactant production,[70] more injurious ventilatory strategies of high tidal volume and low PEEP lead to a reduced pool of functional surfactant and a decreased LA:SA ratio, particularly in injured lungs.[71] Large cyclical alterations in the alveolar surface area and the presence of serum proteins in the airspace may be responsible for these changes.

Lungs can be rendered experimentally deficient in surfactant by saline lavage or detergent aerosolisation, and they may behave in a manner similar to those of premature infants. Strategies that maintain lung recruitment, such as HFOV (with recruitment manoeuvres) and conventional mechanical ventilation at high levels of PEEP, appear to be particularly effective in minimising lung injury in these models.[72–75] Surfactant abnormalities may contribute to VILI in several ways relating to the increase in surface tension:

(1) Alveoli and airways are more prone to collapse with generation of shear stress as they are reopened.

(2) The uneven expansion of lung units increases regional stress forces through interdependence.

(3) The transvascular filtration pressure is increased, promoting oedema formation.[76]

In addition, surfactant is thought to have important immunoregulatory functions[77] which may become impaired through mechanical ventilation.

From the preceding discussion it is logical to propose that increasing the pool of functioning surfactant might lessen lung injury. Surfactant therapy reduces mortality in the neonatal respiratory distress syndrome and may decrease lung injury.[78] In ARDS a role for surfactant supplementation is not established,[79] partly because of difficulties in delivering adequate amounts of active surfactant to damaged and collapsed lung regions.

Activation of aberrant cellular pathways

Physical forces such as stretch play an important role in physiological processes. In fetal life breathing is essential for lung development and in the mature lung ventilation stimulates surfactant production by type II pneumocytes.[70] Central to this is the concept of *mechanotransduction*, whereby physical forces are detected by cells and converted into biochemical signals. There is now good evidence that signalling events activated by injurious ventilation play a role in VILI.[80 81]

The increase in lung vascular permeability induced in isolated perfused rat lungs by high airway pressure ventilation can be blocked by gadolinium in the perfusate.[82] Gadolinium probably exerts this effect through its inhibition of stretch activated cation channels. This indicates that the oedema seen in injurious ventilation is, at least in part, due to the activation of specific cellular processes rather than simply being a reflection of physical disruption of the alveolar-capillary barrier (the "stretched pore" phenomenon).

Considerable attention has focused recently on the release of inflammatory mediators from lung tissue exposed to mechanical forces. A number of studies involving isolated lungs or intact lung injured animals of different species have shown that injurious ventilatory strategies are associated with the release of a variety of proinflammatory mediators, including thromboxane B_2, platelet activating factor, and several cytokines.[83–87] This humoral inflammatory response can precede overt histological damage and appears to be due to stretch activation of specific pathways, in addition to an inflammatory reaction to non-specific injury.[81 87] The importance of these mediators in causing lung injury is unknown, and it is conceivable that they exert a beneficial effect in the injured lung.[88] However, studies using rabbit models of VILI

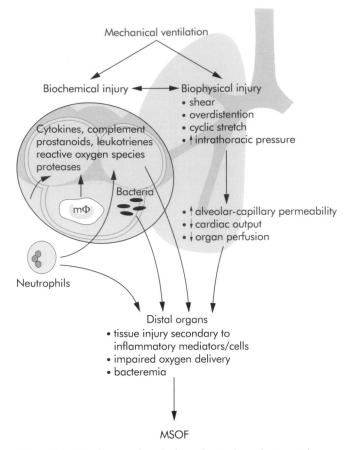

Figure 8.4 Mechanisms by which mechanical ventilation might contribute to multiple system organ failure (MSOF). Reproduced with permission from Slutsky and Tremblay.[93]

have shown that lung damage can be attenuated by administration of anti-tumour necrosis factor (TNF)-α antibodies or interleukin (IL)-1 receptor antagonists, suggesting that these cytokines exert a deleterious effect.[89 90] In the preterm lung cytokines generated by mechanical ventilation may interfere with lung development.[45] The term *biotrauma* has been coined to describe this potentially injurious inflammatory response to physical stress.

Mediators generated in response to injurious ventilation do not remain compartmentalised within the lung. Experiments with perfused mouse lungs and with lung injured rats in vivo have indicated that injurious ventilation leads to increased cytokine levels in the systemic circulation, and recent studies suggest that the same applies in the clinical setting.[85 86 91 92] This has led to the hypothesis that mechanical ventilation can fuel the systemic inflammatory response commonly seen in ARDS and contribute to the development of multiple system organ failure (MSOF).[93]

Ventilation may also influence the systemic inflammatory response through translocation of bacteria or their products from the air spaces into the circulation. In dogs and rats bacteraemia is more likely to develop when lungs that have been inoculated with bacteria are ventilated with high tidal volume/zero PEEP compared with less injurious strategies.[94 95] An analogous effect has been observed in ventilated rabbits following intratracheal administration of lipopolysaccharide (LPS). Injurious ventilation resulted in much higher levels of circulating LPS accompanied by a rise in TNF-α.[96] The possible ways in which ventilation impacts on systemic inflammation and distal organs are summarised in fig 8.4.

CLINICAL CONSEQUENCES OF VILI

Despite the difficulties in distinguishing the effects of mechanical ventilation from those of the underlying condition, there are now clear data showing the clinical impact of

VILI in two conditions—neonatal respiratory distress syndrome and ARDS.

Neonatal chronic lung disease

Most cases of neonatal chronic lung disease (CLD), also known as bronchopulmonary dysplasia, occur in the aftermath of neonatal respiratory distress syndrome. Hyperoxia and mechanical ventilation have been implicated in its aetiology.[97] Evidence for the role of mechanical ventilation in this respect includes the observation that neonatal intensive care units with high rates of intubation and ventilation also have high rates of CLD without improvements in mortality or other morbidity.[98] [99] At two centres with very different rates of mechanical ventilation of low birth weight infants (75% v 29%) and prevalence of CLD (22% v 4%) multivariate regression analysis indicated that the development of CLD was strongly associated with the initiation of mechanical ventilation.[99] Several trials have addressed the use of different ventilatory strategies, particularly HFOV, in neonatal respiratory distress. Despite its theoretical advantages over conventional ventilation in terms of reducing lung injury, the role of HFOV in neonatal respiratory distress remains controversial.[25] [100]

ARDS

The magnitude of the clinical burden of VILI was shown by the recent ARDSnet trial in which 861 patients with ARDS were randomised to receive either a "traditional" tidal volume (12 ml/kg predicted body weight) or a low tidal volume strategy (6 ml/kg).[2] Mortality was 39.8% in the traditional group and 31% in the low volume group. In other words, *at least* 8.8% of the absolute mortality from ARDS is attributable to VILI. A considerable amount of attention is currently directed at the potential clinical benefits of improving and maintaining lung recruitment, based on the theories outlined above, using higher levels of PEEP or HFOV.

It is interesting to speculate on precisely *how* VILI increases mortality. The injury to the lung described in experimental models probably occurs in humans, to a greater or lesser degree. However, most deaths in ARDS are from MSOF rather than respiratory failure.[101] It is therefore likely that mechanical ventilation can influence the development of MSOF, possibly through the release of proinflammatory mediators, as described above. Two recent clinical studies add weight to this hypothesis. Ranieri and coworkers examined the effect of two ventilatory strategies on cytokine levels in ARDS. Forty four patients were randomised either to a "protective" strategy, in which the PEEP and tidal volume were set such that tidal ventilation occurred exclusively between the lower and upper inflection points of the pressure volume curve (see fig 8.1), or a "control" strategy in which the tidal volume was set to obtain normal values of arterial CO_2 and the PEEP set to produce the greatest improvement in arterial oxygen saturation without worsening haemodynamics. The protective group had significantly lower levels of plasma and bronchoalveolar lavage cytokines and significantly less organ failure.[92] [102] Along similar lines, the ARDSnet study found that plasma levels of IL-6 fell significantly more in patients ventilated with the lower than the traditional tidal volume.[2] It therefore seems likely that mechanical ventilation in ARDS can promote systemic inflammation and multiorgan failure. Crucially, however, it is not known which factor(s) are responsible for mediating this detrimental effect and how they exert a toxic effect on distal organs.

In addition to increasing mortality in ARDS, VILI may contribute to the persistent lung function abnormalities (principally a restrictive defect with abnormal transfer factor) seen in a minority of survivors.[103] However, no studies to date have shown that protective ventilatory strategies in ARDS are associated with improved long term lung function.[104]

CONCLUSION

Extensive research over the past 30 years has identified key determinants of VILI. From this, practice has been modified in an attempt to minimise lung damage. In the case of ARDS, ventilation with lower tidal volumes has been shown to reduce mortality.

One of the most exciting developments has been the realisation that VILI may be caused not only by the mechanical disruption of lung tissue, but also by the inappropriate activation of cellular pathways. Such mechanisms may contribute to non-pulmonary organ damage. Future treatments to minimise the impact of VILI may target these mechanisms at the molecular level, in addition to developing less injurious ventilation strategies.

ACKNOWLEDGEMENTS

TW is supported by the Scadding-Morriston-Davies Trust. AS is supported by the Canadian Institutes of Health Research (grant # 8558).

REFERENCES

1 **Fothergill J**. Observations on a case published in the last volume of the medical essays, &c of recovering a man dead in appearance, by distending the lungs with air. *Phil Trans R Soc Med* 1745;**43**:275–81.

2 **The Acute Respiratory Distress Syndrome Network**. Ventilation with lower tidal volumes as compared with traditional tidal volumes for acute lung injury and the acute respiratory distress syndrome. *N Engl J Med* 2000;**342**:1301–8.

3 **Macklin MT**, Macklin CC. Malignant interstitial emphysema of the lungs and mediastinum as an important occult complication in many respiratory diseases and other conditions: an interpretation of the clinical literature in the light of laboratory experiment. *Medicine* 1944;**23**:281–352.

4 **Petersen GW**, Baier H. Incidence of pulmonary barotrauma in a medical ICU. *Crit Care Med* 1983;**11**:67–9.

5 **Weg JG**, Anzueto A, Balk RA, *et al.* The relation of pneumothorax and other air leaks to mortality in the acute respiratory distress syndrome. *N Engl J Med* 1998;**338**:341–6.

6 **Stewart TE**, Meade MO, Cook DJ, *et al.* Evaluation of a ventilation strategy to prevent barotrauma in patients at high risk of acute respiratory distress syndrome. *N Engl J Med* 1998;**338**:355–61.

7 **Brochard L**, Roudot-Thoraval F, Roupie E, *et al.* Tidal volume reduction for prevention of ventilator-induced lung injury in acute respiratory distress syndrome. The Multicenter Trial Group on Tidal Volume reduction in ARDS. *Am J Respir Crit Care Med* 1998;**158**:1831–8.

8 **Downs JB**, Chapman RL Jr. Treatment of bronchopleural fistula during continuous positive pressure ventilation. *Chest* 1976;**69**:363–6.

9 **Webb HH**, Tierney DF. Experimental pulmonary edema due to intermittent positive pressure ventilation with high inflation pressures. Protection by positive end-expiratory pressure. *Am Rev Respir Dis* 1974;**110**:556–65.

10 **Dreyfuss D**, Soler P, Saumon G. Spontaneous resolution of pulmonary edema caused by short periods of cyclic overinflation. *J Appl Physiol* 1992;**72**:2081–9.

11 **John E**, Ermocilla R, Golden J, *et al.* Effects of intermittent positive-pressure ventilation on lungs of normal rabbits. *Br J Exp Pathol* 1980;**61**:315–23.

12 **Kolobow T**, Moretti MP, Fumagalli R, *et al.* Severe impairment in lung function induced by high peak airway pressure during mechanical ventilation. An experimental study. *Am Rev Respir Dis* 1987;**135**:312–5.

13 **Bouhuys A**. Physiology and musical instruments. *Nature* 1969;**221**:1199–204.

14 **Dreyfuss D**, Soler P, Basset G, *et al.* High inflation pressure pulmonary edema. Respective effects of high airway pressure, high tidal volume, and positive end-expiratory pressure. *Am J Respir Crit Care Med* 1988;**137**:1159–64.

15 **Hernandez LA**, Peevy KJ, Moise A, *et al.* Chest wall restriction limits high airway pressure-induced lung injury in young rabbits. *J Appl Physiol* 1989;**66**:2364–8.

16 **Carlton DP**, Cummings JJ, Scheerer RG. Lung overexpansion increases pulmonary microvascular protein permeability in young lambs. *J Appl Physiol* 1990;**69**:577–83.

17 **Slutsky AS**. Mechanical ventilation. American College of Chest Physicians' Consensus Conference. *Chest* 1993;**104**:1833–59.

18 **Ranieri VM**, Brienza N, Santostasi S, *et al.* Impairment of lung and chest wall mechanics in patients with acute respiratory distress syndrome: role of abdominal distension. *Am J Respir Crit Care Med* 1997;**156**:1082–91.

19 **Argiras EP**, Blakeley CR, Dunnill MS, *et al.* High PEEP decreases hyaline membrane formation in surfactant deficient lungs. *Br J Anaesth* 1987;**59**:1278–85.

20 **Sandhar BK**, Niblett DJ, Argiras EP, *et al.* Effects of positive end-expiratory pressure on hyaline membrane formation in a rabbit model of the neonatal respiratory distress syndrome. *Intensive Care Med* 1988;**14**:538–46.

21 **Muscedere JG**, Mullen JB, Gan K, *et al*. Tidal ventilation at low airway pressures can augment lung injury. *Am J Respir Crit Care Med* 1994;**149**:1327–34.

22 **Matamis D**, Lemaire F, Harf A, *et al*. Total respiratory pressure-volume curves in the adult respiratory distress syndrome. *Chest* 1984;**86**:58–66.

23 **Amato MB**, Barbas CS, Medeiros DM, *et al*. Beneficial effects of the "open lung approach" with low distending pressures in acute respiratory distress syndrome. A prospective randomized study on mechanical ventilation. *Am J Respir Crit Care Med* 1995;**152**:1835–46.

24 **McCulloch PR**, Forkert PG, Froese AB. Lung volume maintenance prevents lung injury during high frequency oscillatory ventilation in surfactant-deficient rabbits. *Am Rev Respir Dis* 1988;**137**:1185–92.

25 **Riphagen S**, Bohn D. High frequency oscillatory ventilation. *Intensive Care Med* 1999;**25**:1459–62.

26 **Radford PR**. Static mechanical properties of mammalian lungs. In: Fenn WO, Rahn H, eds. *Handbook of physiology*. Washington DC: American Physiological Society, 1964: 429–49.

27 **Hickling KG**. The pressure-volume curve is greatly modified by recruitment. A mathematical model of ARDS lungs. *Am J Respir Crit Care Med* 1998;**158**:194–202.

28 **Martynowicz MA**, Minor TA, Walters BJ, *et al*. Regional expansion of oleic acid-injured lungs. *Am J Respir Crit Care Med* 1999;**160**:250–8.

29 **Rimensberger PC**, Cox PN, Frndova H, *et al*. The open lung during small tidal volume ventilation: concepts of recruitment and "optimal" positive end-expiratory pressure. *Crit Care Med* 1999;**27**:1946–52.

30 **Gattinoni L**, D'Andrea L, Pelosi P, *et al*. Regional effects and mechanism of positive end-expiratory pressure in early adult respiratory distress syndrome. *JAMA* 1993;**269**:2122–7.

31 **Dreyfuss D**, Saumon G. Pressure-volume curves. Searching for the grail or laying patients with adult respiratory distress syndrome on Procrustes' bed? *Am J Respir Crit Care Med* 2001;**163**:2–3.

32 **Hotchkiss JR**, Blanch L, Murias G, *et al*. Effects of decreased respiratory frequency on ventilator-induced lung injury. *Am J Respir Crit Care Med* 2000;**161**:463–8.

33 **Chabot F**, Mitchell JA, Gutteridge JM, *et al*. Reactive oxygen species in acute lung injury. *Eur Respir J* 1998;**11**:745–57.

34 **Davis WB**, Rennard SI, Bitterman PB, *et al*. Pulmonary oxygen toxicity. Early reversible changes in human alveolar structures induced by hyperoxia. *N Engl J Med* 1983;**309**:878–83.

35 **Hickling KG**, Henderson SJ, Jackson R. Low mortality associated with low volume pressure limited ventilation with permissive hypercapnia in severe adult respiratory distress syndrome. *Intensive Care Med* 1990;**16**:372–7.

36 **Laffey JG**, Kavanagh BP. Biological effects of hypercapnia. *Intensive Care Med* 2000;**26**:133–8.

37 **Nash G**, Bowen JA, Langlinais PC. "Respirator lung": a misnomer. *Arch Pathol* 1971;**91**:234–40.

38 **Bowton DL**, Kong DL. High tidal volume ventilation produces increased lung water in oleic acid-injured rabbit lungs. *Crit Care Med* 1989;**17**:908–11.

39 **Hernandez LA**, Coker PJ, May S, *et al*. Mechanical ventilation increases microvascular permeability in oleic acid-injured lungs. *J Appl Physiol* 1990;**69**:2057–61.

40 **Dreyfuss D**, Soler P, Saumon G Mechanical ventilation-induced pulmonary edema. Interaction with previous lung alterations. *Am J Respir Crit Care Med* 1995;**151**:1568–75.

41 **Gattinoni L**, Pesenti A, Avalli L, *et al*. Pressure-volume curve of total respiratory system in acute respiratory failure. Computed tomographic scan study. *Am Rev Respir Dis* 1987;**136**:730–6.

42 **Goldstein I**, Bughalo MT, Marquette CH, *et al*. Mechanical ventilation-induced air-space enlargement during experimental pneumonia in piglets. *Am J Respir Crit Care Med* 2001;**163**:958–64.

43 **Rouby JJ**, Lherm T, Martin de Lassale E, *et al*. Histologic aspects of pulmonary barotrauma in critically ill patients with acute respiratory failure. *Intensive Care Med* 1993;**19**:383–9.

44 **Desai SR**, Wells AU, Rubens MB, *et al*. Acute respiratory distress syndrome: CT abnormalities at long-term follow-up. *Radiology* 1999;**210**:29–35.

45 **Jobe AH**, Ikegami M. Lung development and function in preterm infants in the surfactant treatment era. *Ann Rev Physiol* 2000;**62**:825–46.

46 **Bjorklund LL**, Ingimarsson J, Curstedt T, *et al*. Manual ventilation with a few large breaths at birth compromises the therapeutic effect of subsequent surfactant replacement in immature lambs. *Pediatr Res* 1997;**42**:348–55.

47 **Dreyfuss D**, Saumon G. Ventilator-induced lung injury: lessons from experimental studies. *Am J Respir Crit Care Med* 1998;**157**:294–323.

48 **Egan EA**. Lung inflation, lung solute permeability, and alveolar edema. *J Appl Physiol* 1982;**53**:121–5.

49 **Kim K J**, Crandall ED. Effects of lung inflation on alveolar epithelial solute and water transport properties. *J Appl Physiol* 1982;**52**:1498–505.

50 **Dreyfuss D**, Basset G, Soler P, *et al*. Intermittent positive-pressure hyperventilation with high inflation pressures produces pulmonary microvascular injury in rats. *Am Rev Respir Dis* 1985;**132**:880–4.

51 **Parker JC**, Townsley MI, Rippe B, *et al*. Increased microvascular permeability in dog lungs due to high airway pressures. *J Appl Physiol* 1984;**57**:1809–16.

52 **Albert RK**, Lakshminarayan S, Kirk W, *et al*. Lung inflation can cause pulmonary edema in zone I of in situ dog lungs. *J Appl Physiol* 1980;**49**:815–9.

53 **Tsuno K**, Miura K, Takeya M, *et al*. Histopathologic pulmonary changes from mechanical ventilation at high peak airway pressures. *Am Rev Respir Dis* 1991;**143**:1115–20.

54 **Hamilton PP**, Onayemi A, Smyth JA, *et al*. Comparison of conventional and high-frequency ventilation: oxygenation and lung pathology. *J Appl Physiol* 1983;**55**:131–8.

55 **Kawano T**, Mori S, Cybulsky M, *et al*. Effect of granulocyte depletion in a ventilated surfactant-depleted lung. *J Appl Physiol* 1987;**62**:27–33.

56 **Mathieu-Costello OA**, West JB. Are pulmonary capillaries susceptible to mechanical stress? *Chest* 1994;**105**:102–7S.

57 **West JB**, Tsukimoto K, Mathieu-Costello O, *et al*. Stress failure in pulmonary capillaries. *J Appl Physiol* 1991;**70**:1731–42.

58 **Tsukimoto K**, Mathieu-Costello O, Prediletto R, *et al*. Ultrastructural appearances of pulmonary capillaries at high transmural pressures. *J Appl Physiol* 1991;**71**:573–82.

59 **Fu Z**, Costello ML, Tsukimoto K, *et al*. High lung volume increases stress failure in pulmonary capillaries. *J Appl Physiol* 1992;**73**:123–33.

60 **Broccard AF**, Hotchkiss JR, Kuwayama N, *et al*. Consequences of vascular flow on lung injury induced by mechanical ventilation. *Am J Respir Crit Care Med* 1998;**157**:1935–42.

61 **Mead J**, Takishima T, Leith D. Stress distribution in lungs: a model of pulmonary elasticity. *J Appl Physiol* 1970;**28**:596–608.

62 **Amato MBP Marini JJ**. Barotrauma, volutrauma, and ventilation of acute lung injury. In: Marini JJ Slutsky AS, eds. *Physiological basis of ventilatory support*. New York: Marcel Dekker, 1998: 1187–245.

63 **Kamm RD**, Schroter RC. Is airway closure caused by a liquid film instability? *Respir Physiol* 1989;**75**:141–56.

64 **Macklem PT**, Proctor DF, Hogg JC. The stability of peripheral airways. *Respir Physiol* 1970;**8**:191–203.

65 **Naureckas ET**, Dawson CA, Gerber BS, *et al*. Airway reopening pressure in isolated rat lungs. *J Appl Physiol* 1994;**76**:1372–7.

66 **Gaver DP**, Samsel RW, Solway J. Effects of surface tension and viscosity on airway reopening. *J Appl Physiol* 1990;**69**:74–85.

67 **Taskar V**, John J, Evander E, *et al*. Healthy lungs tolerate repetitive collapse and reopening during short periods of mechanical ventilation. *Acta Anaesthesiol Scand* 1995;**39**:370–6.

68 **Lewis JF**, Jobe AH. Surfactant and the adult respiratory distress syndrome. *Am Rev Respir Dis* 1993;**147**:218–33.

69 **Vanderzwan J**, McCaig L, Mehta S, *et al*. Characterizing alterations in the pulmonary surfactant system in a rat model of Pseudomonas aeruginosa pneumonia. *Eur Respir J* 1998;**12**:1388–96.

70 **Chander A**, Fisher AB. Regulation of lung surfactant secretion. *Am J Physiol* 1990;**258**:L241–53.

71 **Malloy J**, McCaig L, Veldhuizen R, *et al*. Alterations of the endogenous surfactant system in septic adult rats. *Am J Respir Crit Care Med* 1997;**156**:617–23.

72 **Coker PJ**, Hernandez LA, Peevy KJ, *et al*. Increased sensitivity to mechanical ventilation after surfactant inactivation in young rabbit lungs. *Crit Care Med* 1992;**20**:635–40.

73 **Imai Y**, Kawano T, Miyasaka K, *et al*. Inflammatory chemical mediators during conventional ventilation and during high frequency oscillatory ventilation. *Am J Respir Crit Care Med* 1994;**150**:1550–4.

74 **Taskar V**, Wollmer P, Evander E, *et al*. Effect of detergent combined with large tidal volume ventilation on alveolocapillary permeability. *Clin Physiol* 1996;**16**:103–14.

75 **Taskar V**, John J, Evander E, *et al*. Surfactant dysfunction makes lungs vulnerable to repetitive collapse and reexpansion. *Am J Respir Crit Care Med* 1997;**155**:313–20.

76 **Albert RK**, Lakshminarayan S, Hildebrandt J, *et al*. Increased surface tension favors pulmonary edema formation in anesthetized dogs' lungs. *J Clin Invest* 1979;**63**:1015–8.

77 **Wright JR**. Immunomodulatory functions of surfactant. *Physiol Rev* 1997;**77**:931–62.

78 **Jobe AH**. Pulmonary surfactant therapy. *N Engl J Med* 1993;**328**:861–8.

79 **Anzueto A**, Baughman RP, Guntupalli KK, *et al*. Aerosolized surfactant in adults with sepsis-induced acute respiratory distress syndrome. Exosurf Acute Respiratory Distress Syndrome Sepsis Study Group. *N Engl J Med* 1996;**334**:1417–21.

80 **Liu M**, Tanswell AK, Post M. Mechanical force-induced signal transduction in lung cells. *Am J Physiol* 1999;**277**:L667–83.

81 **Dos Santos CC**, Slutsky AS. Invited review: mechanisms of ventilator-induced lung injury: a perspective. *J Appl Physiol* 2000;**89**:1645–55.

82 **Parker JC**, Ivey CL, Tucker JA. Gadolinium prevents high airway pressure-induced permeability increases in isolated rat lungs. *J Appl Physiol* 1998;**84**:1113–8.

83 **Imai Y**, Kawano T, Miyasaka K, *et al*. Inflammatory chemical mediators during conventional ventilation and during high frequency oscillatory ventilation. *Am J Respir Crit Care Med* 1994;**150**:1550–4.

84 **Tremblay L**, Valenza F, Ribeiro SP, *et al*. Injurious ventilatory strategies increase cytokines and c-fos m-RNA expression in an isolated rat lung model. *J Clin Invest* 1997;**99**:944–52.

85 **von Bethmann AN**, Brasch F, Nusing R, *et al*. Hyperventilation induces release of cytokines from perfused mouse lung. *Am J Respir Crit Care Med* 1998;**157**:263–72.

86 **Chiumello D**, Pristine G, Slutsky AS. Mechanical ventilation affects local and systemic cytokines in an animal model of acute respiratory distress syndrome. *Am J Respir Crit Care Med* 1999;**160**:109–16.

87 **Held H**, Boettcher S, Hamann L, *et al*. Ventilation-induced chemokine and cytokine release is associated with activation of NFκB and is blocked by steroids. *Am J Respir Crit Care Med* 2001;**163**:711–6.

88 **Plotz FB**, van Vught H, Heijnen CJ. Ventilator-induced lung inflammation: is it always harmful? *Intensive Care Med* 1999;**25**:236.

89 **Imai Y**, Kawano T, Iwamoto S, *et al*. Intratracheal anti-tumor necrosis factor-alpha antibody attenuates ventilator-induced lung injury in rabbits. *J Appl Physiol* 1999;**87**:510–5.

90 **Narimanbekov IO**, Rozycki HJ. Effect of IL-1 blockade on inflammatory manifestations of acute ventilator-induced lung injury in a rabbit model. *Exp Lung Res* 1995;**21**:239–54.

91 **Haitsma JJ**, Uhlig S, Goggel R, *et al.* Ventilator-induced lung injury leads to loss of alveolar and systemic compartmentalization of tumor necrosis factor-alpha. *Intensive Care Med* 2000;**26**:1515–22.

92 **Ranieri V**, Suter P, Tortorella C, *et al.* Effect of mechanical ventilation on inflammatory mediators in patients with acute respiratory distress syndrome: a randomized controlled trial. *JAMA* 1999;**282**:54–61.

93 **Slutsky AS**, Tremblay LN. Multiple system organ failure. Is mechanical ventilation a contributing factor? *Am J Respir Crit Care Med* 1998;**157**:1721–5.

94 **Nahum A**, Hoyt J, Schmitz L, *et al.* Effect of mechanical ventilation strategy on dissemination of intratracheally instilled Escherichia coli in dogs. *Crit Care Med* 1997;**25**:1733–43.

95 **Verbrugge SJ**, Sorm V, van't Veen A, *et al.* Lung overinflation without positive end-expiratory pressure promotes bacteremia after experimental Klebsiella pneumoniae inoculation. *Intensive Care Med* 1998;**24**:172–7.

96 **Murphy DB**, Cregg N, Tremblay L, *et al.* Adverse ventilatory strategy causes pulmonary-to-systemic translocation of endotoxin. *Am J Respir Crit Care Med* 2000;**162**:27–33.

97 **Northway WH Jr**. Bronchopulmonary dysplasia: twenty-five years later. *Pediatrics* 1992;**89**:969–73.

98 **Poets CF**, Sens B. Changes in intubation rates and outcome of very low birth weight infants: a population-based study. *Pediatrics* 1996;**98**:24–7.

99 **Van Marter LJ**, Allred EN, Pagano M, *et al.* Do clinical markers of barotrauma and oxygen toxicity explain interhospital variation in rates of chronic lung disease? The Neonatology Committee for the Developmental Network. *Pediatrics* 2000;**105**:1194–201.

100 **Thome U**, Kossel H, Lipowsky G, *et al.* Randomized comparison of high-frequency ventilation with high-rate intermittent positive pressure ventilation in preterm infants with respiratory failure. *J Pediatr* 1999;**135**:39–46.

101 **Ferring M**, Vincent JL. Is outcome from ARDS related to the severity of respiratory failure? *Eur Respir J* 1997;**10**:1297–300.

102 **Ranieri VM**, Giunta F, Suter PM, *et al.* Mechanical ventilation as a mediator of multisystem organ failure in acute respiratory distress syndrome. *JAMA* 2000;**284**:43–4.

103 **Hudson LD**, Steinberg KP. Epidemiology of acute lung injury and ARDS. *Chest* 1999;**116**:74 82S.

104 **Cooper AB**, Ferguson ND, Hanly PJ, *et al.* Long-term follow-up of survivors of acute lung injury: lack of effect of a ventilation strategy to prevent barotrauma. *Crit Care Med* 1999;**27**:2616–21.

9 Ventilatory management of acute lung injury/acute respiratory distress syndrome

J J Cordingley, B F Keogh

The ventilatory management of patients with acute lung injury (ALI) and acute respiratory distress syndrome (ARDS) has evolved in conjunction with advances in understanding of the underlying pathophysiology. In particular, evidence that mechanical ventilation has an influence on lung injury and patient outcome has emerged over the past three decades.[1] The present understanding of optimal ventilatory management is outlined and other methods of respiratory support are reviewed.

PATHOPHYSIOLOGY

The pathophysiology of ARDS is reviewed by Bellingan in chapter 6. However, it is useful to highlight important features relevant to ventilatory management, in particular the anatomical distribution of pulmonary pathology and the potential for ventilator induced lung injury.

The original description of ARDS included the presence of bilateral infiltrates on the chest radiograph.[2] Computerised tomographic (CT) scanning has shown that parenchymal consolidation, far from being evenly distributed, is concentrated in dependent lung regions leaving non-dependent lung relatively spared. This pathological distribution of aerated lung lying over areas of dense consolidation has led to comparisons with ventilation of a much smaller or "baby lung"[3] and has important implications for ventilatory management. Thus, the application of normal physiological tidal volumes can lead to overdistension of the small volume of normally aerated lung, while failing to recruit consolidated dependent regions.

Ventilator induced lung injury can occur by several mechanisms: oxygen toxicity from the use of high Fio_2,[4] (see chapter 8) overdistension of the lung causing local damage and further inflammation,[5] injurious cyclical opening and closing of alveoli from ventilation at low lung volumes,[6] and by increasing systemic levels of inflammatory cytokines.[7]

Ventilatory strategies must therefore be tailored to minimise the risk of inducing or exacerbating lung injury.

RESPIRATORY MECHANICS

Decreased lung compliance is a prominent feature of ARDS. The static compliance of the respiratory system (lung + chest wall) in a ventilated patient is calculated by dividing the tidal volume (Vt) by end inspiratory plateau pressure (Pplat) minus end expiratory pressure + intrinsic PEEP (PEEPi). As the pathology of ARDS is heterogeneous, calculating static compliance does not provide information about regional variations in lung recruitment and varies according to lung volume. Much attention has therefore focused on analysis of the pressure-volume (PV) curve.

The static PV curve of the respiratory system can be obtained by inserting a pause during an inflation-deflation cycle. A number of different methods have been described including the use of a large syringe (super-syringe), or holding a mechanical ventilator at end inspiration of varying tidal volumes. The principles and methods of PV curve measurement have recently been reviewed.[8]

The PV curves thus obtained are sigmoidal and have an inspiratory limb that usually includes a point above which the curve becomes steeper (fig 9.1).[3] Identification of the lower inflection point by clinicians using PV curves is subject to large variability, but is improved by curve fitting.[9] In some patients the lower inflection point may be absent. At higher lung volumes the curve becomes flatter again (upper inflection point), above which further increases in pressure cause little increase in volume. Currently, ventilators used routinely in intensive care units do not have automated functions to obtain a static PV curve. Moreover, the static PV curve only provides information about accessible lung[3] and also includes chest wall compliance. Separating the lung and chest wall components requires the use of oesophageal pressure measurement.[10]

Despite these limitations, many advances in clinical management in patients with ALI/ARDS have been based on consideration of static PV curves. It has recently been suggested that use of the lower and upper inflection points of the static PV curve as indicators of recruitment and overdistension in order to adjust ventilator settings in patients with ARDS is unreliable.[11] It is argued that alveolar recruitment occurs beyond the lower inflection point and that further information, including the deflation PV curve, is required to determine optimal ventilator settings for an individual patient. Analysis of the inspiratory pressure-time curve under conditions of constant flow may also provide useful information about lung recruitment.[12]

VENTILATORY STRATEGIES IN ARDS

The goals of ventilating patients with ALI/ARDS are to maintain adequate gas exchange and avoid ventilator induced lung injury.

Maintenance of adequate gas exchange
Oxygen
High concentrations of inspired oxygen should be avoided to limit the risk of oxygen toxicity and to avoid reabsorption atelectasis. Arterial oxygen saturation (Sao_2) is used as a target in preference to arterial oxygen tension (Pao_2) because oxygen delivery determines tissue oxygenation. Sao_2 values of around 90% are commonly accepted but oxygen delivery decreases quickly below 88%

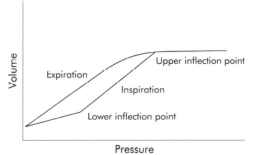

Figure 9.1 Schematic representation of a static pressure-volume curve of the respiratory system from a patient with ARDS. Note the lower and upper inflection points of the inspiratory limb.

because of the shape of the oxyhaemoglobin dissociation curve. However, if a higher Sao_2 can only be obtained by increasing airway pressure to levels that result in haemodynamic compromise, then a lower Sao_2 may have to be accepted.

There is no clinical evidence to support the use of specific Fio_2 thresholds, but it is common clinical practice to decrease Fio_2 below 0.6 as quickly as possible.

Oxygenation can be improved by increased alveolar recruitment through the application of higher airway pressure provided that ventilation-perfusion (V/Q) matching is not adversely affected by the haemodynamic consequences of increased intrathoracic pressure. Lung recruitment is usually obtained by applying extrinsic PEEP, increasing the inspiratory:expiratory (I:E) ratio, or by specific recruitment manoeuvres (discussed below).

Carbon dioxide

Limiting tidal volume and peak pressure to reduce ventilator induced lung injury may cause hypercapnia. Strategies used to manage hypercapnia have included increasing tidal volume and airway pressure, or increasing CO_2 removal with techniques such as tracheal gas insufflation or extracorporeal CO_2 removal. In 1990 it was reported that the alternative of simply allowing CO_2 to rise to a higher level (permissive hypercapnia) and maintaining limits on tidal volume and airway pressure was associated with a significantly lower than predicted mortality from ARDS.[13]

The physiological consequences of hypercapnia are respiratory acidosis, increased cardiac output, and pulmonary hypertension. Neurological changes include increased cerebral blood flow, and cerebral oedema and intracranial haemorrhage have been reported.[14] With severe acidosis there may be myocardial depression, arrhythmias, and decreased response to exogenous inotropes. Renal compensation for the respiratory acidosis occurs slowly.

Unfortunately there are no data to confirm the degree of respiratory acidosis that is safe. Recent studies have allowed hypercapnia as part of lung protective ventilatory protocols.[1 15–18] Arterial pH was lower in the lung protective groups and the ARDSNet study included the use of sodium bicarbonate to correct arterial pH to normal.[1] At present no recommendations can be made concerning the management of respiratory acidosis induced by permissive hypercapnia. However, if bicarbonate is infused, it should be administered slowly to allow CO_2 excretion and avoid worsening of intracellular acidosis.

One method used to increase CO_2 clearance is insufflation of gas into the trachea to flush out dead space CO_2 and reduce rebreathing.[19] Tracheal gas insufflation has been used both continuously and during expiration only. As no commercially available ventilator includes this technique, modifications are required to the ventilator circuit and settings to prevent inadvertent and potentially dangerous increases in intrinsic PEEP, Vt, and peak airway pressure.

In adult patients with ARDS, managed using pressure control ventilation, the introduction of continuous tracheal gas insufflation allowed a decrease in inspiratory pressure of 5 cm H_2O without increasing arterial carbon dioxide tension ($Paco_2$).[20] Tracheal gas insufflation may therefore be useful when permissive hypercapnia is contraindicated. However, managing the appropriate ventilator settings and adjustment is complicated, with real potential for iatrogenic injury.

In practice, $Paco_2$ is allowed to rise during lung protective volume and pressure limited ventilation. $Paco_2$ levels of 2–3 times normal seem to be well tolerated for prolonged periods. Renal compensation for respiratory acidosis occurs over several days. Many clinicians infuse sodium bicarbonate slowly if arterial pH falls below 7.20.

Avoidance of ventilator induced lung injury

Traditional mechanical ventilation (as applied during routine general anaesthesia) involves tidal volumes that are relatively large (10–15 ml/kg) in order to reduce atelectasis. PEEP levels are adjusted to maintain oxygenation but high levels are generally avoided to prevent cardiovascular instability related to increased intrathoracic pressure. Present understanding of ventilator induced lung injury suggests that traditional mechanical ventilation, using high tidal volumes and low PEEP, is likely to enhance lung injury in patients with ARDS. Five randomised studies of "lung protective" ventilation in ARDS have recently been published, four of which investigated limitation of tidal volume to prevent injury from over-distension (table 9.1).

In these studies the protective ventilatory strategy was directed at preventing lung overdistension and was not designed to look at differences in ventilation at low lung volumes. Only the largest study (ARDSNet)[1] showed an advantage of such a protective strategy. The ARDSNet study had the largest difference in Vt and Pplat between the groups, the highest power, and was the only study to correct respiratory acidosis (table 9.2).

Other studies have addressed the issue of adjustment of ventilatory support based on PV curve characteristics. Amato et al[18] randomised 53 patients with early ARDS to either traditional ventilation (volume cycled, Vt 12 ml/kg, minimum PEEP guided by Fio_2, normal $Paco_2$) or a lung protective strategy (PEEP adjusted to above the lower inflection point of a static PV curve, Vt <6 ml/kg, permissive hypercapnia, and pressure limited ventilatory mode with PIP limited to <40 cm H_2O). Patients in the lung protective group had improved indices of oxygenation, compliance, and weaning rates. Mortality in the traditional ventilation group was worse at 28 days (71% v 45%, p<0.001) and hospital discharge (71% v 45%, p=0.37). By using the static PV curve to adjust PEEP in the protective ventilation group, this study also addressed the issue of ventilator induced damage by cyclical opening and closure of alveoli. The hospital mortality was very high in the traditional ventilation group, making this study difficult to interpret. Further clinical investigation into the role of higher levels of PEEP in combination with recruitment manoeuvres has been undertaken by the ARDSNet group. Patients with ALI or ARDS were randomised to a high PEEP/low Fio_2 or low PEEP/high Fio_2 strategy. The study (ALVEOLI) was stopped after 550 patients were enrolled because an interim analysis demonstrated lack of efficacy.

Considerable controversy over clinical trials of low tidal volume for ventilation in ARDS has arisen following the publication of a meta-analysis suggesting that differences in patient survival in the five studies included could be explained by variations in the conventional ventilation protocols.[21] These criticisms were rejected by the ARDS Network.[22]

Pressure and volume limited ventilation

Invasive ventilation of adult patients has traditionally been provided by delivering a set tidal volume at a set rate and

Table 9.1 Randomised prospective studies of ventilatory strategies to limit lung overdistension in patients with ARDS

Reference	n	"Protective"	Control	Mortality
Stewart (1998)[15]	120	• Vt <8 ml/kg • PIP <30 cm H_2O • PEEP levels similar in both groups	• Vt 10–15 ml/kg • PIP <50 cm H_2O	No difference
Brochard (1998)[16]	116	• Vt <10 ml/kg • Pplat <25 cm H_2O • PEEP levels similar in both groups	• Vt 10 ml/kg • Normocapnia	No difference
Brower (1999)[17]	52	• Vt 5–8 ml/kg • Pplat <30 cm H_2O	• Vt 10–12 ml/kg • Pplat <45–55 cm H_2O	No difference
ARDSNet (2000)[1]	861	• Vt 6 ml/kg • PIP <30 cm H_2O	• Vt 12 ml/kg • PIP <50 cm H_2O	Lower in "protective" group (31% v 40%)

Vt=tidal volume; PIP=peak inspiratory pressure; Pplat=end inspiratory plateau pressure; PEEP=positive end expiratory pressure.

Table 9.2 Protective lung ventilation protocol from the ARDSNet study[1]

Variable	Setting
Ventilator mode	Volume assist-control
Tidal volume (initial) (ml/kg)	6 (adjusted according to plateau pressure)
Plateau pressure (cm H_2O)	<30
Rate (breaths/min)	6–35
I:E ratio	1:1–1:3
Oxygenation target	
Pao_2 (kPa)	7.3–10.7
Spo_2 (%)	88–95
PEEP and Fio_2	Set according to predetermined combinations (PEEP range 5–24 cm H_2O)

inspiratory flow. This technique has the advantage of maintaining a constant minute volume and $Paco_2$ under conditions of changing respiratory system compliance providing that preset limits of airway pressure are not reached. Another strategy that has been used increasingly over the last 10 years is to use pressure controlled ventilation in which a decelerating inspiratory flow profile is applied to a set pressure limit. Changes in compliance during pressure control ventilation will result in variable minute volume and $Paco_2$, but this mode has the advantage of limiting pressure to a set level. More sophisticated mechanical ventilators have allowed adjustment of more parameters in each mode and have made the distinction between these two types of ventilation blurred. Studies of volume versus pressure controlled ventilation in ARDS have been reported but have been too small to detect any important outcome differences.[23–25] The largest study of ventilation in ARDS reported an outcome difference between two protocols using volume controlled ventilation, suggesting that settings rather than the mode is the important issue.[1]

Whatever mode of ventilation is used, it is now clear that tidal volume should be set in the region of 6 ml/kg rather than the traditional 10–12 ml/kg and the peak pressure should be limited to 30–35 cm H_2O to prevent lung overdistension—that is, inspiration should be terminated before the upper inflection point on the PV curve.

PEEP

The application of PEEP improves oxygenation by providing movement of fluid from the alveolar to the interstitial space, recruitment of small airways and collapsed alveoli, and an increase in functional residual capacity (FRC). In addition, cyclical collapse and low volume lung injury is attenuated. Increased Pao_2 induced by PEEP was found to be correlated with the volume of lung recruited.[26]

In theory, setting PEEP above the lower inflection point may prevent derecruitment and low lung volume ventilator associated injury. As discussed above, adjusting the level of PEEP to 2 cm H_2O above the lower inflection point was part of a lung ventilatory strategy that was advantageous.[18] In a crossover study of 15 patients mechanically ventilated because of ALI, lung volume recruitment and Pao_2 were increased with the combination of lower Vt (6 ml/kg) and increased PEEP at constant Pplat.[27]

It has been suggested that the effect of PEEP on recruitment in ARDS varies according to the regional distribution of consolidation. Hence, PEEP had little effect on lobar consolidation but induced the greatest reduction in non-aerated lung in patients with diffuse CT abnormalities.[28] Current clinical practice in the absence of static PV curve measurement is to set PEEP at a relatively high level such as 15 cm H_2O in patients with ARDS.

Inspiratory time

Prolongation of the inspiratory time with an increased I:E ratio is commonly used as a method of recruitment. Mean airway pressure is increased. Shortening of expiratory time can cause hyperinflation and increase intrinsic PEEP (PEEPi). Providing that ventilation is pressure limited, PEEPi can be manipulated to increase recruitment further. In volume control modes of ventilation without pressure limitation, PEEPi levels can cause overdistension and haemodynamic compromise. No clinical outcome studies have specifically addressed inspiratory time or levels of PEEPi. It is common practice during pressure control ventilation to increase the I:E ratio to 1:1 or 2:1 (inverse ratio ventilation) with close monitoring of PEEPi and haemodynamics.

Recruitment manoeuvres

There has been renewed interest recently in manoeuvres aimed at increasing alveolar recruitment following the recognition that higher levels of PEEP are necessary to sustain any benefit obtained by such manoeuvres, and that any sudden reduction such as ventilator disconnection for suctioning leads to derecruitment.

The sigh function involves the delivery of intermittent breaths of larger tidal volume, administered either via the mechanical ventilators or by hand. Sighs delivered to patients with ARDS increase alveolar recruitment but the benefit is short lived, lasting less than 30 minutes.[29] The same authors also suggest that secondary ARDS (ARDS as a result of non-pulmonary disease) is more responsive to sighs than primary ARDS.

Sustained inflation or continuous positive airway pressure (CPAP) is another form of recruitment manoeuvre. Several investigators have reported the effects of different manoeuvres in patients with ARDS (table 9.3).

Table 9.3 Reported lung recruitment manoeuvres

Reference	n	Pressure (cm H₂O)	Time (s)	Effective	Duration
Amato (1998)[18]	29	35–40	40	–	–
Lapinsky (1999)[53]	14	30–45	20	Yes	4 hours
Medoff (2000)[54]	1	40+20 PS	120	Yes	–

PS=pressure support.

Recruitment manoeuvres may be more effective in patients ventilated with relatively low levels of PEEP. Conversely, they may be less effective and cause lung overdistension in patients with already optimally recruited lungs—that is, with higher levels of PEEP. Recruitment manoeuvres all involve increasing intrathoracic pressure and therefore the risk of barotrauma and cardiovascular instability. At present there are no published data from randomised studies to indicate whether recruitment manoeuvres, of whatever form, influence outcome.

Spontaneous breathing during positive pressure ventilation (BiPAP, APRV)

Two modes of ventilation commonly available on mechanical ventilators—biphasic airway pressure (BiPAP) and airway pressure release ventilation (APRV)—allow spontaneous breathing to occur at any stage of the respiratory cycle. In these modes the ventilator cycles between an upper and lower pressure at preset time intervals. Spontaneous breathing during mechanical ventilation decreases intrathoracic pressure and improves V/Q matching and cardiac output.[30] These theoretical benefits have resulted in more widespread use of the BiPAP mode, which provides a range of I:E ratios (APRV applies a very short expiratory time), but again no data exist concerning any influence on outcome.

PRONE VENTILATION

Prone position was reported to improve oxygenation in patients with ARDS as long ago as 1976.[31] The mechanism of the improvement in oxygenation on turning prone, seen in about two thirds of patients with ARDS, is complex. The intuitive explanation that regional lung perfusion is primarily dependent on gravity leading to improved perfusion of non-consolidated lung on turning is not substantiated by research. In fact, perfusion to dorsal lung regions predominates whatever the patient's position,[32] and gravity accounts for less than half the perfusion heterogeneity seen in either the supine or prone position.[33] Changes in regional pleural pressure are more important. The gradient of pleural pressure from negative ventrally to positive dorsally in the supine position is not completely reversed on turning prone, so that the distribution of positive pressure ventilation is more homogenous in the prone position.[34] Thus, recruitment of dorsal lung appears to be the predominant mechanism of improved oxygenation.

Potential problems associated with prone positioning are pressure-induced skin damage, increased venous pressure in the head (facial oedema), eye damage (corneal abrasions, retinal and optic nerve ischaemia), dislodgment of endotracheal tubes and intravascular catheters, and increased intra-abdominal pressure.

A multicentre prospective randomised study of the prone position for adult patients with acute respiratory failure was undertaken in Italy.[35] Patients randomised to prone positioning were assessed daily for the first 10 days and turned prone for at least 6 hours if severity criteria were met. There were no differences in clinical outcome.

Prone positioning is a useful adjunct to ventilation and may help to improve oxygenation and pulmonary mechanics but, as yet, has not been shown to alter outcome in ARDS.

HIGH FREQUENCY VENTILATION

There has been a resurgence of interest in high frequency ventilation (HFV, rate >60/min) over the last few years. Initial enthusiasm had been tempered by practical difficulties and the lack of clinical outcome data showing any advantage over conventional mechanical ventilation. The recent clinical studies of conventional ventilation demonstrating the advantages of limited Vt and maintenance of lung volume have helped to promote interest in HFV. The very low Vt (1–5 ml/kg) provided by HFV offers the possibility of maintaining lung volume at a higher point on the PV curve with less risk of causing overdistension.[36] High frequency jet ventilation (HFJV) and high frequency oscillatory ventilation (HFOV) have been the two most commonly used methods.

High frequency jet ventilation (HFJV)

HFJV uses a high pressure gas jet delivered into an endotracheal tube at high frequency (1–10 Hz). Other gas in the ventilator circuit is entrained producing a Vt of 2–5 ml/kg that can be adjusted by altering the inspiratory time and/or driving pressure. During HFJV, expiration occurs passively. Practical problems encountered are inadequate humidification, potential for gas trapping, difficulty in adjusting ventilator settings, and the need for a specialised endotracheal tube.

HFJV has been investigated in two large prospective randomised studies. In a study of 309 patients being ventilated for different causes of respiratory failure, the use of HFJV resulted in no significant outcome differences.[37] Similarly, a study of 113 patients at risk of ARDS had similar clinical outcomes in both patients ventilated conventionally and in those in whom HFJV was used.[38] These studies did not include recruitment manoeuvres that are now recognised to be important[39] and were underpowered with respect to clinical outcomes such as mortality.[40]

High frequency oscillatory ventilation (HFOV)

HFOV differs from HFV in a number of important aspects. Tidal volume (1–3 ml/kg) is generated by the excursion of an oscillator within a ventilator circuit similar to that used for CPAP and is varied by altering the frequency, I:E ratio, and oscillator amplitude. The use of an oscillator to generate Vt results in active expiration. Mean airway pressure is adjusted by altering the fresh gas flow (bias flow) into the circuit or the expiratory pressure valve. Oxygenation is controlled by altering mean airway pressure or Fio₂.

On initiation of HFOV, lung recruitment is achieved by increasing mean airway pressure and monitoring arterial oxygenation. Once optimal recruitment has occurred, mean airway pressures are reduced, taking advantage of the hysteresis of the lung pressure-volume relationship in order to prevent alveolar overdistension. This process needs to be repeated after each episode of derecruitment.[40]

HFOV has been used extensively in neonates, and studies suggest that it is associated with a lower incidence of chronic lung disease than conventional ventilation.[41] HFOV (with a recruitment protocol) was compared with conventional mechanical ventilation in 70 paediatric patients with respiratory failure secondary to diffuse alveolar disease or large air leaks using a crossover (for treatment failure) study design.[42] Overall outcomes were similar with the exception that patients randomised to HFOV had a lower requirement for supplemental oxygen at 30 days. After subgroup analysis, mortality was lower in patients treated with HFOV than in those treated with conventional mechanical ventilation only (6% v 40%).

There are few data on the use of HFOV in adult patients. In an observational study of 17 patients with ARDS, HFOV was reported to be effective and safe.[43] A prospective randomised controlled trial (Multicentre Oscillator ARDS Trial, MOAT) of HFOV versus conventional ventilation in 148 adults with ARDS was recently reported.[44] The HFV group had an early non-sustained improvement in Pao_2/Fio_2 ratio but there were no significant differences in mortality at 30 days or 6 months. The authors concluded that HFOV was a safe and effective alternative to conventional ventilation.

LIQUID VENTILATION

ARDS is associated with loss of surfactant, a consequent rise in surface tension, and alveolar collapse. Filling the lung with liquid removes the air-liquid interface and supports alveoli, thus preventing collapse. Perfluorocarbons have been used in this approach because they have low surface tension and dissolve oxygen and carbon dioxide readily.

Total liquid ventilation involves filling the entire lung with liquid and using a special ventilator to oxygenate the perfluorocarbon, a technique that is both difficult and expensive. Partial liquid ventilation is a much more practical alternative. The lung is filled to FRC with liquid and ventilated with a conventional mechanical ventilator. Although partial liquid ventilation is practical and safe, no randomised prospective studies against conventional management have yet been published.[45] Further information on liquid ventilation can be obtained from a recent review by Leonard.[46]

OTHER RESPIRATORY SUPPORT
Inhaled vasodilators

The use of inhaled vasodilators in patients with ALI/ARDS is described in chapter 10 and is not discussed further here.

Extracorporeal gas exchange

During extracorporeal membrane oxygenation (ECMO) venous blood is removed via a cannula in the inferior vena cava or right atrium, passed through a heart/lung machine, and is returned to either the right atrium (veno-venous bypass) or aorta (veno-arterial bypass). In veno-venous bypass, pulmonary and systemic haemodynamics are maintained by the patient's own cardiovascular function. Veno-arterial bypass allows systemic haemodynamic support as well as gas exchange. Institution of ECMO allows ventilator pressures and volumes to be decreased to prevent further ventilator induced lung injury. In addition, the reduction in intrathoracic pressure allows fluid removal to be carried out with less risk of haemodynamic instability. A pumpless form of extracorporeal gas exchange using arteriovenous cannulation has recently been described.[47]

ECMO has proven mortality benefit in neonatal ARDS. In adults a single prospective randomised study failed to show a survival advantage over conventional support.[48] However, overall survival in both groups was extremely low and the results are not applicable to current practice. Extracorporeal CO_2 removal (ECCOR) involves use of an extracorporeal veno-venous circuit with lower blood flows and oxygenation still occurring via the patient's lungs. A randomised prospective study of ECCOR compared with conventional support in patients with severe ARDS reported no significant difference in survival.[49] Several centres have recently reported observational studies showing high survival rates in adult patients managed with extracorporeal support (table 9.4). These encouraging survival rates should be interpreted, however, in the context of improved survival without ECMO.[50 51] A

Table 9.4 Recent observational studies reporting survival of patients with ARDS managed with extracorporeal membrane oxygenation (ECMO)

Reference	n	Survival (%)
Lewandowski (1997)[55]	122	75*
Ullrich (1999)[56]	13	62*
Bartlett (2000)[57]	86	61
Linden (2000)[58]	16	76

*Patients managed with a protocol that included ECMO if necessary.

randomised prospective controlled study of ECMO in adult patients is currently underway in Leicester, UK (CESAR trial).

CONCLUSION

The current data relating to conventional ventilation in ARDS suggest that high tidal volumes (12 ml/kg) with high plateau pressure (more than 30–35 cm H_2O) are deleterious and that a strategy aimed at preventing overdistension by decreasing tidal volume to 6 ml/kg and limiting peak pressure to <30 cm H_2O is associated with lower mortality.[52] In addition, ventilation directed at preventing cyclical opening and closing of alveoli by adjusting PEEP according to the PV curve to maintain recruitment may have a role in preventing lung injury. There may also be a role for recruitment manoeuvres, particularly after episodes of derecruitment. High frequency ventilation, including a recruitment protocol, may offer the ultimate lung protective ventilation, but further clinical studies are required.

REFERENCES

1 **Acute Respiratory Distress Syndrome Network (ARDSNet)**. Ventilation with lower tidal volumes as compared with traditional tidal volumes for acute lung injury and the acute respiratory distress syndrome. N Engl J Med 2000;**342**:1301–8.
2 **Ashbaugh DG**, Bigelow DB, Petty T, et al. Acute respiratory distress in adults. Lancet 1967;ii:319–23.
3 **Gattinoni L**, Pesenti A, Avalli L, et al. Pressure-volume curve of total respiratory system in acute respiratory failure. Computed tomographic scan study. Am Rev Respir Dis 1987;**136**:730–6.
4 **Singer MM**, Wright F, Stanley LK, et al. Oxygen toxicity in man. A prospective study in patients after open-heart surgery. N Engl J Med 1970;**283**:1473–8.
5 **Dreyfuss D**, Sauman G. Ventilator-induced lung injury: lessons from experimental studies. Am J Respir Crit Care Med 1998;**157**:294–323.
6 **Muscedere JG**, Mullen JB, Gan K, et al. Tidal ventilation at low airway pressures can augment lung injury. Am J Respir Crit Care Med 1994;**149**:1327–34.
7 **Ranieri VM**, Suter PM, Tortorella C, et al. Effect of mechanical ventilation on inflammatory mediators in patients with acute respiratory distress syndrome: a randomised controlled trial. JAMA 1999;**282**:54–61.
8 **Brochard L**. Respiratory pressure-volume curves. In: Tobin MJ, ed. Principles and practice of intensive care monitoring. New York: McGraw-Hill, 1998: 597–616.
9 **Harris RS**, Hess DR, Venegas JG. An objective analysis of the pressure-volume curve in the acute respiratory distress syndrome. Am J Respir Crit Care Med 2000;**161**:432–9.
10 **Hall JB**. Respiratory system mechanics in adult respiratory distress syndrome. Stretching our understanding. Am J Respir Crit Care Med 1998;**158**:1–2.
11 **Hickling KG**. Reinterpreting the pressure-volume curve in patients with the acute respiratory distress syndrome. Curr Opin Crit Care 2002;**8**:32–8.
12 **Ranieri VM**, Zhang H, Mascia L, et al. Pressure-time curve predicts minimally injurious ventilatory strategy in an isolated rat lung model. Anesthesiology 2000;**93**:1320–8.
13 **Hickling KG**, Henderson SJ, Jackson R. Low mortality associated with low volume pressure limited ventilation with permissive hypercapnia in severe adult respiratory distress syndrome. Intensive Care Med 1990;**16**:372–7.
14 **Rodrigo C**, Rodrigo G. Subarachnoid haemorrhage following permissive hypercapnia in a patient with severe acute asthma. Am J Emerg Med 1999;**17**:697–9.
15 **Stewart TE**, Meade MO, Cook DJ, et al. Evaluation of a ventilation strategy to prevent barotrauma in patients at high risk for acute respiratory distress syndrome. N Engl J Med 1998;**338**:355–61.
16 **Brochard L**, Roudot-Thoraval F, Roupie E, et al. Tidal volume reduction for prevention of ventilator-induced lung injury in acute respiratory distress syndrome. Am J Respir Crit Care Med 1998;**158**:1831–8.

17 **Brower RG**, Shanholtz CB, Fessler HE, et al. Prospective, randomised, controlled clinical trial comparing traditional versus reduced tidal volume ventilation in acute respiratory distress syndrome patients. *Crit Care Med* 1999;**27**:1492–8.

18 **Amato MBP**, Barbas CSV, Medeiros DM, et al. Effect of a protective-ventilation strategy on mortality in the acute respiratory distress syndrome. *N Engl J Med* 1998;**338**:347–54.

19 **Nahum A**, Ravenscraft SA, Nakos G, et al. Tracheal gas insufflation during pressure-control ventilation. Effect of catheter position, diameter, and flow rate. *Am Rev Respir Dis* 1992;**146**:965–73.

20 **Hoffman LA**, Miro AM, Tasota FJ, et al. Tracheal gas insufflation. Limits of efficacy in adults with acute respiratory distress syndrome. *Am J Respir Crit Care Med* 2000;**162**:387–92.

21 **Eichacker PQ**, Gerstenberger FP, Banks SM, et al. Meta-analysis of acute lung injury and acute respiratory distress syndrome trials testing low tidal volumes. *Am J Respir Crit Care Med* 2002;**166**:1510–4.

22 **Brower RG**, Mathay M, Schoenfeld D. Meta-analysis of acute lung injury and acute respiratory distress syndrome trials [letter]. *Am J Respir Crit Care Med* 2002;**166**:1515–7.

23 **Rappaport SH**, Shpiner R, Yoshihara G, et al. Randomized, prospective trial of pressure-limited versus volume-controlled ventilation in severe respiratory failure. *Crit Care Med* 1994;**22**:22–32.

24 **Lessard MR**, Guerot E, Lorino H, et al. Effects of pressure-controlled ventilation on respiratory mechanics, gas exchange and haemodynamics in patients with adult respiratory distress syndrome. *Anesthesiology* 1994;**80**:983–91.

25 **Esteban A**, Alia I, Gordo F, et al. Prospective randomised trial comparing pressure-controlled ventilation and volume-controlled ventilation in ARDS. Spanish Lung Failure Collaborative Group. *Chest* 2000;**117**:1690–6.

26 **Ranieri VM**, Eissa NT, Corbeil et al. Effects of positive end-expiratory pressure on alveolar recruitment and gas exchange in patients with the adult respiratory distress syndrome. *Am Rev Respir Dis* 1991;**144**:544–51.

27 **Richard JC**, Brochard L, Vandelet P, et al. Respective effects of end-expiratory and end-inspiratory pressures on alveolar recruitment in acute lung injury. *Crit Care Med* 2003;**31**:89–92.

28 **Puybasset L**, Gusman P, Muller JC, et al. Regional distribution of gas and tissue in acute respiratory distress syndrome. III. Consequences for the effects of positive end-expiratory pressure. CT Scan ARDS Study Group. Adult Respiratory Distress Syndrome. *Intensive Care Med* 2000;**26**:1215–27.

29 **Pelosi P**, Cadringher P, Bottino N, et al. Sigh in acute respiratory distress syndrome. *Am J Respir Crit Care Med* 1999;**159**:872–80.

30 **Putensen C**, Mutz NJ, Putensen-Himmer G, et al. Spontaneous breathing during ventilatory support improves ventilation perfusion distributions in patients with acute respiratory distress syndrome. *Am J Respir Crit Care Med* 1999;**159**:1241–8.

31 **Piehl MA**, Brown RS. Use of extreme position changes in respiratory failure. *Crit Care Med* 1976;**4**:13–4.

32 **Glenny RW**, Lamm WJ, Albert RK, et al. Gravity is a minor determinant of pulmonary blood flow distribution. *J Appl Physiol* 1991;**71**:620–9.

33 **Jones AT**, Hansell DM, Evans TW. Pulmonary perfusion in supine and prone positions: an electron-beam computed tomography study. *J Appl Physiol* 2001;**90**:1342–8.

34 **Lamm WJ**, Graham MM, Albert RK. Mechanism by which the prone position improves oxygenation in acute lung injury. *Am J Respir Crit Care Med* 1994;**150**:184–93.

35 **Gattinoni L**. Presentation at the European Society of Intensive Care Medicine 13th Annual Congress, Rome 2000.

36 **Froese AB**, McCullough PR, Siguria M, et al. Optimizing alveolar expansion prolongs the effectiveness of exogenous surfactant therapy in the adult rabbit. *Am Rev Respir Dis* 1993;**148**:569–77.

37 **Carlon GC**, Howland WS, Ray C, et al. High frequency jet ventilation: a prospective, randomised evaluation. *Chest* 1983;**84**:551–9.

38 **Hurst JM**, Branson RD, Davis K, et al. Comparison of conventional mechanical ventilation and high-frequency ventilation: a prospective randomised trial in patients with respiratory failure. *Ann Surg* 1990;**211**:486–91.

39 **Herridge MS**, Slutsky AS, Colditz GA. Has high-frequency ventilation been inappropriately discarded in adult acute respiratory distress syndrome? *Crit Care Med* 1998;**26**:2073–7.

40 **Froese AB**. High-frequency oscillatory ventilation for adult respiratory distress syndrome: let's get it right this time. *Crit Care Med* 1997;**25**:906–8.

41 **Riphagen S**, Bohn D. High frequency oscillatory ventilation. *Intensive Care Med* 1999;**25**:1459–62.

42 **Arnold JH**, Hanson JH, Toro-Figuero LO, et al. Prospective, randomised comparison of high-frequency oscillatory ventilation and conventional mechanical ventilation in pediatric respiratory failure. *Crit Care Med* 1994;**22**:1530–9.

43 **Fort P**, Farmer C, Westerman J, et al. High-frequency oscillatory ventilation for adult respiratory distress syndrome: a pilot study. *Crit Care Med* 1997;**25**:937–47.

44 **Derdak S**, Mehta S, Stewart TE, et al. High-frequency oscillatory ventilation for acute respiratory distress syndrome in adults: a randomised, controlled trial. *Am J Respir Crit Care Med* 2002;**6**:801–8.

45 **Hirschl RB**, Conrad S, Kaiser R, et al. Partial liquid ventilation in adult patients with ARDS: a multicenter phase I-II trail. *Ann Surg* 1998;**228**:692–700.

46 **Leonard RC**. Liquid ventilation. *Anaesth Int Care* 1998;**26**:11–21.

47 **Reng M**, Philipp A, Kaiser M, et al. Pumpless extracorporeal lung assist and adult respiratory distress syndrome. *Lancet* 2000;**356**:219–20.

48 **Zapol WM**, Snider MT, Hill JD, et al. Extracorporeal membrane oxygenation in severe acute respiratory failure. A randomised prospective study. *JAMA* 1979;**242**:2193–6.

49 **Morris AH**, Wallace CJ, Menlove RL, et al. Randomized clinical trial of pressure-controlled inverse ratio ventilation and extracorporeal CO_2 removal for adult respiratory distress syndrome. *Am J Respir Crit Care Med* 1994;**149**:295–305.

50 **Abel SJ**, Finney SJ, Brett SJ, et al. Reduced mortality in association with the acute respiratory distress syndrome (ARDS). *Thorax* 1998;**53**:292–4.

51 **Millberg JA**, Davis DR, Steinberg KP, et al. Improved survival of patients with acute respiratory distress syndrome (ARDS): 1983–1993. *JAMA* 1995;**273**:306–9.

52 **International consensus conferences in intensive care medicine**. Ventilator-associated lung injury in ARDS. *Intensive Care Med* 1999;**25**:1444–52.

53 **Lapinsky SE**, Aubin M, Mehta S, et al. Safety and efficacy of a sustained inflation for alveolar recruitment in adults with respiratory failure. *Intensive Care Med* 1999;**25**:1297–301.

54 **Medoff BD**, Harris RS, Kesselman H, et al. Use of recruitment maneuvers and high-positive end-expiratory pressure in a patient with acute respiratory distress syndrome. *Crit Care Med* 2000;**28**:1210–6.

55 **Lewandowski K**, Rossaint R, Pappert D, et al. High survival rate in 122 patients managed according to a clinical algorithm including extra-corporeal membrane oxygenation. *Intensive Care Med* 1997;**23**:819–35.

56 **Ullrich R**, Larber C, Roder G, et al. Controlled airway pressure therapy, nitric oxide inhalation, prone position, and ECMO as components of an integrated approach to ARDS. *Anesthesiology* 1999;**91**:1577–86.

57 **Bartlett RH**, Roloff DW, Custer JR, et al. Extracorporeal life support. The University of Michigan Experience. *JAMA* 2000;**283**:904–8.

58 **Linden V**, Palmer K, Reinhard J, et al. High survival in adult patients with acute respiratory syndrome treated by extracorporeal membrane oxygenation, minimal sedation, and pressure supported ventilation. *Intensive Care Med* 2000;**26**:1630–7.

10 Non-ventilatory strategies in acute respiratory distress syndrome

J Cranshaw, M J D Griffiths, T W Evans

Our understanding of the pathophysiology and management of the acute respiratory distress syndrome (ARDS) has improved immensely since its original description, but pharmacotherapies have proved disappointing in clinical trials. Several reasons have been proposed for this failure.

- There are no good experimental models of ARDS so that drugs may not have the desired effect or produce unacceptable side effects when used clinically.

- The inflammatory cascades that cause sepsis and ARDS are characterised by widespread redundancy so it is unlikely that a single agent could reverse or terminate such complex processes.

- Although a drug may improve pulmonary function, it may not alter outcome. Fewer than 5% of patients with ARDS die of respiratory failure; the majority suffer from multiple organ failure and succumb after withdrawal of support.

- Enrolling patients with ARDS in clinical trials using the American-European Consensus Conference definition[1] ignores the heterogeneity of the disease. In pathological terms, the acute exudative and fibroproliferative phases present distinct targets for intervention, making the timing of drug administration (after disease onset) crucial. The primary cause(s) of ARDS, the patient's age and medical history all affect prognosis and possibly drug responsiveness of the condition.

Recent reports suggest that the mortality associated with ARDS may be falling, probably because of advances in supporting critically ill patients.[2] This trend may increase the number of potential survivors and the window of opportunity for pharmacological manipulation of lung injury. Thus, drugs that have been apparent failures in terms of mortality may still have a useful role to play, either in combination with other agents or in subgroups of ARDS patients defined either by their underlying condition or by their stage of lung injury. This chapter reviews the major pharmacological approaches to treating ARDS in the context of modern supportive care (fig 10.1). We conclude with a proposal for future strategies in the non-ventilatory management of ARDS.

INTRAVENOUS FLUID MANAGEMENT

Patients with ARDS often have cardiovascular dysfunction caused by systemic inflammation that is commonly associated with sepsis. Hence, myocardial depression, abnormal vascular tone, and permeability contribute to abnormal tissue oxygenation and ultimately organ failure. In practice, achieving adequate organ perfusion may occur at the cost of increasing extravascular water manifesting as an exacerbation of pulmonary oedema. Low extravascular lung water levels are associated with better oxygenation and a lower mortality in patients with ARDS in retrospective studies.[3 4] There is limited prospective evidence that targeting lower extravascular lung water using diuretics with vasopressors to support organ perfusion reduces the time required on a ventilator.[5 6] Our policy is to keep the intravascular volume as low as possible while maintaining an adequate cardiac index and mean arterial pressure.

INHALED VASODILATORS

Nitric oxide (NO) is a free radical gas produced constitutively in the lung by nitric oxide synthase from L-arginine, NADPH, and oxygen. Endothelial cells constitutively release NO, causing pulmonary vasodilation primarily via the secondary messenger cyclic guanosine monophosphate. ARDS is characterised by ventilation-perfusion mismatching which produces arterial hypoxaemia that may in part be caused by disordered endogenous NO activity. Patients with ARDS commonly have mild pulmonary hypertension. Any inhaled vasodilator can augment hypoxic pulmonary vasoconstriction by selectively vasodilating vessels associated with ventilated alveoli to improve oxygenation (fig 10.2).

Improved oxygenation and direct vascular smooth muscle relaxation by NO also reduce pulmonary vascular resistance (PVR). Vasoconstriction by hypoxia, hypercapnia, thromboxane A_2, and angiotensin II can all be partially reversed by inhaled NO, although the PVR of normal volunteers is not affected.[7] Reducing PVR and consequential improvements in right ventricular function may benefit some patients with ARDS. However, NO does not increase cardiac output in the majority.[8] Reduced arteriolar and venous tone may lower capillary pressure, reducing leakage and further improving gas exchange. Unfortunately, in patients with pulmonary hypertension associated with impaired left ventricular function, pulmonary vascular relaxation may also increase pulmonary oedema.

Endothelial NO also inhibits platelet aggregation and neutrophil adhesion that are likely mediators of lung injury. Although the importance of these actions in ARDS is uncertain, inhaled NO has been used immediately after lung transplantation to reduce ischaemia-reperfusion injury.[9] NO quickly scavenges reactive oxygen species (ROS) including the superoxide anion to produce a less reactive but still potentially harmful product, namely peroxynitrite. Although ROS

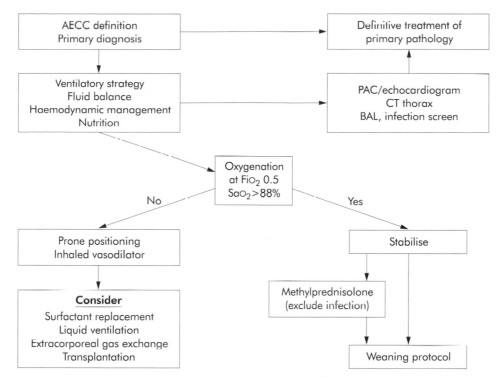

Figure 10.1 Suggested treatment algorithm for acute lung injury (ALI) and ARDS. AECC=American-European Consensus Conference 1993; PAC=pulmonary artery catheter; CT=computed tomography; BAL=bronchoalveolar lavage; FiO_2=fractional inspired oxygen concentration; SaO_2=arterial oxygen saturation.

are usually kept at low levels in lung tissue by antioxidants and dismutases, these protective systems may be overwhelmed during ARDS.[10] Peroxynitrite oxidises and nitrosylates proteins, nucleic acids and lipids, including essential components of the surfactant system. However, the clinical significance of peroxynitrite production is unknown.

Approximately 60% of patients with ARDS or acute lung injury (ALI) of all causes respond to inhaled NO, increasing their PaO_2 by more than 20%.[11] The effect can frequently be seen in less than 10 minutes or may take several hours.[12 13] However, in several trials the oxygenation of control groups has risen to meet that of NO treated patients between 24 hours and 4 days.[11 13 14] The dose-response relationship between inhaled NO and arterial oxygenation shows considerable interindividual variation.[15] Currently there are no indicators that will predict the response. Maximal improvement in oxygenation is sometimes achieved with 1–2 parts per million (ppm) and occurs at less than 10 ppm in most patients. Maximal reduction in pulmonary artery pressure is usually obtained between 10 and 40 ppm, with no benefit and possible toxicity at doses greater than 80 ppm. United Kingdom guidelines suggest a maximum dose of 40 ppm.[16] Intraindividual variation in response with time is also significant and may be influenced by lung recruitment, co-existent pathology, or the resolution of inflammation. Clinically, it is sometimes difficult to stop inhaled NO without "rebound" pulmonary hypertension and hypoxaemia. The last 1–2 ppm may have to be weaned especially slowly.

The systemic effects of inhaled NO are negligible due to the rapid strong combination of NO with haemoglobin to form methaemoglobin. This is normally reduced to functional haemoglobin and NO is ultimately converted to soluble NO_3. Methaemoglobinaemia produces a functional anaemia and a left shift in the dissociation curve, but rarely causes a clinical problem. Normal levels of methaemaglobin are less than 2% and values less than 5% usually do not need treatment. NO reacts slowly with oxygen and water to form toxic NO_2, nitrous and nitric acids. These damage the lung at concentrations as low as 2 ppm. The reaction rate is proportional to the fractional inspired oxygen concentration (FiO_2) and the square

of the NO concentration. Thus, the contact time and concentrations of the gases should be kept to a minimum. With proper monitoring, delivery systems, and NO doses of less than 40 ppm, NO_2 is not a significant problem. Delivery systems that add NO "upstream" of the ventilator allow longer mixing with oxygen and are not recommended. Continuous "downstream" addition of NO may allow NO to collect in the inspiratory limb of the circuit during the expiratory phase of some systems. Synchronised NO delivery during inspiration may be the optimum mode of delivery. NO contained in exhaled gas should be absorbed before release.

Randomised controlled trials in patients with ARDS have shown that, while inhaled NO temporarily improves oxygenation and reduces pulmonary artery pressure in the majority, its use is not associated with an improved outcome (table 10.1). Inhaled NO is therefore not a standard treatment for ARDS. However, patients with severe refractory hypoxaemia and inadequate right ventricular function secondary to pulmonary hypertension may benefit from inhaled NO. NO may also protect patients whose oxygenation might otherwise depend upon a potentially damaging ventilatory strategy. In small studies the pulmonary vasoconstrictor almitrine improved oxygenation in patients with ARDS.[17] It has been suggested that low dose intravenous almitrine potentiates hypoxic pulmonary vasoconstriction and the combination of almitrine and inhaled NO may improve oxygenation synergistically in patients with ARDS.[18]

Prostacyclin (PGI_2) is an endothelium-derived prostaglandin vasodilator that inhibits platelet aggregation and neutrophil adhesion. Its mechanism of action differs from NO in that smooth muscle relaxation is associated with a rise in cytoplasmic cyclic adenosine monophosphate. Its half life is only 2–3 minutes but it is not metabolised by the lung, so when administered intravenously, PGI_2 lowers pulmonary vascular resistance but may also increase intrapulmonary shunting and cause systemic hypotension.[15] However, nebulised PGI_2 (0–50 ng/kg/min)[19 20] or alprostadil (PGE_1, 20–80 µg/h)[21] produce equivalent effects to inhaled NO with minimal systemic side effects and without measurable platelet dysfunction, but there have been no large randomised trials of

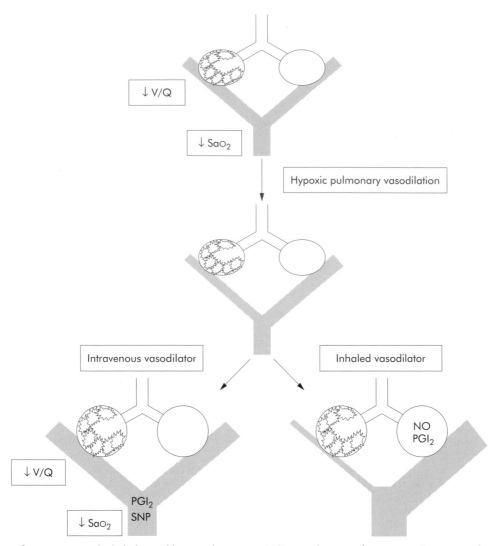

Figure 10.2 Effect of intravenous and inhaled vasodilators in lung injury. V/Q=ventilation:perfusion ratio; Sao_2=arterial oxygen saturation; PGI_2=prostacyclin; SNP=sodium nitroprusside; NO=nitric oxide.

these therapies. Nevertheless, the relatively simple delivery system, harmless metabolites, and no requirement for special monitoring make nebulised PGI_2 an attractive alternative to inhaled NO, despite its expense.

CORTICOSTEROIDS

Corticosteroids reduce the production of a great number of inflammatory and profibrotic mediators by many mechanisms. The importance of steroid therapy to the resolution of

Table 10.1 Randomised controlled trials of inhaled nitric oxide (NO) in patients with ARDS

Author	No of patients	Diagnosis	Blinded	Inhaled NO dose (ppm)	Duration	Outcome
Lundin et al (1999)[76]	260	ALI (American-European Consensus Conference) and 18–96 hours ventilation with Pao_2/Fio_2 <22 kPa, PEEP at least 5 cm H_2O, mean airway pressure >10 cm H_2O and I:E 1:2–2:1	No	2–40	30 days	180 randomised responded to NO. The frequency of reversal of ALI did not differ from controls. Development of severe respiratory failure less (2.2% v 10.3%) in NO treated group. Mortality not altered (44% v 40% control).
Dellinger et al (1998)[11]	177	ARDS (American-European Consensus Conference) within 72 hours of onset and PEEP at least 8 cm H_2O and Fio_2 >0.5	Yes	1.25–80	28 days	Pao_2 increased >20% in first 4 hours in 60% of patients treated with NO and 24% of controls. Fio_2 and intensity of ventilation could be reduced in first 4 days. No difference in mortality (30% v 32–38% in NO treated groups).
Michael et al (1998)[13]	40	ARDS (American-European Consensus Conference) and Fio_2 at least 0.8 for 12 hours or 0.65 for 24 hours	No	5–20	3 days	NO improved Pao_2/Fio_2 by at least 20% and allowed a decrease in Fio_2 of at least 0.15 only in the first 24 hours in more treated patients than controls.
Troncy (1998)[14]	30	Murray score at least 2.5	No	0.5–40	30 days	NO improved oxygenation only in the first 24 hours in more treated patients than controls. Mortality (60% v 67% in control) not altered.

Table 10.2 Published trials of short term, high dose steroid therapy in patients with ARDS

Author	No of patients	Diagnosis	Randomised	Control group	Prospective	Blinded	Methylprednisolone dose	Duration	Outcome
Meduri et al (1998)[28]	24	Late ARDS	Yes	Yes	Yes	Yes	2 mg/kg load then 0.5 mg/kg 6 hrly reduced weekly to 1 mg/kg/day, 0.5 mg/kg/day then 0.15 mg/kg/day	32 days	Improvement in LIS, MODS, reduced mortality
Hooper et al (1996)[77]	26	Established ARDS of >3 days with cause resolved	No	No	Yes	No	125–250 mg 6 hrly for 3–4 days reducing by 50% every 2–3 days	3–6 weeks	81% survival
Meduri et al (1995)[78]	9	Late ARDS	No	No	Yes	No	200 mg bolus, 2–3 mg/kg/day	Until extubation (average 6 weeks)	Reduction in plasma and BAL inflammatory cytokines
Biffl et al (1995)[79]	6	Prolonged ARDS failing conventional therapy	No	No	Yes	No	1–2 mg/kg 6 hrly	13–42 days	83% survival; improved LIS and PaO_2/FiO_2
Meduri et al (1994)[80]	25	Late ARDS	No	No	Yes	No	200 mg bolus, 2–3 mg/kg/day	Until extubation	Reduction in LIS, improved $PaCO_2/FiO_2$
Meduri et al (1991)[81]	8	Late ARDS	No	No	No	No	2 mg/kg bolus, 2–3 mg/kg 6 hrly	Until extubation	Reduction in LIS
Luce et al (1988)[82]	75	Culture positive septic shock	Yes	Yes (mannitol placebo)	Yes	Yes	30 mg/kg 6 hrly	24 h	Terminated early after publication of 26, no alteration in LIS
Bone et al (1987)[26]	381	Severe sepsis and septic shock	Yes	Yes	Yes	Yes	30 mg/kg 6 hrly	24 h	No change in incidence of ARDS; mortality of ARDS higher; less frequent ARDS reversal
Bernard et al (1987)[25]	99	ARDS	Yes	Yes	Yes	Yes	30 mg/kg 6 hrly	24 h	No mortality benefit
Weigelt et al (1985)[24]	81	ARDS	Yes	Yes	Yes	Yes	30 mg/kg 6 hrly	48 h	No mortality benefit; increased infection rate
Lucas et al (1981)[23]	114	Post-injury hypovolaemic shock lung	Yes	Yes	Yes	No	30 mg/kg 6 hrly	3 days	Increased mortality
Sladen (1976)[22]	10	Shock lung	No	No	Yes	No	30 mg/kg 6 hrly	48 h	Improved mortality

LIS=lung injury score; MODS=multiple organ dysfunction syndrome.

lung inflammation in animal models became apparent in the 1980s. Unfortunately, trials of short term, high dose steroid therapy (for example, methylprednisolone 30 mg/kg 6 hourly for 24 hours) failed to show an improvement in mortality of patients at risk of or with early ARDS associated with sepsis, aspiration, and trauma (table 10.2).[22–26] In fact, some trials showed increased risk of infection, lower rates of reversal of ARDS, and increased mortality associated with the use of high dose steroids. Meta-analyses of available trials emphasise the adverse effects of these agents in patients with sepsis.

However, the use of steroids in patients with late ARDS (7–14 days from diagnosis) has not been abandoned. Recent data suggest that inflammation and fibrosis in the lung are distinct and thus independently manipulable processes.[27] There is also clinical evidence that steroids favourably modify the fibroproliferative phase of ARDS. In the 1990s lower dose (2–8 mg/kg/day methyprednisolone), longer term (2–6 weeks) corticosteroid treatment was used in patients with ARDS of over 10 days duration. Mortality fell to approximately 20% in some uncontrolled series but complications attributable to steroids were not infrequent and included sepsis, pneumonia, wound infection, gastric ulceration, and diabetes. A trial using this approach randomised 24 patients with "unresolving" ARDS of more than 7 days duration to methylprednisolone (2 mg/kg load then 2 mg/kg/day in four divided doses reducing weekly to 1 mg/kg/day, then 0.5 mg/kg/day, then 0.15 mg/kg/day).[28] None of the 16 patients in the steroid group died compared with five of eight originally given placebo. Steroid therapy was associated with improved oxygenation and successful extubation. Eligible patients were examined for pulmonary infection by bronchoalveolar lavage at day 5 and all febrile patients received a broad septic screen before trial entry. Documented infections were treated with appropriate antibiotics for at least 3 days before steroids were administered. Despite these precautions, 75% of patients in both arms of the trial suffered new sepsis. Although the results are promising, the design and interpretation of this trial have proved contentious.[29] The larger NIH ARDS Network Late Steroid Rescue Study may provide sounder evidence for prescribing low dose steroids in late ARDS.

SURFACTANT

Type II alveolar cells synthesise and recycle surfactant phospholipids and proteins. Surfactant lowers alveolar surface tension and prevents collapse at low lung volumes. The same effects reduce the hydrostatic pressure gradient favouring fluid movement into the alveolar space. Surfactant also has anti-inflammatory and antimicrobial properties. During ARDS, surfactant activity may be deficient because of reduced production, increased removal with recurrent alveolar collapse during ventilation, abnormal composition and, importantly, dysfunction caused by plasma proteins,[30] ROS, and proteases in the flooded alveolar space.[31]

Various preparations, doses, administration regimens, and delivery techniques have been proposed. Phospholipids alone are inferior to composites of lipid and surfactant proteins. The amount of drug required varies with the type of administration technique—intratracheal delivery, aerosolisation in ventilator gas, and direct bronchoscopic instillation. Simultaneous segmental lavage has been combined with the latter approach and this process itself may benefit some patients. The optimum timing and duration of surfactant therapy is still to be determined.

A phase III clinical trial of one aerosolised preparation in sepsis induced ARDS has been conducted on a background of improved oxygenation in previous reports.[32] No significant effect was seen on oxygenation, duration of ventilation, or survival with up to 5 days of continuous treatment beginning within 48 hours of ventilation. However, this study has been criticised because the compound used contained no protein and aerosolisation may have delivered less than 5 mg/kg/day of phospholipid when investigations suggest instillation of 300 mg/kg/day may be required. Bovine surfactant administered intratracheally in a smaller trial has shown that higher doses (100 mg/kg qds) are required to alter alveolar surfactant composition.[33] This dose improved oxygenation over 120 hours and a trend was observed towards reduced mortality at 28 days. Total bronchopulmonary segmental lavage with 30 ml per segment of a synthetic protein containing surfactant was safe and effective at improving oxygenation within 72 hours of the onset of sepsis induced ARDS.[34] Despite these trials, the use of surfactant in ARDS remains experimental. Successful use of surfactant in animal models of lung injury and in neonatal respiratory distress syndrome suggests that efficient administration of an effective substitute could be beneficial in ARDS. The goals of treatment would include both improved gas exchange and protection against ventilator induced lung injury.

IMMUNONUTRITION

Avoiding nutritional depletion while delivering a high fat, low carbohydrate diet to reduce carbon dioxide production and ventilatory demand is appropriate for patients with ARDS.[35] Immunonutrition aims to influence inflammation positively and to protect gastrointestinal integrity. However, supplying enteral nutrition of any type may stimulate gastrointestinal and pulmonary IgA defence mechanisms.[36] In vitro, dietary additives improve depressed immune cell function from some critically ill patients and attenuate the production of proinflammatory mediators in others.

The amino acids glutamine and arginine may be useful dietary additives for patients at risk of or with established ARDS.[37] Enterocytes metabolise glutamine in a manner that enhances intestinal mucosal integrity and reduces translocation of bacteria and toxins into the portal circulation that may fuel a systemic inflammatory response. Glutamine and arginine also augment lymphocyte function, and arginine improves monocyte function in critically injured patients. L-arginine supplementation may also increase NO production, alter vascular tone, and augment free radical mediated antibacterial defences. Similarly, omega-3 fatty acids such as eicosapentaenoic acid and the unsaturated oil gammalinolenic acid reduce proinflammatory cytokine and eicosanoid production.[38] Less biologically active eicosanoids such as prostaglandin PGE_1, thromboxane TXA_3, and leukotriene LTB_5 are produced from these unsaturated fats by cyclo-oxygenase (COX) and 5-lipoxygenase during inflammation. Animal experiments suggest that polyunsaturated fatty acids can reduce pulmonary vascular resistance, lung neutrophil infiltration, and microvascular permeability, thereby improving gas exchange.

In patients with ARDS, enteral immunonutrition supplemented with antioxidants for at least 4 days was associated with reduced pulmonary neutrophil recruitment, improved oxygenation, a shortened duration of mechanical ventilation, and reduced morbidity in terms of new organ failure.[39] However, there was no difference in mortality between the control and treatment groups. A meta-analysis of 12 randomised controlled trials comparing critically ill medical, surgical, and trauma patients given standard enteral nutrition with patients receiving immunonutrition suggested reduced rates of infection including nosocomial pneumonia, but again no effect on mortality.[40] With some reservations, the authors concluded that their data suggested real benefits of immunonutrition in surgical and trauma patients, but that a large double blind, multicentre, randomised controlled trial was still required.

PROSTAGLANDIN E₁

Intravenous PGE_1 causes both pulmonary and systemic vasodilation and, in some critically ill patients, increases cardiac output and oxygen delivery.[41] Although the effect on the pulmonary circulation is usually small, vasodilation is more marked under hypoxic conditions, and the nebulised drug improves ventilation-perfusion matching.[21] PGE_1 also inhibits platelet aggregation and neutrophil adhesion. The initial trial of PGE_1[42] showed improved survival in trauma patients with respiratory failure. However, this benefit could not be reproduced in a subsequent multicentre trial[43] in patients suffering from lung injury precipitated by surgery, trauma, or sepsis. The dose of PGE_1 was limited by side effects, particularly systemic hypotension. More recent trials have used liposome technology to increase drug delivery while mitigating side effects.[44 45] The use of a liposome itself is associated with immune modulating effects including downregulation of neutrophil adhesion molecules. A combined PGE_1-liposome preparation in a rodent model of ALI reduced pulmonary neutrophil infiltration and capillary leak.[46] However, although the phase II and III trials of liposomal PGE_1 showed that patients with ARDS receiving the drug had more rapid improvements in the Pao_2/Fio_2 ratio, neither a survival benefit nor a reduced requirement for ventilatory support was found in the treatment group.[44 45] Retrospective subgroup analysis suggested that high dose therapy might reduce the time to extubation.

THROMBOXANE SYNTHASE AND 5-LIPOXYGENASE INHIBITORS

Thromboxane and leukotrienes are in part responsible for the pulmonary hypertension and hypoxaemia of ARDS. Pulmonary vascular smooth muscle cells, endothelial cells, platelets, and neutrophils all release TXA_2 on stimulation. TXA_2 can initiate microvascular thromboses consisting of neutrophil and platelet aggregates that are responsible for perfusion abnormalities and recurrent ischaemia-reperfusion injury to the lung. The vasoconstrictive effect of TXA_2 similarly contributes to impaired gas exchange.[47] In animal models of lung injury thromboxane synthase inhibition reduced pulmonary oedema formation and inhibited microembolism, but pulmonary hypertension was only partially relieved.[48] Similarly, improved oxygenation and reduced pulmonary hypertension have been found in small trials of a thromboxane receptor antagonist in patients with ARDS.

Leukotrienes (LT) are derived from arachidonic acid by 5-lipoxygenase. LTB_4 is a potent neutrophil chemokine while LTC_4 and LTD_4 cause pulmonary vasoconstriction, capillary leak, and pulmonary oedema. The role of leukotrienes in ARDS has been less well researched but bronchoalveolar lavage fluid from patients with ARDS contains increased concentrations of LTB_4, LTC_4 and LTD_4, which may be markers for developing ARDS.[49] Ketoconazole is an imidazole antifungal agent that inhibits thromboxane synthase and 5-lipoxygenase without inhibiting COX. Ketoconazole may therefore have a dual anti-inflammatory action in ARDS by inhibiting inflammatory eicosanoid synthesis and directing COX products down other less inflammatory metabolic paths such as those synthesising prostacyclin or PGE_2.[50] Four trials have used enteral ketoconazole in patients at risk of or with ARDS. The incidence of acute respiratory failure was reduced in high risk surgical patients and other critically ill patients.[51–53] However, an ARDS Network trial (http://hedwig.mgh.harvard.edu/ardsnet) in patients with established ARDS of medical and surgical aetiology found no differences in in-hospital mortality, ventilator free days at day 28, organ failure-free days, or markers of gas exchange between patients given ketoconazole or placebo.[54] This trial achieved plasma levels of ketoconazole higher than targeted previously but could not demonstrate a reduction in thromboxane production in vivo. The effect of decreasing thromboxane synthesis in ARDS is therefore still unknown. It is still possible that ketoconazole in surgical and trauma patients at risk of or with incipient pulmonary injury may be beneficial.

ANTIOXIDANTS

The damage caused by ROS to matrix and cellular proteins, lipids and nucleic acids and ROS mediated signalling contribute to the pathogenesis of ARDS.[55] The thiol groups of glutathione concentrated in the lower respiratory tract normally provide physiological antioxidant protection. However, the concentration and activity of glutathione in bronchoalveolar lavage fluid of patients with ARDS is reduced.[56] Intravenous administration does not reliably raise glutathione levels, but glutathione synthesis is stimulated by N-acetylcysteine (NAC) and procysteine (L-2 oxothiazolidine-4-carboxylate). Administration of these precursors increases plasma, erythrocyte, neutrophil, and BAL fluid concentrations of glutathione in patients with ARDS, although a complete effect may require 10 days of treatment.[57] Early results of NAC therapy were promising, but several trials have found no difference in mortality, length of ventilatory support, or improvement in oxygenation in patients with established ARDS,[58–61] and a large, as yet unpublished, phase III trial of procysteine was stopped early because of concerns about mortality in the treatment arm of the study. Currently, there is little evidence that intravenous NAC or procysteine are of benefit to patients with ARDS.

Dietary antioxidants such as ascorbic acid, tocopherol, and flavonoids have ROS scavenging ability and the capacity to reduce oxidised antioxidants as well as binding ROS producing catalysts such as free iron. Although reports of a significant action of these supplements on pulmonary inflammation are lacking, they are already components of some "immunonutrition" preparations.[39]

PHOSPHATIDIC ACID INHIBITION

Phosphatidic acids are liberated in response to inflammatory stimuli by lysophosphatidic acyl transferase and, like arachidonic acid, are a source of inflammatory mediators. Pentoxifylline and its more potent metabolite lisofylline are lysophosphatidic acyl transferase inhibitors. These compounds reduce serum free fatty acids in humans and lower cytokine production, neutrophil activation, pulmonary neutrophil sequestration, and attenuate lung injury in animal models. However, a study of lisofylline in 235 patients with ALI and ARDS was stopped at the first interim analysis because the pre-specified level of improvement for the treatment arm of the trial was not achieved.[62]

PHOSPHOLIPASE INHIBITION

The enzymes of the secretory phospholipase A_2 group are capable of releasing biologically active polyunsaturated lipids, including arachidonic acid, from cell membranes and circulating plasma lipoprotein complexes. The liberated free fatty acids and their metabolites, including prostaglandins and other eicosanoids, are proinflammatory and may contribute to the pathophysiology of the sepsis syndrome and multiple organ failure.[63] Furthermore, secretory phospholipases have the capacity to damage type II alveolar cells directly and degrade surfactant.[64 65] Raised secretory phospholipase A_2 activity is found in bronchoalveolar lavage fluid from patients with ARDS and correlates with the severity of lung injury as measured using the Murray lung injury score.[66] Serum secretory phospholipase A_2 concentrations are elevated in patients with sepsis and correlate with the development of ARDS in patients with septic shock and trauma.[67 68]

The positive effects of secretory phospholipase A_2 inhibition in animal models of sepsis and lung injury led to preliminary trials of two concentrations of a selective inhibitor of group IIa secretory phospholipase A_2, namely LY315920Na/S-5920, infused for 7 days in patients presenting within 36 hours with severe sepsis.[69] In the phase II study the treatment group showed a non-significant reduction in the development of ARDS and time spent on the ventilator. The principal mortality benefit occurred in patients who received the drug within 18 hours of their first organ failure. Prospective trials are required to confirm that early administration of LY315920Na/S-5920 protects lung function and improves mortality in patients with severe sepsis.

CONCLUSION

Most pharmacological strategies used in ARDS have targeted the inflammatory response. Many agents not mentioned here—cytokine inhibitors, anti-inflammatory cytokines, antiproteases, and anti-endotoxin agents—alone and in combination are in the early phases of drug development. Between 18% and 41% of patients with sepsis will develop ARDS and post mortem examination reveals evidence of infection, particularly pneumonia, in almost all patients with ARDS.[70] This overlap between sepsis and ARDS means that improvements in the treatment of sepsis may influence the incidence and outcome of ARDS. Large clinical trials of anti-inflammatory agents for sepsis such as ibuprofen,[71] anti-endotoxin,[72 73] and anti-tumour necrosis factor alpha antibodies[74] have had no human impact on the mortality associated with ARDS so far. At the time of writing recombinant activated protein C has been shown to decrease the mortality of patients with sepsis and may improve the outlook of patients with sepsis induced ARDS.[75]

If the future of ARDS treatment lies in improvements in the management of multiorgan failure, then the pharmacological approach to treating lung injury may change. Previous attempts at simply dampening or halting the whole acute inflammatory process may be replaced by targeted therapies directed at elements of the pathological process that produce specific clinical problems. For example, reducing pathological fibrosis may be possible when more is understood about the regulation of collagen turnover in the normal and injured lung. Similarly, the protection, stimulation or suppression of alveolar cell division, migration, and secretion may be possible. This may enhance the repair of the alveolar epithelial cell barrier, the clearance of intra-alveolar exudate, and the normal turnover and function of surfactant.

REFERENCES

1 **Bernard GR**, Artigas A, Brigham KL, et al. The American-European Consensus Conference on ARDS. Definitions, mechanisms, relevant outcomes, and clinical trial coordination. Am J Respir Crit Care Med 1994;**149**(3 Pt 1):818–24.

2 **Abel SJ**, Finney SJ, Brett SJ, et al. Reduced mortality in association with the acute respiratory distress syndrome (ARDS). Thorax 1998;**53**:292–4.

3 **Davey-Quinn A**, Gedney J, Whiteley S, et al. Extravascular lung water and acute respiratory distress syndrome: oxygenation and outcome. Anaesth Intensive Care 1999;**27**:357–62.

4 **Humphrey H**, Hall J, Sznajder I, et al. Improved survival in ARDS patients associated with a reduction in pulmonary capillary wedge pressure. Chest 1990;**97**:1176–80.

5 **Mitchell JP**, Schuller D, Calandrino FS, et al. Improved outcome based on fluid management in critically ill patients requiring pulmonary artery catheterization. Am Rev Respir Dis 1992;**145**:990–8.

6 **Schuller D**, Mitchell JP, Calandrino FS, et al. Fluid balance during pulmonary edema. Is fluid gain a marker or a cause of poor outcome? Chest 1991;**100**:1068–75.

7 **Payen D**. Inhaled nitric oxide and acute lung injury. Clin Chest Med 2000;**21**:519–29.

8 **Rossaint R**, Slama K, Steudel W, et al. Effects of inhaled nitric oxide on right ventricular function in severe acute respiratory distress syndrome. Intensive Care Med 1995;**21**:197–203.

9 **Murakami S**, Bacha EA, Mazmanian GM, et al. Effects of various timings and concentrations of inhaled nitric oxide in lung ischemia-reperfusion. The Paris-Sud University Lung Transplantation Group. Am J Respir Crit Care Med 1997;**156**(2 Pt 1):454–8.

10 **Chabot F**, Mitchell J, Gutteridge J, et al. Reactive oxygen species in acute lung injury. Eur Respir J 1998;**11**:745–57.

11 **Dellinger RP**, Zimmerman JL, Taylor RW, et al. Effects of inhaled nitric oxide in patients with acute respiratory distress syndrome: results of a randomized phase II trial. Inhaled Nitric Oxide in ARDS Study Group. Crit Care Med 1998;**26**:15–23.

12 **Gerlach H**, Rossaint R, Pappert D, et al. Time-course and dose-response of nitric oxide inhalation for systemic oxygenation and pulmonary hypertension in patients with adult respiratory distress syndrome. *Eur J Clin Invest* 1993;**23**:499–502.

13 **Michael JR**, Barton RG, Saffle JR, et al. Inhaled nitric oxide versus conventional therapy: effect on oxygenation in ARDS. *Am J Respir Crit Care Med* 1998;**157**(5 Pt 1):1372–80.

14 **Troncy E**, Collet JP, Shapiro S, et al. Inhaled nitric oxide in acute respiratory distress syndrome: a pilot randomized controlled study. *Am J Respir Crit Care Med* 1998;**157**(5 Pt 1):1483–8.

15 **Rossaint R**, Falke KJ, Lopez F, et al. Inhaled nitric oxide for the adult respiratory distress syndrome. *N Engl J Med* 1993;**328**:399–405.

16 **Cuthbertson BH**, Dellinger P, Dyar et al. UK guidelines for the use of inhaled nitric oxide therapy in adult ICUs. American-European Consensus Conference on ALI/ARDS. *Intensive Care Med* 1997;**23**:1212–8.

17 **Reyes A**, Roca J, Rodriguez-Roisin R, et al. Effect of almitrine on ventilation-perfusion distribution in adult respiratory distress syndrome. *Am Rev Respir Dis* 1988;**137**:1062–7.

18 **Gallart L**, Lu Q, Puybasset L, et al. Intravenous almitrine combined with inhaled nitric oxide for acute respiratory distress syndrome. The NO Almitrine Study Group. *Am J Respir Crit Care Med* 1998;**158**:1770–7.

19 **Walmrath D**, Schneider T, Schermuly R, et al. Direct comparison of inhaled nitric oxide and aerosolized prostacyclin in acute respiratory distress syndrome. *Am J Respir Crit Care Med* 1996;**153**:991–6.

20 **Zwissler B**, Kemming G, Habler O, et al. Inhaled prostacyclin (PGI2) versus inhaled nitric oxide in adult respiratory distress syndrome. *Am J Respir Crit Care Med* 1996;**154**(6 Pt 1):1671–7.

21 **Meyer J**, Theilmeier G, Van Aken H, et al. Inhaled prostaglandin E1 for treatment of acute lung injury in severe multiple organ failure. *Anesth Analg* 1998;**86**:753–8.

22 **Sladen A**. Methylprednisolone. Pharmacologic doses in shock lung syndrome. *J Thorac Cardiovasc Surg* 1976;**71**:800–6.

23 **Lucas CE**, Ledgerwood AM. Pulmonary response of massive steroids in seriously injured patients. *Ann Surg* 1981;**194**:256–61.

24 **Weigelt JA**, Norcross JF, Borman KR, et al. Early steroid therapy for respiratory failure. *Arch Surg* 1985;**120**:536–40.

25 **Bernard GR**, Luce JM, Sprung CL, et al. High-dose corticosteroids in patients with the adult respiratory distress syndrome. *N Engl J Med* 1987;**317**:1565–70.

26 **Bone RC**, Fisher CJ Jr, Clemmer TP, et al. A controlled clinical trial of high-dose methylprednisolone in the treatment of severe sepsis and septic shock. *N Engl J Med* 1987;**317**:653–8.

27 **Kaminski N**, Allard JD, Pittet JF, et al. Global analysis of gene expression in pulmonary fibrosis reveals distinct programs regulating lung inflammation and fibrosis. *Proc Natl Acad Sci USA* 2000;**97**:1778–83.

28 **Meduri GU**, Headley AS, Golden E, et al. Effect of prolonged methylprednisolone therapy in unresolving acute respiratory distress syndrome: a randomized controlled trial. *JAMA* 1998;**280**:159–65.

29 **Brun-Buisson C**, Brochard L. Corticosteroid therapy in acute respiratory distress syndrome: better late than never? *JAMA* 1998;**280**:182–3.

30 **Manalo E**, Merritt TA, Kheiter A, et al. Comparative effects of some serum components and proteolytic products of fibrinogen on surface tension-lowering abilities of beractant and a synthetic peptide containing surfactant KL4. *Pediatr Res* 1996;**39**:947–52.

31 **Amirkhanian JD**, Merritt TA. Inhibitory effects of oxyradicals on surfactant function: utilizing in vitro Fenton reaction. *Lung* 1998;**176**:63–72.

32 **Anzueto A**, Baughman RP, Guntupalli KK, et al. Aerosolized surfactant in adults with sepsis-induced acute respiratory distress syndrome. Exosurf Acute Respiratory Distress Syndrome Sepsis Study Group. *N Engl J Med* 1996;**334**:1417–21.

33 **Gregory TJ**, Steinberg KP, Spragg R, et al. Bovine surfactant therapy for patients with acute respiratory distress syndrome. *Am J Respir Crit Care Med* 1997;**155**:1309–15.

34 **Wiswell TE**, Smith RM, Katz LB, et al. Bronchopulmonary segmental lavage with Surfaxin (KL(4)-surfactant) for acute respiratory distress syndrome. *Am J Respir Crit Care Med* 1999;**160**:1188–95.

35 **Al-Saady NM**, Blackmore CM, Bennett ED. High fat, low carbohydrate, enteral feeding lowers PaCO₂ and reduces the period of ventilation in artificially ventilated patients. *Intensive Care Med* 1989;**15**:290–5.

36 **King BK**, Kudsk KA, Li J, et al. Route and type of nutrition influence mucosal immunity to bacterial pneumonia. *Ann Surg* 1999;**229**:272–8.

37 **Chang DW**, DeSanti L, Demling RH. Anticatabolic and anabolic strategies in critical illness: a review of current treatment modalities. *Shock* 1998;**10**:155–60.

38 **Zaloga GP**. Dietary lipids: ancestral ligands and regulators of cell signaling pathways. *Crit Care Med* 1999;**27**:1646–8.

39 **Gadek JE**, DeMichele SJ, Karlstad MD, et al. Effect of enteral feeding with eicosapentaenoic acid, gamma-linolenic acid, and antioxidants in patients with acute respiratory distress syndrome. Enteral Nutrition in ARDS Study Group. *Crit Care Med* 1999;**27**:1409–20.

40 **Beale RJ**, Bryg DJ, Bihari DJ. Immunonutrition in the critically ill: a systematic review of clinical outcome. *Crit Care Med* 1999;**27**:2799–805.

41 **Silverman HJ**, Slotman G, Bone RC, et al. Effects of prostaglandin E1 on oxygen delivery and consumption in patients with the adult respiratory distress syndrome. Results from the prostaglandin E1 multicenter trial. The Prostaglandin E1 Study Group. *Chest* 1990;**98**:405–10.

42 **Holcroft JW**, Vassar MJ, Weber CJ. Prostaglandin E1 and survival in patients with the adult respiratory distress syndrome. A prospective trial. *Ann Surg* 1986;**203**:371–8.

43 **Bone RC**, Slotman G, Maunder R, et al. Randomized double-blind, multicenter study of prostaglandin E1 in patients with the adult respiratory

distress syndrome. Prostaglandin E1 Study Group. *Chest* 1989;**96**:114–9.

44 **Abraham E**, Park YC, Covington P, et al. Liposomal prostaglandin E1 in acute respiratory distress syndrome: a placebo-controlled, randomized, double-blind, multicenter clinical trial. *Crit Care Med* 1996;**24**:10–5.

45 **Abraham E**, Baughman R, Fletcher E, et al. Liposomal prostaglandin E1 (TLC C-53) in acute respiratory distress syndrome: a controlled, randomized, double-blind, multicenter clinical trial. TLC C-53 ARDS Study Group. *Crit Care Med* 1999;**27**:1478–85.

46 **Leff JA**, Baer JW, Kirkman JM, et al. Liposome-entrapped PGE1 posttreatment decreases IL-1 alpha-induced neutrophil accumulation and lung leak in rats. *J Appl Physiol* 1994;**76**:151–7.

47 **Petrak RA**, Balk RA, Bone RC. Prostaglandins, cyclo-oxygenase inhibitors, and thromboxane synthetase inhibitors in the pathogenesis of multiple systems organ failure. *Crit Care Clin* 1989;**5**:303–14.

48 **Hechtman HB**, Valeri CR, Shepro D. Role of humoral mediators in adult respiratory distress syndrome. *Chest* 1984;**86**:623–7.

49 **Pittet JF**, Mackersie RC, Martin TR, et al. Biological markers of acute lung injury: prognostic and pathogenetic significance. *Am J Respir Crit Care Med* 1997;**155**:1187–205.

50 **Beetens JR**, Loots W, Somers Y, et al. Ketoconazole inhibits the biosynthesis of leukotrienes in vitro and in vivo. *Biochem Pharmacol* 1986;**35**:883–91.

51 **Slotman GJ**, Burchard KW, D'Arezzo A, et al. Ketoconazole prevents acute respiratory failure in critically ill surgical patients. *J Trauma* 1988;**28**:648–54.

52 **Yu M**, Tomasa G. A double-blind, prospective, randomized trial of ketoconazole, a thromboxane synthetase inhibitor, in the prophylaxis of the adult respiratory distress syndrome. *Crit Care Med* 1993;**21**:1635–42.

53 **Sinuff T**, Cook DJ, Peterson JC, et al. Development, implementation, and evaluation of a ketoconazole practice guideline for ARDS prophylaxis. *J Crit Care* 1999;**14**:1–6.

54 **The ARDS Clinical Trials Network**. Ketoconazole for early treatment of acute lung injury and acute respiratory distress syndrome: a randomized controlled trial. The ARDS Network. *JAMA* 2000;**283**:1995–2002.

55 **Quinlan G**, Upton R. Oxidant-antioxidant balance in acute respiratory distress syndrome. In: Evans T, Griffiths M, Keogh B, eds. *European Respiratory Monograph: ARDS*. Sheffield: European Respiratory Journals Ltd, 2002.

56 **Pacht ER**, Timerman AP, Lykens MG, et al. Deficiency of alveolar fluid glutathione in patients with sepsis and the adult respiratory distress syndrome. *Chest* 1991;**100**:1397–403.

57 **Bernard GR**. N-acetylcysteine in experimental and clinical acute lung injury. *Am J Med* 1991;**91**:54–9S.

58 **Ortolani O**, Conti A, De Gaudio AR, et al. Protective effects of N-acetylcysteine and rutin on the lipid peroxidation of the lung epithelium during the adult respiratory distress syndrome. *Shock* 2000;**13**:14–8.

59 **Jepsen S**, Herlevsen P, Knudsen P, et al. Antioxidant treatment with N-acetylcysteine during adult respiratory distress syndrome: a prospective, randomized, placebo-controlled study. *Crit Care Med* 1992;**20**:918–23.

60 **Domenighetti G**, Suter PM, Schaller MD, et al. Treatment with N-acetylcysteine during acute respiratory distress syndrome: a randomized, double-blind, placebo-controlled clinical study. *J Crit Care* 1997;**12**:177–82.

61 **Bernard GR**, Wheeler AP, Arons MM, et al. A trial of antioxidants N-acetylcysteine and procysteine in ARDS. The Antioxidant in ARDS Study Group. *Chest* 1997;**112**:164–72.

62 **The ARDS Clinical Trials Network**. Randomized, placebo-controlled trial of lisofylline for early treatment of acute lung injury and acute respiratory distress syndrome. *Crit Care Med* 2002;**30**:1–6.

63 **Anderson BO**, Moore EE, Banerjee A. Phospholipase A₂ regulates critical inflammatory mediators of multiple organ failure. *J Surg Res* 1994;**56**:199–205.

64 **Durham SK**, Selig WM. Phospholipase A₂-induced pathophysiologic changes in the guinea pig lung. *Am J Pathol* 1990;**136**:1283–91.

65 **Kuwabara K**, Furue S, Tomita Y, et al. Effect of methylprednisolone on phospholipase A₂ activity and lung surfactant degradation in acute lung injury in rabbits. *Eur J Pharmacol* 2001;**433**:209–16.

66 **Kim DK**, Fukuda T, Thompson B, et al. Bronchoalveolar lavage fluid phospholipase A₂ activities are increased in human adult respiratory distress syndrome. *Am J Physiol* 1995;**269**:109–18.

67 **Endo S**, Inada K, Nakae H, et al. Plasma levels of type II phospholipase A₂ and cytokines in patients with sepsis. *Res Commun Mol Pathol Pharmacol* 1995;**90**:413–21.

68 **Buchler M**, Deller A, Malfertheiner P, et al. Serum phospholipase A₂ in intensive care patients with peritonitis, multiple injury, and necrotizing pancreatitis. *Klin Wochenschr* 1989;**67**:217–21.

69 **Abraham E**, Naum C, Bandi V, et al. Efficacy and safety of LY315920Na/S-5920, a selective inhibitor of 14-kDa group IIA secretory phospholipase A₂, in patients with suspected sepsis and organ failure. *Crit Care Med* 2003;**31**:718–28.

70 **Fein AM**, Calalang-Colucci MG. Acute lung injury and acute respiratory distress syndrome in sepsis and septic shock. *Crit Care Clin* 2000;**16**:289–317.

71 **Bernard GR**, Wheeler AP, Russell JA, et al. The effects of ibuprofen on the physiology and survival of patients with sepsis. The Ibuprofen in Sepsis Study Group. *N Engl J Med* 1997;**336**:912–8.

72 **McCloskey RV**, Straube RC, Sanders C, et al. Treatment of septic shock with human monoclonal antibody HA-1A. A randomized, double-blind, placebo-controlled trial. CHESS Trial Study Group. *Ann Intern Med* 1994;**121**:1–5.

73 **Ziegler EJ**, Fisher CJ, Jr., Sprung CL, *et al.* Treatment of gram-negative bacteremia and septic shock with HA-1A human monoclonal antibody against endotoxin. A randomized, double-blind, placebo-controlled trial. The HA-1A Sepsis Study Group. *N Engl J Med* 1991;**324**:429–36.

74 **Cohen J**, Carlet J. INTERSEPT: an international, multicenter, placebo-controlled trial of monoclonal antibody to human tumor necrosis factor-alpha in patients with sepsis. International Sepsis Trial Study Group. *Crit Care Med* 1996;**24**:1431–40.

75 **Bernard GR**, Vincent JL, Laterre PF, *et al.* Efficacy and safety of recombinant human activated protein C for severe sepsis. *N Engl J Med* 2001;**344**:699–709.

76 **Lundin S**, Mang H, Smithies M, *et al.* Inhalation of nitric oxide in acute lung injury: results of a European multicentre study. The European Study Group of Inhaled Nitric Oxide. *Intensive Care Med* 1999;**25**:911–9.

77 **Hooper RG**, Kearl RA. Established ARDS treated with a sustained course of adrenocortical steroids. *Chest* 1990;**97**:138–43.

78 **Meduri GU**, Headley S, Tolley E, *et al.* Plasma and BAL cytokine response to corticosteroid rescue treatment in late ARDS. *Chest* 1995;**108**:1315–25.

79 **Biffl WL**, Moore FA, Moore EE, *et al.* Are corticosteroids salvage therapy for refractory acute respiratory distress syndrome? *Am J Surg* 1995;**170**:591–5; discussion 595–6.

80 **Meduri GU**, Chinn AJ, Leeper KV, *et al.* Corticosteroid rescue treatment of progressive fibroproliferation in late ARDS. Patterns of response and predictors of outcome. *Chest* 1994;**105**:1516–27.

81 **Meduri GU**, Belenchia JM, Estes RJ, *et al.* Fibroproliferative phase of ARDS. Clinical findings and effects of corticosteroids. *Chest* 1991;**100**:943–52.

82 **Luce JM**, Montgomery AB, Marks JD, *et al.* Ineffectiveness of high-dose methylprednisolone in preventing parenchymal lung injury and improving mortality in patients with septic shock. *Am Rev Respir Dis* 1988;**138**:62–8.

11 Difficult weaning

J Goldstone

Difficulty in weaning from mechanical ventilation is associated with intrinsic lung disease and/or a prolonged critical illness. After critical illness the incidence of weaning failure varies with 20% of all admissions failing initial weaning.[1][2] The incidence of weaning failure increases in patients who have been ventilated for many weeks but is low (<5%) in patients who undergo elective surgery such as after cardiopulmonary bypass.[3] In a recent audit in our intensive care unit (ICU) of patients who had received mechanical ventilation for more than 72 hours, weaning was the dominant clinical problem during recovery and accounted for over half of the total time spent on the ICU. The mean number of weaning episodes was 5 per patient.

When assessing patients clinically, it is useful to determine whether the patient has yet to start weaning, is in the middle of a weaning attempt, is not yet ready to wean, or will never be able to wean. A simple assessment screen consisting of the concentration of inspired oxygen relative to the arterial oxygen tension, the level of positive end expiratory pressure (PEEP), the amount of sedation, and the inotropic requirements can be performed every day in patients receiving mechanical ventilation. The screen identifies patients who may be successfully weaned and reduces the number of patients receiving mechanical ventilation for more than 21 days.[4] Furthermore, passing the screening test is associated with reduced in-hospital mortality.[4] This chapter concentrates on patients who are difficult to wean from mechanical ventilation, many of whom will have made repeated attempts at weaning.

PREDICTING THE LIKELY SUCCESS OF WEANING

Although much has been written about the assessment of weaning, many studies do not set a numerical threshold for a score which is then tested *prospectively*. This important element of study design has resulted in many papers using retrospective analysis and may in part explain the variability of study results. For example, tachypnoea is an indicator of weaning failure in some studies[5] but not in others.[2]

Apart from study design, other influences are important when interpreting the ability of a test to predict weaning success. Tests should be standardised and reproducible.[6] Although many tests are standardised in the laboratory or in normal subjects, few studies have been performed on standardisation of weaning parameters in the critically ill.[7] Similarly, their reproducibility in the ICU environment is crucial. A further problem is that many studies have been performed on a heterogeneous group of patients.

SIMPLE BEDSIDE TESTS

Spirometric tests of lung function have been used frequently and are often quoted as predictors of weaning. Although early reports suggested that minute ventilation, maximal pressure generation, and the ability to increase minute ventilation (maximal voluntary ventilation) were useful, further studies have not reproduced these findings. Indeed, although some of the commonly used tests have high sensitivity, their specificity is often surprisingly low (table 11.1).

Rapid shallow breathing

A common finding in patients who fail to wean is the early development of rapid shallow breathing when the ventilator is disconnected.[5] This represents the coordinated response of the patient to the ventilatory load applied. The attractive features of this assessment are that it tests the whole ventilatory system and requires that the patient be disconnected from the ventilator, thus indicating whether or not the patient can breathe in a controlled environment. Rapid shallow breathing (frequency divided by tidal volume, f/Vt) is best assessed with the patient breathing with continuous positive airway pressure (CPAP) at the level of PEEP used during mechanical ventilation. Rapid shallow breathing has a sensitivity of 0.97 with a specificity of 0.64.[8] Weaning parameters with a low specificity result in some patients, who are able to breathe independently, being prevented from weaning. By encouraging all patients to be disconnected from the ventilator this may in part be avoided.

Combined tests

Combining measurements may improve one's ability to predict weaning outcome. Sassoon and Mahutte[9] repeated the analysis of rapid shallow breathing but combined it with the occlusion pressure in the first 100 ms ($P_{0.1}$), an index of central drive. At this early phase of respiration, where little length has changed, the pressure generated is related to the degree of stimulation to the respiratory muscles. Although the combination of f/Vt and $P_{0.1}$ provided the most sensitive and specific predictor, receiver operator curve (ROC) analysis showed only a modest gain with the addition of $P_{0.1}$.

Table 11.1 Commonly quoted predictive variables of weaning[8]

Variable	Threshold value	Sensitivity	Specificity
Minute ventilation	15 l/min	0.78	0.18
Maximum inspiratory pressure	−15 cm H_2O	0.97	0.36
Tidal volume	4 ml/kg	1.00	0.11

Threshold value=value beyond which weaning is predicted to fail.

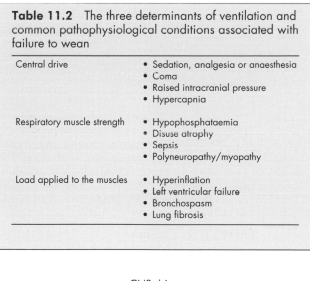

Table 11.2 The three determinants of ventilation and common pathophysiological conditions associated with failure to wean

Central drive	• Sedation, analgesia or anaesthesia • Coma • Raised intracranial pressure • Hypercapnia
Respiratory muscle strength	• Hypophosphataemia • Disuse atrophy • Sepsis • Polyneuropathy/myopathy
Load applied to the muscles	• Hyperinflation • Left ventricular failure • Bronchospasm • Lung fibrosis

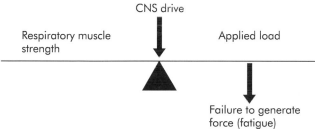

Figure 11.1 Key components of spontaneous breathing. Drive from the central nervous system acts on the peripheral respiratory muscles. The balance between the components can be disordered, leading to fatigue of the respiratory muscles, failure to generate force, and a decrease in alveolar ventilation.

Yang and Tobin[8] devised the CROP index (($Cdyn \times Pimax \times [Pao_2/Pao_2]$)/rate) which consisted of dynamic compliance (Cdyn), maximum mouth pressure (Pimax), oxygenation (Pao_2/Pao_2), and respiratory rate. This was no better than f/Vt alone when assessed prospectively. Measurements integrating ventilatory endurance and the efficiency of gas exchange yield the most successful results but are complex and difficult to use.[10]

COMPONENTS OF WEANING FAILURE

Weaning from mechanical ventilation depends on the strength of the respiratory muscles, the load applied to the muscles, and the central drive (table 11.2). Respiratory failure may result from disorders in one of these three areas—for example, a myopathy reducing strength, acute bronchospasm suddenly increasing load, or opiates acting on the central nervous system. However, it is also possible that disorders of strength and load occur together.

The relationship between these three key components of spontaneous breathing may be visualised as a balance (fig 11.1). If the muscles are heavily loaded, spontaneous contraction cannot be maintained and the muscles may fail acutely. Such acute reversible failure of force generation is termed fatigue. This has been shown in studies of both electromyography (EMG)[11][12] and changes in the relaxation rate of respiratory muscles during weaning.[13] The pathophysiology of weaning failure has been studied in small groups of patients.[13-15] It seems likely that the dominant feature is high levels of load relative to the strength of the respiratory muscles. As weaning progresses, load increases compared with those who succeed a weaning trial. In most cases the drive to breathe is high.[15]

Respiratory muscle strength

Originally the tension of the respiratory muscles was tested in normal subjects by taking maximum pressure measurements at the mouth (Pimax),[16][17] while oesophageal and gastric balloon catheters allow the study of diaphragmatic strength. Contractions of the diaphragm can be obtained by electric or magnetic stimulation of the phrenic nerves.[18][19]

In the intubated patient maximal pressure generation can be assessed during occluded maximal manoeuvres and this can be simply performed as the endotracheal tube is easily accessible. Pimax was originally measured in intubated patients being weaned from mechanical ventilation by Sahn and Lakshminarayan.[1] Patients with severe weakness (Pimax <20 cm H_2O) were unable to wean. However, as a sole indicator of the ability to breathe spontaneously, muscle strength alone may not predict success or failure. Severely weak muscles can only sustain spontaneous breathing if all other factors are entirely normal.

The measurement of respiratory muscle strength on the ICU presents more challenges.[20] Firstly, generating maximal pressure with an artificial airway leads to movement of the endotracheal tube which inhibits maximal pressure generation. Secondly, many patients cannot sustain the one second plateau pressure demanded by the original Pimax protocol.[16] Lastly, few patients can coordinate respiration to ensure that they reach residual volume before maximum inspiratory effort.

In order to improve the ability of patients and normal subjects to perform a maximal inspiratory manoeuvre, brief inspiratory efforts were investigated during gasping against a closed airway with pressure measured in the endotracheal tube.[13][21] Inspiration against an occluded airway is well tolerated by patients provided the technique is well explained and that the gasping does not continue for longer than 20 seconds. An advantage of the gasp is that maximal efforts build up over the 3–8 inspiratory efforts. This technique has been used to measure strength in patients who are not fully conscious, enabling a voluntary estimate to be made in a group of patients who were previously unable to comply with a volitional protocol.[21]

When the reproducibility of the measurement of inspiratory strength was assessed in intubated patients, the between observer, within day, and between day variability of inspiratory efforts were very variable.[22] The observation of a low (weak) inspiratory pressure has to be treated with caution. However, a strong effort is reassuring and unlikely to be an artifact. Finally, non-volitional magnetic stimulation of the diaphragm has been applied to the critically ill. This technique may enable studies to be performed that will address the time course and extent of respiratory and skeletal muscle weakness in critically ill patients.[23]

Aetiology of respiratory muscle weakness in the critically ill

Although most patients are weak, the precise cause of weakness is not always known. Causes of acute weakness include electrolyte disturbances such as hypophosphataemia and hypomagnesaemia. Although electrolyte abnormalities are relatively common on the ICU, their significance in this context is unknown. Long term weakness may be due to critical illness itself. Disuse of skeletal muscles leads to atrophy, where the reduced cross section of the muscle decreases maximum tension. This process is rapid and 7–10 days of disuse may decrease maximum pressure generation by the diaphragm by 50%.[24] Critical illnesses are commonly associated with a polyneuropathy,[25] with or without a myopathy.[26] Such patients may present with extreme weakness, mainly in the legs, and tetraplegia is possible.[27]

If the muscles are weak, can we improve strength with exercise or training? Skeletal muscle responds to training regimens by increasing mass and cross sectional area. For a training regimen to be effective it must be controlled, such that the task is repetitive and supramaximal with periods of rest between training exercises.[28] In addition, strength training differs conceptually and in practice from endurance training.[29] For the respiratory muscles, training is ill defined and although it is felt that the respiratory muscles should behave in a similar manner to other muscle groups, definitive studies have yet to show how they may be trained. It is likely that the response to training will in part be genetically determined. The general observation that some individuals are responsive to and have ability at certain types of exercise has led to studies showing genetic differences in the response to training according to genotype.[30] A genetic polymorphism of the angiotensin converting enzyme (ACE) gene has been described with a 256 base pair deletion or insertion, termed DD or II.[31] In de-trained subjects there is an 11-fold difference between homozygous subgroups in response to performing a repetitive biceps exercise.[30] Recently, respiratory muscle strength and endurance was studied in de-trained subjects who underwent general non-specific training. Respiratory muscle endurance was increased fivefold in the II subgroup.[32]

Central nervous system drive

Although central respiratory drive is not often measured on the ICU, it is possible to measure $P_{0.1}$, an index of drive.[33] $P_{0.1}$ is raised when respiratory drive is artificially increased during a hypercapnic challenge and is also high in patients suffering ventilatory failure.[34] In intubated patients it is often the case that little or no gas flows in the early part of inspiration, if valves are required to open and the speed of response is slow. In such circumstances, patients may be making occluding breathing efforts and $P_{0.1}$ may be measured within the airway automatically by the ventilator.[35]

Can $P_{0.1}$ be used to assess weaning from mechanical ventilation? It is easy to apply the technique to ventilated patients and, when respiratory drive is raised, the measured pressure exceeds 5.5 cm H_2O. A raised $P_{0.1}$ is associated with failure to wean.[36] Interestingly, patients who are able to breathe during weaning trials not only have a low $P_{0.1}$ but are also able to increase drive and minute ventilation during a hypercapnic challenge.[37] Patients who are able to breathe spontaneously do so with a lower central drive and also have some ventilatory reserve, contrasting with the fixed capacity of patients who fail to wean.

Respiratory drive has been measured in patients receiving pressure support ventilation where the level of pressure support was decreased in stages.[38] It would follow that, as the amount of support decreases, there will be a moment when drive to the muscles increases. In patients who were able to breathe spontaneously, the level of drive remained low. Conversely, in patients who fail to wean, drive increased, often above the level seen previously. It is possible that the level of ventilatory support could be titrated in this manner, keeping the level of drive within the "normal" range for patients on the ICU. A similar approach was used to adjust the level of external PEEP applied to patients with varying degrees of intrinsic PEEP.[39] As the level of external PEEP increased, the ability of the patients to achieve gas flow reduced until the optimum balance of internal and external PEEP was reached (fig 11.2). Respiratory drive increased if external PEEP achieved hyperinflation, enabling the adjustment of external PEEP to the correct level without requiring the difficult measurement of internal PEEP in the spontaneously breathing patient.

Load applied to the muscles

Work is performed when a force moves through a distance and is termed "external" as it may be easily measured. Internal work is performed when there is no movement, when the muscle contracts and produces tension and heat. To calculate external work in the respiratory system, the tidal volume must be integrated with respect to the transpleural pressure generated during the breath. This requires some measure of pleural

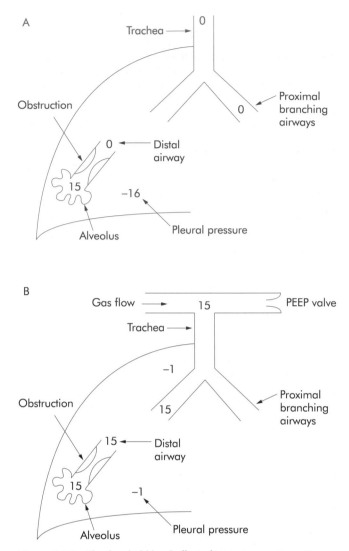

Figure 11.2 The threshold load effect of intrinsic or auto-positive end expiratory pressure (PEEP). When auto-PEEP is high, no gas flow will occur at the mouth until the pressure generated within the chest exceeds the level of intrinsic PEEP. (A) The pressure within the alveolus cannot fall to zero because of the obstruction to expiratory flow. The pressure to begin gas flow must be less than the level of intrinsic PEEP, in this case −16 cm H_2O. (B) External PEEP is applied, balancing the intrinsic PEEP. This has the effect of reducing the pressure required to begin inspiratory flow, in this case from −16 to −1 cm H_2O.

pressure, usually obtained from oesophageal balloon catheters, and simultaneous measurement of volume at the mouth. Internal work can be imagined if there is no gas flow, as occurs in complete obstruction. In this circumstance, energy is dissipated against distortions of the chest wall and no ventilation occurs.

Work is often increased in weaning failure[40][41] and successful weaning occurs when work is reduced. It is possible to monitor work continuously and, in those who fail to wean, pressure generation is significantly higher at the end of the weaning trial, inspiration as a fraction of the respiratory cycle lengthens, and patients are tachypnoeic.

CLINICAL IMPLICATIONS

Exhaustive breathing may damage skeletal muscle fibres and cause a reduction in the ability to generate pressure. Indeed, in healthy volunteers the strength of the diaphragm as judged by magnetic twitch transdiaphragmatic pressure is substantially reduced up to 24 hours after breathing to exhaustion through an inspiratory resistance of 60% of maximal.[42]

Failure to wean from mechanical ventilation does not exclusively affect respiratory muscle performance. The oxygen consumption of muscles can rise considerably and changes in gut mucosal pH indicate that an oxygen debt occurs during failed weaning attempts.[43][44] More organ specific disorders occur when the level of respiratory work is high. In patients at risk of coronary artery disease, weaning precipitates ischaemia[45] which may not be detected at the bedside, particularly if three lead ECG monitoring is used. Weaning is less likely to succeed if myocardial ischaemia occurs.[46] Furthermore, mechanical ventilation supports left ventricular function in patients with incipient heart failure.[47] Hence, invasive haemodynamic measurements and radionuclide imaging in patients showed decreased left ventricular performance and oesophageal pressure, and a 2–3-fold increase in pulmonary artery occlusion pressure when weaning failed. Re-ventilation reversed this effect and subsequent treatment to support the myocardium led to successful weaning. Heart failure in patients who fail to disconnect from mechanical ventilation is an important differential diagnosis.

Triggering mechanical ventilation is an important aspect of setting the ventilator when patients are breathing spontaneously. Triggering from the inspiratory flow reduces work involved in triggering compared with pressure triggering.[48] If the trigger sensitivity is set inappropriately, it is difficult to breathe through the ventilator and, in weak patients, it is possible that no breath is delivered and de-synchrony occurs. Improvements in trigger methodology have decreased inspiratory work, with flow triggering becoming the standard. In health, ventilators can now be set such that almost no work is performed to initiate a breath. Mechanical ventilation in severe lung disease is a greater challenge, especially in obstructive lung diseases where the transmission of the inspiratory effort to the upper airway may be delayed. When the time delay is prolonged, the ventilator senses inspiration at a point when the inspiratory muscles are contracting. Thus, persistent respiratory muscle contraction leads to occult internal work being performed. Instead of conventional triggering at the ventilator end of the airway, sensing inspiration at the distal tip of the endotracheal tube would avoid some of the time delay in patients with chronic obstructive pulmonary disease (COPD). Experimentally, it is possible to compare conventional triggering with triggering at the ventilator, and substantial reductions in the work can be achieved. It is possible to move the inspiratory trigger even closer to the respiratory muscles, offsetting the delay in triggering if pressure is sensed within the chest. Oesophageal triggering has recently been found to reduce total inspiratory work in normal volunteers.[49]

RECENT ADVANCES IN MECHANICAL VENTILATION
Proportional assist ventilation (PAV)
A conventional ventilator has one variable that is determined by the user. For example, in the pressure control mode the airway pressure can be manipulated. During the breath the volume delivered to the patient depends on the mechanics of the lung and chest wall. With PAV the ventilator measures the compliance and resistance of the system during each breath. The ventilator can then be set to deliver the pressure required for a given tidal volume, or a proportion of it, depending on the gain of the system set by the operator. PAV can unload the respiratory muscles to a greater extent than other modes of ventilation. It can compensate for dynamic changes in resistance and compliance and allow the patient to vary tidal breathing, maintaining the amount of intrinsic muscle effort set by the operator.[50][51] Similar technology can be applied to the work required to breathe through an endotracheal tube. By measuring the resistance and compliance of a standard endotracheal tube, automatic tube compensation (the amount of assistance relative to the inspiratory flow rate) can be provided.[52]

Hyperinflation
Expiratory flow limitation causes hyperinflation and increased resting end expiratory pressure. This is termed auto or intrinsic PEEP,[53] and it acts as a load during inspiration as the patient must generate a negative pressure equal to the level of auto-PEEP in order to generate gas flow at the mouth that triggers inspiration. Asynchrony with the ventilator may be caused by excessive auto-PEEP and may be resolved by matching the external applied PEEP to balance the system.[54] In normal subjects, such a load would be easily borne. For example, an average level of intrinsic PEEP of 11 cm H_2O is a small fraction of the total pressure generating ability. However, many intubated patients generate a maximum of –30 cm H_2O. In this context, overcoming the threshold load effect of intrinsic PEEP uses 33% of available pressure generation and may contribute to fatigue.

Techniques of weaning
Important studies in the 1990s established that the mode of ventilation has a major influence on the success of weaning. Brochard *et al*[55] compared weaning by pressure support (PS), T-piece trials, and synchronised intermittent mandatory ventilation (SIMV) in a group of patients who had failed to wean and in whom it was predicted that weaning would be problematic. Over a period of 28 days SIMV was clearly inferior to the other techniques, with an advantage in favour of the PS group. This study also emphasised the importance of a weaning protocol. The Spanish Lung Failure Collaborative Group reported contrasting findings.[56] While SIMV was clearly less favourable, T-piece weaning was advantageous overall. Although both studies showed that SIMV was disadvantageous, the explanation for the differing findings between PS and T-piece weaning may relate to differences in study design. For example, the duration of mechanical ventilation was different between the two studies, with fewer longer term patients in the Spanish study.

Non-invasive ventilation (NIV)
NIV has several advantageous features for weaning patients, including the absence of sedative drugs, early removal of the endotracheal tube, a decrease in ventilator associated pneumonia, and better compliance with chest physiotherapy.[57] These advantages have seldom been studied in a controlled manner and to date the majority of studies have been performed in patients with chronic respiratory failure in an effort to avoid endotracheal intubation.

In 22 patients referred to a specialist chronic ventilation unit for weaning from mechanical ventilation, NIV was rapidly tolerated in 20 and many were extubated quickly.[58] Ten patients required nasal ventilation at night when discharged home. Although this study was not controlled, it certainly shows that patients who are difficult to wean can be extubated and may be managed in a high dependency area using NIV support.

Psychological support
Psychological disturbance occurs during weaning trials and feelings of hopelessness affect performance.[59] Clinically, there appears to be a gap between the physiological testing performed at the bedside and the actual performance of the patient, some of which may be attributable to other factors including personality, fear, agitation, depression, and empowerment.[60] Weaning is associated with depression and treatment may be helpful.[61] An important element of the care of patients during weaning is to devise methods of psychological support.[62] One example is to ask the patient to imagine a particularly strong memory and through rehearsal this fantasy is strengthened. The memory is then used during weaning to allay anxiety and increase tolerance of reductions in ventilatory support.

Specialist weaning units

The demand for ICU beds has led to the development of facilities specialising in weaning.[63 64] Weaning units tend to admit patients with single organ failure who do not require complex organ support. Such units are more cost effective, with dramatic reductions in both the fixed overheads and the consumable cost associated with weaning. Moreover, by concentrating effort in a specialist area and through the development of protocols to guide the weaning effort, it is possible to decrease the time spent on mechanical ventilation.[63 65 66]

REFERENCES

1 **Sahn SA**, Lakshminarayan S. Bedside criteria for discontinuation of mechanical ventilation. *Chest* 1973;**63**:1002–5.
2 **Tahvanainen J**, Salmenpera M, Nikki P. Extubation criteria after weaning from intermittent mandatory ventilation and continuous positive airway pressure. *Crit Care Med* 1983;**11**:702–7.
3 **Demling RH**, Read T, Lind LJ, et al. Incidence and morbidity of extubation failure in surgical intensive care patients. *Crit Care Med* 1988;**16**:573–7.
4 **Ely EW**, Baker AM, Evans GW, et al. The prognostic significance of passing a daily screen of weaning parameters. *Intensive Care Med* 1999;**25**:581–7.
5 **Tobin MJ**, Peres W, Guenther SM, et al. The pattern of breathing during successful and unsuccessful trials of weaning from mechanical ventilation. *Am Rev Respir Dis* 1986;**134**:1111–8.
6 **Yang KL**. Reprodcibility of weaning parameters a need for standerdization. *Chest* 1992;**102**:1829–32.
7 **Yang KL**, Tobin MJ. Measurement of minute ventilation in ventilator dependent patients: need for standardization. *Crit Care Med* 1991;**19**:49–53.
8 **Yang KL**, Tobin MJ. A prospective study of indexes predicting the outcome of trials of weaning from mechanical ventilation. *N Engl J Med* 1991;**324**:1445–50.
9 **Sassoon CSH**, Mahutte CK. Airway occlusion pressure and breathing pattern as predictors of weaning outcome. *Am Rev Respir Dis* 1993;**148**:860–6.
10 **Jabour ER**, Rabil DM, Truwit J, et al. Evaluation of a new weaning index based on ventilatory endurance and the efficiency of gas excahnge. *Am Rev Respir Dis* 1991;**144**:531–7.
11 **Cohen CA**, Zagelbaum G, Gross D, et al. Clinical manifestations of inspiratory muscle fatigue. *Am J Med* 1982;**73**:308–16.
12 **Brochard L**, Harf A, Lorino H, et al. Inspiratory pressure support prevents diaphragmatic fatigue during weaning from mechanical ventilation. *Am Rev Respir Dis* 1989;**139**:513–21.
13 **Goldstone JC**, Green M, Moxham J. Maximum relaxation rate of the diaphragm during weaning from mechanical ventilation. *Thorax* 1994;**49**:54–60
14 **Jubran A**, Tobin MJ. Pathophysiologic basis of acute respiratory distress in patients who fail a trial of weaning from mechanical ventilation. *Am J Respir Crit Care Med* 1997;**155**:906–15.
15 **Purro A**, Appendini L, de Gaetano A, et al. Pathophysiologic determinants of weaning. *Am J Respir Crit Care Med* 2000;**161**:1115–23.
16 **Black LF**, Hyatt RE. Maximal respiratory pressures: normal values and relationship to age and sex. *Am Rev Respir Dis* 1969;**99**:696–702.
17 **Kim MJ**, Druz WS, Danon J, et al. Mechanics of the canine diaphragm. *J Appl Physiol* 1976;**41**:369–82.
18 **Similowski TB**, Fleury S, Launois HP, et al. Cervical magnetic stimulation: a new painless method for bilateral phrenic nerve stimulation in conscious humans. *J Appl Physiol* 1989;**67**:1311–8.
19 **Polkey MI**, Duguet A, Luo Y, et al. Anterior magnetic phrenic nerve stimulation: laboratory and clinical evaluation. *Intensive Care Med* 2000;**26**:1065–75.
20 **Moxham J**, Goldstone JC. Assessment of respiratory muscle strength in the intensive care unit. *Eur Respir J* 1994;**7**:2057–61.
21 **Marini JJ**, Smith TC, Lamb V. Estimation of inspiratory muscle strength in mechanically ventilated patients: measurement of maximum inspiratory pressure. *J Crit Care* 1988;**1**:32–8.
22 **Multz AS**, Aldrich TK, Prezant DJ, et al. Maximal inspiratory pressure is not a reliable test of inspiratory muscle strength in mechanically ventilated patients. *Am Rev Respir Dis* 1990;**142**:529–32.
23 **Watson AC**, Hughes PD, Harris L, et al. Measurement of twitch transdiaphragmatic, esophageal and endo-tracheal tube pressure with bilateral anterolateral magnetic phrenic nerve stimulation in patients in the intensive care unit. *Crit Care Med* 2001;**29**:1476–8.
24 **Anzueto A**, Peters JI, Tobin MJ, et al. Effects of prolonged controlled mechanical ventilation on diaphragmatic function in healthy adult baboons. *Crit Care Med* 1997;**25**:1187–90.
25 **Bolton CF**. Neuromuscular complications of sepsis. *Intensive Care Med* 1993;**19**:S58–63.
26 **Coakley JH**, Nagendran K, Yarwood GD, et al. Patterns of neurophysiological abnormality in prolonged critical illness. *Intensive Care Med* 1998;**24**:801–7.
27 **Kennedy DD**, Fletcher SN, Ghosh IR, et al. Reversible tetraplegia due to polyneuropathy in a diabetic patient with hyperosmolar non-ketotic coma. *Intensive Care Med* 1999;**25**:1437–9.

28 **Rochester DF**, Arora NS. Respiratory muscle failure. *Med Clin North Am* 1983;**67**:573–97.
29 **Leith DE**, Bradley M. Ventilatory muscle strength and endurance training. *J Appl Physiol* 1976;**41**:508–16.
30 **Williams AG**, Rayson MP, Jubb M, et al. The ACE gene and muscle performance. *Nature* 2000;**403**:614.
31 **Woods DR**, Humphries SE, Montgomery HE. The ACE I/D polymorphism and human physical performance. *Trends Endocrinol Metab* 2000;**11**:416–20.
32 **Chieveley-Williams S**, Field D, Woods D, et al. Genetic determinants of respiratory muscle training. *Am J Respir Crit Care Med* 2001;**163**:A287.
33 **Whitelaw WA**, Derenne JP, Milic-Emili J. Occlusion pressure as a measure of respiratory center output in conscious man. *Respir Physiol* 1975;**23**:181–99.
34 **Murciano D**, Boczkowski J, Lecocguic Y, et al. Tracheal occlusion pressure: a simple index to monitor respiratory muscle failure in patients with chronic obstructive pulmonary disease. *Ann Intern Med* 1988;**108**:800–5.
35 **Kuhlen R**, Hausmann S, Pappert D, et al. A new method for $P_{0.1}$ measurement using standard respiratory equipment. *Intensive Care Med* 1995;**21**:545–6.
36 **Sassoon CSH**, Te TT, Mahutte CK, et al. Airway occlusion pressure: an important indicator for successful weaning in patients with chronic obstructive pulmonary disease. *Am Rev Respir Dis* 1987;**135**:107–13.
37 **Montgomery AB**, Holle RHO, Neagley SR, et al. Prediction of successful ventilator weaning using airway occlusion pressure and hypercapnic challenge. *Chest* 1987;**91**:496–9.
38 **Alberti A**, Gallo F, Fongaro A, et al. $P_{0.1}$ is a useful parameter in setting the level of pressure support ventilation. *Intensive Care Med* 1995;**21**:547–53.
39 **Mancebo J**, Albaladejo P, Touchard D, et al. Airway occlusion pressure to titrate positive end-expiratory pressure in patients with dynamic hyperinflation. *Anesthesiology* 2000;**93**:81–90.
40 **Fiastro JF**, Habib MP, Shon BY, et al. Comparison of standard weaning parameters and the mechanical work of breathing in mechanically ventilated patients. *Chest* 1988;**94**:232–8.
41 **Shikora A**, Bistrian BR, Borlase BC, et al. Work of breathing: reliable predictor of weaning and extubation. *Crit Care Med* 1990;**18**:157–62.
42 **Laghi F**, D'Alfonso N, Tobin MJ. Pattern of recovery from diaphragmatic fatigue over 24 hours. *J Appl Physiol* 1995;**79**:539–46.
43 **Hurtado FJ**, Beron M, Olivera W, et al. Gastric intramucosal pH and intraluminal PCO_2 during weaning from mechanical ventilation. *Crit Care Med* 2001;**29**:70–6.
44 **Maldonado A**, Bauer TT, Ferrer M, et al. Capnometric recirculation gas tonometry and weaning from mechanical ventilation. *Am J Respir Crit Care Med* 2000;**161**:171–6.
45 **Abalos A**, Leibowitz AB, Distefano D, et al. Myocardial ischemia during the weaning period. *Am J Crit Care* 1992;**1**:32–6.
46 **Srivastava S**, Chatila W, Amoateng-Adjepong Y, et al. Myocardial ischemia and weaning failure in patients with coronary artery disease: an update. *Crit Care Med* 1999;**27**:2109–12.
47 **Lemaire F**, Teboul JL, Cinotti L, et al. Acute left ventricular dysfunction during unsuccessful weaning from mechanical ventilation. *Anesthesiology* 1988;**69**:171–9.
48 **Polese G**, Massara A, Poggi R, et al. Flow triggering reduces inspiratory effort during weaning from mechanical ventilation. *Intensive Care Med* 1995;**21**:682–6.
49 **Barnard M**, Shukla A, Lovell T, et al. Esophageal-directed pressure support ventilation in normal volunteers. *Chest* 1999;**115**:482–9.
50 **Ranieri VM**, Giuliani R, Mascia L, et al. Patient-ventilator interaction during acute hypercapnia: pressure-support vs. proportional assist ventilation. *J Appl Physiol* 1996;**81**:426–36.
51 **Grasso S**, Puntillo F, Mascia L, et al. Compensation for increase in respiratory workload during mechanical ventilation: pressure-support versus proportional-assist ventilation. *Am J Respir Crit Care Med* 2000;**161**:819–26.
52 **Fabry B**, Haberthur C, Zappe D, et al. Breathing pattern and additional work of breathing in spontaneously breathing patients with different ventilatory demands during inspiratory pressure support ventilation and automatic tube compensation. *Intensive Care Med* 1997;**23**:545–52.
53 **Pepe PE**, Marini JJ. Occult positive end-expiratory pressure in mechanically ventilated patients with airflow obstruction: the auto-PEEP effect. *Am Rev Respir Dis* 1982;**126**:166–70.
54 **Tobin M**. PEEP, auto-PEEP and waterfalls. *Chest* 1989;**96**:449–51.
55 **Brochard L**, Rauss A, Benito S, et al. Comparison of three methods of gradual withdrawal from ventilatory support during weaning from mechanical ventilation. *Am J Respir Crit Care Med* 1994;**150**:896–903.
56 **Esteban A**, Frutos F, Tobin MJ, et al. A comparison of four methods of weaning patients from mechanical ventilation. *N Engl J Med* 1995;**332**:345–50.
57 **Goldstone JC**. Non invasive ventilation in the intensive care unit and operating theatre. In: Simonds AK, ed. *Non invasive respiratory support*. London: Chapman & Hall, 1996.
58 **Udwadia ZF**, Santis GK, Steven MH, et al. Nasal ventilation to facilitate weaning in patients with chronic respiratory insufficiency. *Thorax* 1992;**47**:715–8.
59 **Moody LE**, Lowry L, Yarandi H, et al. Psychophysiologic predictors of weaning from mechanical ventilation in chronic bronchitis and emphysema. *Clin Nurs Res* 1997;**6**:311–30.
60 **Engstrom CP**, Persson LO, Larsson S, et al. Health-related quality of life in COPD: why both disease-specific and generic measures should be used. *Eur Respir J* 2001;**18**:69–76.

61 **Rothenhausler HB**, Ehrentrault S, von Gegenfeld G, *et al*. Treatment of depression with methylphenidate in patients difficult to wean from mechanical ventilation in the intensive care unit. *J Clin Psychiatry* 2000;**61**:750–5.

62 **Miller JF**. Hope-inspiring strategies of the critically ill. *Appl Nurs Res* 1989;**2**:23–9.

63 **Dasgupta A**, Rice R, Mascha E, *et al*. Four-year experience with a unit for long-term ventilation (respiratory special care unit) at the Cleveland Clinic Foundation. *Chest* 1999;**116**:447–55.

64 **Seneff MG Wagner D**, Thompson D, *et al*. The impact of long-term acute-care facilities on the outcome and cost of care for patients undergoing prolonged mechanical ventilation. *Crit Care Med* 2000;**28**:342–50.

65 **Henneman E**, Dracup K, Ganz T, *et al*. Effect of a collaborative weaning plan on patient outcome in the critical care setting. *Crit Care Med* 2001;**29**:297–303.

66 **Marelich GP**, Murin S, Battistella F, *et al*. Protocol weaning of mechanical ventilation in medical and surgical patients by respiratory care practitioners and nurses: effect on weaning time and incidence of ventilator-associated pneumonia. *Chest* 2000;**118**:459–67.

12 Critical care management of respiratory failure resulting from chronic obstructive pulmonary disease

A C Davidson

Acute episodes of respiratory failure in patients with chronic obstructive pulmonary disease (COPD) account for 5–10% of emergency medical admissions to hospital and failure of first line treatment is a common reason for referral to the intensive care unit (ICU). In recent years such patients have become better characterised and the driving force in this has been the need to define those suitable for treatment by non-invasive ventilation (NIV) rather than intubation. Bacterial infection has traditionally been considered aetiologically dominant but its importance has been over stressed. Heart failure, cardiac arrhythmia, pulmonary embolism, and "uncertain causes" are common.[1] Acute deterioration precipitated by viral infection is increasingly recognised.[2] Consideration of all the ways in which the co-morbidity of COPD influences ICU management is beyond the scope of this chapter. Its presence affects both ventilator strategy and the outcome of patients after elective or emergency surgery. COPD also contributes to delay in the weaning of patients from mechanical ventilation.[3–5] This chapter focuses on the common problem of the patient with respiratory failure arising from an exacerbation of chronic airflow obstruction.

In the past the perception that survival of patients with COPD was poor, especially long term, combined with insufficient provision of critical care facilities in the UK has limited access to the ICU. This was especially so when "end stage" COPD was considered to be present. This might be inferred if there is no apparent precipitating cause such as pneumonia or pneumothorax. In these circumstances, as there is no apparent reversible cause, it could be argued that recovery is unlikely. Survival following mechanical ventilation (MV) is, however, better in the absence of a major precipitating cause.[1] This apparent paradox probably arises because patients who require a longer period of ventilatory support—which will be the case if, for instance, pneumonia is present—are exposed to the secondary complications of ICU admission. Just as survival in the acute respiratory distress syndrome is more closely related to associated multiorgan failure or nosocomial infection than to the severity of the initial lung injury,[6] so the complications that arise during the ICU stay of a patient with COPD may have a greater influence on outcome than the severity of airflow obstruction. Nevertheless, age, severity of airflow obstruction, co-morbidity, and general pre-admission health status are important in determining survival.[1 7–10]

There are national and international differences in both the institution and withdrawal of MV in COPD. The prevalence of COPD in the community and admission practices will determine how costly ICU management of COPD will be locally. For instance, in one patient simulation study there was considerable variation in prognostic estimates by respondents for identical clinical scenarios.[11] The prognosis predicted markedly affected willingness to offer hypothetical ICU admission and the estimates were uniformly worse than US outcome prediction data would suggest. In one UK report withdrawal of treatment was the most common cause of death,[12] while in an Italian study two thirds of patients were still being actively weaned 60 days after admission.[13] The European Human Rights Act[14] might increase the pressure to admit patients to the ICU and there is some evidence that this is occurring. This is probably desirable in the UK where, in the past, respiratory physicians may not have sufficiently championed the cause of the patient with COPD. Short term survival following invasive MV can be expected in 63–86%,[1 7–10 15] a figure well above that for unplanned medical admissions. Although long term survival is less good—in one study 52%, 42%, and 37% at 1, 2 and 3 years, respectively[15]—this is similar to survival following myocardial infarction when left ventricular dysfunction is present. A better long term outcome is reported following an episode of respiratory failure managed with NIV.[16–18] It is also possible that survival may subsequently be improved by domiciliary NIV in selected patients,[19] although interim results of controlled trials of domiciliary ventilation have been negative.

Despite reasonable survival to hospital discharge, the decision to admit to the ICU in advanced cases is frequently difficult[20] and involves balancing health status with an estimate of expectation of survival and quality of life issues. This often needs to be established on the basis of scant information and in the face of sometimes unreasonable expectations from distraught relatives. Furthermore, these difficult decisions commonly fall on the least experienced doctors as hospital presentation is often "out of hours". A recent report found that co-morbidity, need for MV beyond 72 hours, and failure following extubation were strong predictors of a poor outcome.[10] Survival to discharge for the whole group (166 patients) was 72% and increased to 88% in those without co-morbidity. This report therefore suggests that an active policy, with early review once MV has been initiated, may be appropriate. Ideally, the value and complications of MV should be discussed prior to the medical emergency.[21] Such discussion may be difficult to initiate in the outpatient clinic and primary care is probably a better setting. The recovery period following a period of MV is an ideal opportunity and it is well suited for inclusion in rehabilitation programmes,[22] but resistance to such discussion is common, at least in the UK.[23]

Box 12.1 Mechanisms involved in decompensated COPD

Increased resistive load
- Widespread airflow obstruction

Decreased respiratory system compliance
- High lung volume

Dynamic hyperinflation
- Shortened expiratory time
- Poorly emptying lung units

Reduced power of respiratory pump
- Impaired mechanical efficiency
- Effects of acidosis and hypoxaemia

Impaired drive
- Sleep deprivation
- CO_2 narcosis

Box 12.2 Contraindications to NIV

- Impaired consciousness (except O_2 induced)
- Uncooperative patient
- Significant vomiting risk
- Cardiac arrythmia or hypotension (if severe)
- Profound hypoxaemia (unless in ICU)
- Excessive secretions

RECOGNISING THE NEED FOR VENTILATORY SUPPORT

The recognition that MV is required is commonly an "end of the bed" assessment by an experienced clinician. No one clinical feature or investigation is absolute except respiratory arrest or loss of consciousness.[20] In most cases failure to improve with medical treatment in the hours following admission triggers ICU referral. Late failure several days after admission to hospital is less common and may indicate a worse prognosis.[24] In many, a downward spiral of increasing carbon dioxide retention and sleep deprivation eventually leads to impaired consciousness as the ventilatory pump fails to cope with the increased respiratory "load". The mechanisms involved in decompensated COPD (box 12.1) are an increase in airflow resistance related to widespread bronchial wall inflammation and progressive dynamic hyperinflation that maximises expiratory flow at the cost of increasing inspiratory muscle work.[25] [26]

In addition to this resistive work, reduced respiratory system compliance associated with operating towards the top of the pressure-volume curve is combined with decreased mechanical efficiency of the diaphragm at high lung volumes. Premature expiratory closure of small airways, either because of lack of support in emphysema or functional narrowing from airway inflammation or smooth muscle contraction, results in impaired gas exchange. Positive end expiratory intrathoracic pressure—so called intrinsic PEEP—further loads the inspiratory muscles. Recruitment of abdominal muscles during expiration is common. This may not increase expiratory airflow as dynamic expiratory resistance, the choke effect, may occur and will then only accentuate gas trapping. Sudden relaxation of abdominal muscle contraction at end expiration, a feature of the failing patient, may be employed to unload the inspiratory muscles by natural recoil at the start of inspiration.[25] Additionally, as respiratory rate increases, gas exchange is further impaired by increased dead space ventilation and further muscle loading is the result of additional dynamic hyperinflation as expiratory time shortens. Increased pulmonary vascular resistance and reduced venous return impair right heart function and decrease cardiac output. Inadequate systemic oxygen delivery to meet energy requirements then adds a metabolic component to the respiratory acidosis. Hypoxaemia and acidosis further impair respiratory muscle function.[27] Unless controlled oxygen therapy, bronchodilators, and fluid replacement can both improve gas exchange and reduce the load on the respiratory muscles, mechanical ventilatory support will be required.

At what stage in this process should intervention occur and how can this state be recognised? The need for MV is better predicted by arterial pH and carbon dioxide ($Paco_2$) levels than the degree of hypoxaemia. For instance, in a study investigating the value of NIV in acute COPD, 74% of patients randomised to management without NIV (mean pH 7.26) reached the a priori criteria for tracheal intubation.[16] The use of uncontrolled oxygen therapy may have precipitated further deterioration in this study, resulting in a high frequency of ventilatory support. In a similar study which included less severely affected patients,[17] 27% of patients with a ward admission pH of 7.25–7.35 progressed to fulfil intubation criteria compared with 36% of those with a pH of <7.25. Soo Hoo et al[9] found a higher overall need for intubation at 54% with a 70% risk in those with an initial pH <7.2. Subsequent multivariate analysis from the study by Plant et al[28] reveals that both pH and $Paco_2$ levels contribute to risk, although the sensitivity and specificity of these factors alone do not allow sufficiently accurate prediction on an individual basis. For instance, the odds ratio for reaching intubation criteria for a patient with an arterial pH of 7.30 and $Paco_2$ 8 kPa was 3.84 compared with 16.8 for pH 7.25 and $Paco_2$ 10 kPa. Data from this study also showed that pH often improves between arrival in the emergency department and ward admission with conventional non-ventilator management. Accordingly, in the absence of a clear need for tracheal intubation such as a Glasgow coma score of <8 or respiratory rate >40 or <10, conservative therapy or the use of NIV may be used initially. Usually, it is the failure to improve that signals the need for assisted ventilation.[20] [29]

MODES OF VENTILATORY SUPPORT
Non-invasive ventilation

Several studies have demonstrated the superiority of NIV over tracheal intubation and MV in acute COPD.[16] [17] [28] [30] NIV is indicated after initial treatment if the pH remains <7.30 and after exclusion of reversible precipitating causes such as a pneumothorax, the depressant effect of uncontrolled oxygen therapy, or the excessive use of sedatives. Depending on the circumstances, NIV may be delivered either in the admissions ward, HDU, or the respiratory ward.[29] Generally accepted exclusions to the use of NIV (box 12.2) are impaired consciousness (with uncontrolled oxygen therapy as an exception), vomiting, cardiovascular compromise, and the uncooperative patient.

The benefit of NIV in patients with more profound acidosis (pH <7.25) is unclear.[17] In such patients NIV should, ideally, only be used in the ICU so that tracheal intubation can be rapidly performed. The decision about the appropriateness of resuscitation, which necessarily includes intubation, should be made at the start of ventilatory support. In some patients NIV may be the "ceiling" of therapy, depending on co-morbidity, the presence of reversible factors, and consideration of health status or advance directives. It should be remembered that NIV fails in up to 30% of patients,[16] [29] with a significant proportion being late failures.[24] Failure with NIV may result from a number of causes including patient intolerance because there is inadequate offloading of the respiratory muscles. This may arise when there is a failure of triggering with the spontaneous mode of ventilatory support. Alternatively, there may be inadequate augmentation of tidal volume because of insufficient pressure, autotriggering arising from excessive trigger sensitivity with bi-level ventilators, or machine delivered breaths that are not synchronised with glottic opening. In the patient naïve to NIV, a full face mask is

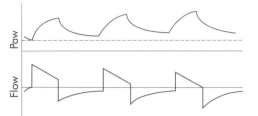

Figure 12.1 Progressive hyperinflation results from either excessive tidal volume or insufficient expiratory time, or both. If machine delivered breath occurs before flow has ceased (positive end expiratory pressure, PEEP), peak airway pressure (Paw) will increase and tidal volume will fall as progressive hyperinflation develops. If this results from premature airway collapse, externally applied PEEP will increase tidal volume without an increase in Paw.

usually required but leaking is then more problematic and this may also affect ventilator triggering. Not uncommonly, apparent early success is not matched by a fall in the $Paco_2$. Rebreathing with the increased dead space of a face mask may be the cause, but an ineffective cough and retained bronchial secretions are more commonly responsible. In these situations a nose mask and chin strap may be beneficial by allowing spontaneous coughing. Excessive secretions may also cause impairment of gas exchange resulting in refractory hypoxaemia.

Monitoring the impact of NIV is essential. A greater expansion of the chest during assisted breathing should be the primary aim with good matching of the patient's breathing effort with the ventilator or effective ventilation with machine timed breaths. Whichever mode is employed, a reduction in respiratory distress is an important prognostic feature and both cardiac and respiratory rate will fall with a gradual reversal of respiratory acidosis when NIV is effective. In our experience the need for frequent arterial blood gas analysis and appropriate monitoring of physiological variables is best provided in the HDU or level 2 facility. In some hospitals, where specialist medical wards are available, NIV may be provided in level 1 beds. This is particularly the case when used in patients with less physiological disturbance such as a higher pH, using spontaneous mode only ventilators.[17] With increased recognition of the value of NIV in such patients, greater availability of equipment and the necessary skill mix of staff required, NIV will hopefully be effectively used outside the ICU. Excellent reviews and comprehensive guidelines for NIV are available.[29 30]

Tracheal intubation and mechanical ventilation

Impending cardiorespiratory arrest is indicated by profound hypoxaemia on disconnection from oxygen or NIV, significant hypotension, or an altered mental state. Immediate intubation may then be required. As cardiovascular collapse is common after intubation, transfer of the spontaneously breathing patient to the ICU may, however, be safer. Collapse arises from a combination of reduced venous return secondary to positive intrathoracic pressure, and direct vasodilation and reduced sympathetic tone induced by sedative agents. Before intubation pre-oxygenation is essential. Intubation with the rapid sequence induction and cricoid pressure to reduce the risk of aspiration should ideally be performed by an experienced clinician. Suxamethonium is classically used for muscle relaxation as its short effect makes it safer in the event of a failure to intubate. Concerns about hyperkalaemic cardiac arrest[31] have led to the increased use of short acting non-depolarising agents such as rocuronium. Doubts about the effectiveness of cricoid pressure in preventing aspiration[32] have also resulted in a move to "head up" non-paralytic intubation. This is a high risk period in which profound hypotension may result in cardiac arrhythmia or arrest. Unless hypotension resolves rapidly

with fluid replacement, cardiac tamponade induced by hyperinflation (bagging) should be suspected. In these circumstances, temporary disconnection of the endotracheal tube from positive pressure will lead to a return in cardiac output.

Controlled mechanical ventilation

Having secured the airway and corrected hypoxaemia, management is aimed at correcting the respiratory acidosis while avoiding further hyperinflation. This is best achieved by a combination of slow MV with a prolonged expiratory time and a limited tidal volume. A degree of permissive hypercapnia is well tolerated,[33] while bronchial toilet and bronchodilation—usually with a combination of intravenous and nebulised agents—will improve alveolar ventilation. The benefit of steroids has been established in acute COPD,[34] but these probably take hours to effect an improvement. Inotropes such as epinephrine (adrenaline) are well known to cause a metabolic acidosis but this may also occur with β_2 stimulants, largely by stimulating metabolism.[35] In the first 12–24 hours of MV, paralysis is normally required. This reduces the chest and abdominal wall contributions to the reduced respiratory system compliance and prevents patient ventilator dysynchrony or fighting, which will impair alveolar ventilation and result in high airway pressures. Airflow resistance and hyperinflation both contribute to the need for high inflation pressures to achieve an effective tidal volume and these may progressively increase if the set ventilatory parameters are causing further hyperinflation (see fig 12.1). The immediate complications of high airway pressures are impaired cardiac output, pneumothorax, and mediastinal and subcutaneous emphysema.

The ventilator may be set either to control volume or pressure. In volume controlled ventilation, conventional settings would be a tidal volume of 8–12 ml/kg at a frequency of 10–14 breaths/minute and an inspiratory:expiratory (I: E) ratio of 1:2.5 or 3.0. The disadvantage of volume control is the potential for high airway pressures; pressure limitation provides protection and is available on most modern machines. Alternatively, pressure controlled ventilation may be preferred as high airway pressures are avoided and the inspiratory flow pattern, which better resembles normal breathing, tends to equalise ventilation between lung units rather than preferentially ventilating, and possibly overinflating, the less obstructed (or faster filling and emptying) lung units (fig 12.2). This mode of ventilation has gained favour as it has become recognised that additional lung injury may result from relatively high tidal volumes that accompany the use of high ventilatory pressures rather than from high airway pressure per se.[36] Although the importance of this concept has so far only been demonstrated in ARDS where a reduced mortality accompanies limited tidal volume ventilation,[37] the same mechanisms probably operate in other indications for MV.

The use of PEEP when ventilating patients with airflow obstruction is controversial. It was argued that externally applied positive airway pressure (PEEPe) would be harmful as it would increase hyperinflation. When small airway collapse develops during expiration from the structural changes associated with emphysema, the application of PEEPe will reduce gas trapping by stenting open the airways. The value of PEEPe to offset intrinsic PEEP is also important when supporting spontaneous breathing and is considered below. In controlled ventilation, a practical method to judge its use is to monitor tidal volume and airway pressure (PEEPi). As PEEPe is applied, tidal volume will increase without an increase in airway pressure until PEEPe exceeds PEEPi . Intrinsic PEEP can be measured by measuring plateau pressure following a prolonged expiratory pause, so called static PEEPi (see fig 12.3).[38] Intrinsic PEEP will, however, be overestimated if there is active abdominal expiratory effort. Accurate measurement of dynamic PEEP (PEEPi dyn) in spontaneously breathing

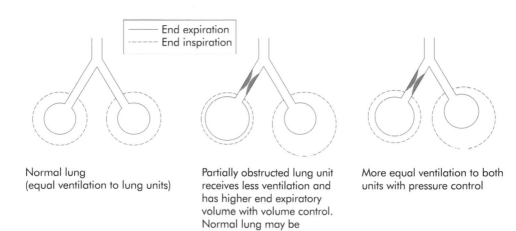

Figure 12.2   Improved distribution of ventilation with pressure controlled mandatory ventilation.

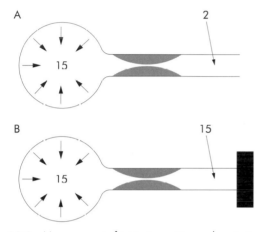

Figure 12.3   Measurement of intrinsic positive end expiratory pressure (PEEPi). (A) Tracheal end expiratory pressure is low with open expiratory port. (B) Measurement of auto-PEEP or intrinsic PEEP by occlusion of expiratory port at end expiration. The balloon represents the ventilated lung with expiratory flow obstruction. Intrinsic PEEP will be overestimated if there is active abdominal muscle contraction.

patients is more difficult and requires simultaneous measurement of gastric pressure (Pga) when PEEPi = PEEPi dyn – Pga.[39]

Assisted modes of ventilatory support

In many patients correction of acidosis and the need for a high inspired oxygen concentration (Fio$_2$) rapidly resolves. Spontaneous breathing may still be inadequate but partial ventilatory support is possible with synchronised intermittent mandatory ventilation (SIMV). It provides a background of machine delivered breaths whilst spontaneous breathing effort is enhanced by positive pressure (pressure support) acting to increase the tidal volume of such triggered breaths. These breaths then delay the next machine delivered breath (synchronisation). It would seem an attractive mode during the weaning period. Excessive amounts of respiratory work may, however, occur with SIMV[40] unless attention is paid to optimise triggering by adjustment of PEEPe, and to titrate the degree of pressure support. At this point, knowing the level of PEEPi is useful but more difficult to measure.[39] By adjusting PEEPe to approximate PEEPi, the inspiratory pressure required to trigger a breath can be reduced (gas flow cannot begin until a negative deflection in airway pressure is registered by the ventilator). Flow triggers are more sensitive than pressure triggers but are only available on newer ventilators. A bias flow, usually 1–5 l/min, is provided by the ventilator during expiration. When the flow signal changes with the onset of inspiration, the ventilator is triggered to deliver pressure support.

An additional cause of patient distress may, however, occur before the ventilator begins to provide flow. If the inspiratory flow rate, which commonly has a default setting of 60–80 l/min, is insufficient for patient demand (which may be up to 120 l/min), a sense of "air hunger" occurs which may result in premature cessation of inspiratory effort. On the other hand, if the mandatory machine delivered breaths are too large or too long, expiratory effort will occur before the end of inspiration and result in unnecessary work and patient distress. This phenomenon also occurs if the level of support is excessive (to ensure a "normal" tidal volume). Disentangling the primary problem leading to patient-ventilator dysynchrony versus more straightforward causes such as the discomfort of the endotracheal tube or anxiety may be difficult.[41] Accordingly, accepting a high respiratory rate and small tidal volume with pressure support may be preferable to SIMV. With either mode, examination of the real time pressure and volume traces, available on modern ventilators, will provide clues to the setting of PEEPe, the presence of inspiratory effort that fails to produce triggering or of expiratory effort before the end of inspiration. Occasionally, however, direct measurement of the oesophageal or gastric pressure is necessary.

One disadvantage of pressure support occurs during sleep when prolonged apnoeic periods, potentiated by lowering Paco$_2$ below normal, may result in repeated ventilator alarms. It is our preference to ensure adequate ventilatory support and allow restorative sleep at night using a controlled mode and then progressively reduce the degree of pressure support during the day. An alternative is to use timed bi-level pressure support[42] which ensures adequate ventilation during sleep and, if adjusted appropriately, comfortable pressure support by day. As this method does not involve triggered breathing (it can be conceptualised as CPAP with a timed higher pressure period superimposed), inadvertent triggering during suctioning or coughing is avoided—another mechanism for patients becoming distressed. With bi-level pressure support (BiPAP) there is the potential for increasing hyperinflation if inappropriate timing results in expiratory effort during the high pressure period.

Although conventional extubation criteria[43] such as an Fio$_2$ of <0.4 and tidal volume >10 ml/kg can be encountered soon after admission to the ICU, up to 30% of patients with COPD meeting such criteria fail in the period following extubation.[44] A significant delay in the weaning process or failure following extubation may result from airflow obstruction, continued hypersecretion, impaired left ventricular function, or over-sedation.[45] Propofol, a short acting sedative, may allow good titration of sedation in the period leading up to extubation and permit good synchrony between patient and ventilator, an essential requirement when deciding upon the likelihood of successful extubation. Nava et al[13] have provided evidence that early extubation is possible in patients who would be at high risk of post extubation failure by using NIV as a bridge. Although another study was unable to confirm more successful weaning with this approach, the use of NIV had some benefits.[46] It is our practice to aim for extubation at the 48–72 hours "window of opportunity" before secondary infections or other complications occur. Should this then fail, especially if stridor from glottic or supraglottic oedema is present after extubation, we proceed immediately to percutaneous tracheostomy on days 3–4 (see below).

NON-VENTILATORY CONSIDERATIONS

Steroids are useful in speeding the resolution of airway inflammation but are implicated in the myopathy associated with critical illness[47] and our practice is to taper the dose rapidly. The value of nebulised steroids has not been established in this situation. Adequate nutritional support is essential but should not be excessive. There is no convincing evidence that manipulation of the metabolic costs of feeding by energy substitution with fats speeds weaning. The risk of nosocomial pneumonia increases with longer ventilatory support. Nursing in the head up position may reduce the incidence,[48] while the risk/benefits of ulcer prophylaxis[49] and gut sterilisation[50] continue to be debated. Adequate hydration is clearly important in mobilising tenacious secretions. Inhaled or nebulised β_2 stimulants are more effective than saline in aiding sputum clearance, and mucolytics such as N-acetyl cysteine or DNase may occasionally be helpful. High inspired oxygen (>50%) inactivates N-acetyl cysteine but is rarely required in COPD. The value of cough assist devices (Exsufflator; Emerson & Co) is increasingly recognised in neuromuscular causes of respiratory failure when cough is ineffective and may prove to be of use in COPD.

In the past the morbidity and inconvenience of surgical tracheostomies often resulted in prolonged ventilation with an endotracheal tube. The advantages of the percutaneous technique and the recognition that the resulting comfort of a tracheostomy allows less sedation has resulted in percutaneous tracheostomy being performed earlier in the clinical course. It allows intermittent ventilatory support and access to the lower respiratory tract for suctioning when ventilatory support is no longer required. A further advantage is that rehabilitation can be more active without the risk of inadvertent extubation. Fenestrated tracheostomy tubes will provide phonation, which improves communication and is an important milestone when weaning. One-way speaking valves (Passey Muir) provide an even better voice and can be inserted into the single lumen ventilation circuits employed with bi-level ventilators when used to support patients during the weaning process.

WEANING FAILURE

This aspect of management is considered in the chapter by Goldstone. Weaning protocols[51] may be helpful, principally by identifying patients who no longer require ventilatory support. COPD accounts for approximately 25% of weaning failures, defined as those still ventilator dependent 3 weeks or more after recovery from the condition precipitating ICU admission.[3-5] The negative aspects of a continued stay in the modern ICU environment, especially when only single organ (respiratory) failure persists, justifies considering referral to specialist weaning centres[4 5] which may be regionally provided in the future. On the other hand, sensitivity to the wishes of patients and/or judicious withholding of an escalation in therapy when deterioration occurs is also good practice in the irreversibly ventilator dependent patient.[14]

REFERENCES

1 **Seneff MG**, Wagner DP, Wagner RP, et al. Hospital and 1 year survival of patients admitted to intensive care units with acute exacerbations of chronic obstructive disease. JAMA 1995;**274**:1852–7.

2 **Seemungal TA**, Harper-Owen R, Bhowmik A, et al. Detection of rhinovirus in induced sputum at exacerbations of chronic obstructive pulmonary disease. Eur Respir J 2000;**16**:677–83.

3 **Hamid S**, Noonan YM, Williams AJ, et al. An audit of weaning from mechanical ventilation in a UK weaning centre. Thorax 1999;**54**:86P.

4 **Scheinhorn DJ**, Chao DC, Stearn-Hassenpflug M, et al. Outcomes in post ICU mechanical ventilation. Treatment of 1123 patients at a regional weaning centre. Chest 1997;**111**:1654–9.

5 **Pilcher DV**, Hamid S, Williams AJ, et al. Outcomes, cost and long term survival of patients referred to a regional centre for weaning from mechanical ventilation. Br J Anaesth 2002;**89**:361–2P.

6 **Squara P**, Dhainaut JF, Artigas A, et al. Hemodynamic profile in severe ARDS: results of the European Collaborative ARDS study. Intensive Care Med 1998;**24**:1018–28.

7 **Hudson LD**. Survival data in patients with acute or chronic lung disease requiring mechanical ventilation. Am Rev Respir Dis 1989;**140**:519–24.

8 **Gracey DR**, Naessens JM, Krishan I, et al. Hospital and post hospital survival among patients with COPD who require mechanical ventilation for acute respiratory failure. Chest 1989;**101**:211–4.

9 **Soo Hoo GW**, Hakiman I, Santiago SM. Hypercapnic respiratory failure in COPD patients. Response to therapy. Chest 2000;**117**:169–77.

10 **Nevins ML**, Epstein SK. Predictors of outcome for patients with COPD requiring invasive mechanical ventilation. Chest 2001;**119**:1840–9.

11 **Wildman MJ**, Odea J, Kostopoulou O, et al. Variation in intubation decisions for patients with COPD in one critical care network. QJM 2003;**96**:583–91.

12 **Hill AT**, Hopkinson RB, Stapleforth DE. Ventilation in a Birmingham intensive care unit 93–95: outcome for patients with chronic obstructive pulmonary disease. Respir Med 1998;**92**:156–61.

13 **Nava S**, Ambrosino N, Clini E, et al. Non invasive mechanical ventilation in the weaning of patients with respiratory failure due to chronic obstructive pulmonary disease. A randomised controlled trial. Ann Intern Med 1998;**128**:721–8.

14 Withholding and withdrawing life prolonging treatment. Guidance for decision-making. London: BMJ Publishing, 2001.

15 **Breen D**, Churches T, Hawker F, et al. Acute respiratory failure secondary to chronic obstructive pulmonary disease treated in the intensive care unit: a long term follow up study. Thorax 2002;**57**:29–33.

16 **Brochard L**, Moncebo J, Wysocki M, et al. Non invasive ventilation for acute exacerbations of chronic obstructive pulmonary disease. N Engl J Med 1995;**333**:817–22.

17 **Plant P**, Owen J, Elliott M. A multi centre randomised control trial of the early use of non invasive ventilation for acute exacerbations of chronic obstructive pulmonary disease. Lancet 2000;**355**:1931–5.

18 **Confalonieri M**, Perigi P, Scartabellati A, et al. Non invasive mechanical ventilation improves the immediate and long term outcome of COPD patients with acute respiratory failure. Eur Respir J 1996;**9**:422–30.

19 **Jones SE**, Packham S, Hebden M, et al. Domiciliary nocturnal intermittent positive pressure ventilation in patients with respiratory failure due to severe COPD: long term follow up and effect on survival. Thorax 1998;**53**:495–8.

20 **Aldrich TK**, Prezant DJ. Indications for mechanical ventilation. In: Tobin MJ, ed. Principles and practice of mechanical ventilation. New York: McGraw Hill, 1994: 155–89.

21 **Dales RE**, O'Connor A, Hebert P, et al. Intubation and mechanical ventilation for COPD: development of an instrument to elicit patient preferences. Chest 1999;**116**:792–800.

22 **British Thoracic Society Standards of Care Subcommittee on Pulmonary Rehabilitation**. Pulmonary rehabilitation. Thorax 2001;**56**:827–35.

23 **Morgan D**, Evans S, Steele K, et al. Prognosis in COPD. Ignorance is bliss? ERJ 2002;**20**(Suppl 38):1694

24 **Moretti C**, Cilione, C, Tampieri A, et al. Incidence and causes of non-invasive mechanical ventilation failure after initial success. Thorax 2000;**55**:819–25.

25 **Ninane V**, Yernault JC, De Troyer A. Intrinsic PEEP in patients with chronic obstructive pulmonary disease: role of expiratory muscles. Am Rev Respir Dis 1993;**148**:1037–42.

26 **Rochester DF**. Respiratory muscle weakness, pattern of breathing and CO_2 retention in chronic obstructive pulmonary disease. Am Rev Respir Dis 1991;**143**:901–3.

27 **Decramer M**, Aubier M. The respiratory muscles: cellular and molecular physiology. Eur Respir J 1997;**10**:1943–5.

28 **Plant PK**, Owen JL, Elliott MW. Non-invasive ventilation in acute exacerbations of chronic obstructive pulmonary disease: long term survival and predictors of in-hospital outcome. Thorax 2001;**56**:708–12.

29 **British Thoracic Society Standards of Care Subcommittee**. Non-invasive ventilation in acute respiratory failure. Thorax 2002;**57**:192–211.

30 **Brochard L**. Non invasive ventilation for acute exacerbations of COPD: a new standard of care. Thorax 2000;**55**:817–8.

31 **Yentis SM**. Suxamethonium and hyperkalaemia. Anaesth Intensive Care 1990;**18**:92–101.

32 **Brimacombe JR**, Berry AM. Cricoid pressure: a review article. Can J Anaesth 1997;**44**:414–25.

33 **Feihl F**, Perrett C. Permissive hypercapnoea. How permissive should we be? Am J Respir Crit Care Med 1994;**150**:1722–37.

34 **Davies L**, Angus RM, Calverley PMA. Oral steroids in patients admitted to hospital with exacerbations of chronic obstructive pulmonary disease: a prospective randomised controlled trial. *Lancet* 1999;**354**:456–60.

35 **Rabbat A**, Laaban JP, Boussairi A, *et al*. Hyperlactatemia during acute severe asthma. *Intensive Care Med* 1998;**24**:304–12.

36 **Ranieri VM**, Suter PM, Tortorella C, *et al*. Effect of mechanical ventilation on inflammatory mediators in patients with acute respiratory distress syndrome. A randomised controlled trial. *JAMA* 1999;**282**:54–61.

37 **Adult Respiratory Distress Syndrome Network**. Ventilation with lower tidal volumes compared with traditional lung injury in ARDS. *N Engl J Med* 2000;**342**:1301–8.

38 **Rossi A**, Gottfried SB, Zocchi L, *et al*. Measurement of static compliance of the total respiratory system in patients with acute respiratory failure during mechanical ventilation. The effect of intrinsic positive end-expiratory pressure. *Am Rev Respir Dis* 1985;**131**:672–7.

39 **Zakynthinos SG**, Vassilakopoulos T, Zakynthinos E, *et al*. Measuring dynamic PEEP. *Am J Respir Crit Care Med* 2000;**162**:1633–40.

40 **Marini JJ**, Smith TC, Lamb VJ. External work output and force generation during synchronised intermittent mechanical ventilation. Effect of machine assistance on breathing effort. *Am Rev Respir Dis* 1988;**138**:1169–79.

41 **Rossi RA**, Appendini L. Wasted effort and dyssynchrony: is the patient-ventilator battle back? *Intensive Care Med* 1995;**21**:867–70.

42 **Hormann CH**, Baum M, Putensen CH, *et al*. Bi-phasic positive airway pressure (BIPAP) a new mode of ventilatory support. *Eur J Anaesthesiol* 1993;**11**:37–42.

43 **Yang KL**, Tobin MJ. A prospective study of indices predicting the outcome of trials of weaning from mechanical ventilation. *N Engl J Med* 1991;**324**:1445–50.

44 **Jubran A**, Tobin MJ. Pathophysiologic basis of acute respiratory distress in patients who fail a trial of weaning from mechanical ventilation. *Am J Respir Crit Care Med* 1997;**155**:906–15.

45 **Kollef MH**, Levy NT, Ahrens TS, *et al*. The use of continuous IV sedation is associated with prolongation of mechanical ventilation. *Chest* 1998;**114**:541–8.

46 **Girault C**, Daudenthoni, Chevron V, *et al*. Non invasive ventilation as a systematic extubation and weaning technique in acute or chronic respiratory failure. *Am J Respir Crit Care Med* 1999;**160**:186–92.

47 **Hanson P**, Dive A, Brucher JM, *et al*. Acute corticosteroid myopathy in intensive care patients. *Muscle Nerve* 1997;**20**:1371–80.

48 **Drakulovic MB**, Torres A, Bauer TT, *et al*. Supine body position as a risk factor for nosocomial pneumonia in mechanically ventilated patients, a randomised trial. *Lancet* 1999; **354**:1851–8.

49 **Messori A**, Trippoli S, Vaiani M, *et al*. Breathing and pneumonia in intensive care patients given rinitadine and sucralfate for prevention of stress ulcer: meta-analysis of randomised trials. *BMJ* 2000;**321**:1103–6.

50 **D'Amico R**, Pifferi S, Leuretti C, *et al*. Effectiveness of antibiotic prophylaxis in critically ill adult patients: systematic review of randomised controlled trials. *BMJ* 1998;**316**:1275–85.

51 **Ely EW**, Baker A, Dungan D, *et al*. Effect of the duration of mechanical ventilation of identifying patients capable of breathing spontaneously. *N Engl J Med* 1996;**335**:1864–9.

13 Acute severe asthma

P Phipps, C S Garrard

Most asthma exacerbations are managed in the community or emergency department while the more severe cases that fail to respond to bronchodilator and anti-inflammatory therapy require admission to high dependency (HDU) or intensive care units (ICU).

Worldwide asthma prevalence is increasing, and with that the total number of admissions to hospital and intensive care. Although the time between the onset of symptoms and the requirement for ventilation is becoming shorter, the outcome is improving with fewer deaths and lower complication rates.[1]

MORTALITY

A history of mechanical ventilation or ICU admission is a well documented indicator of subsequent near fatal asthma.[2 3] Women and smokers are also over-represented in both life threatening attacks and asthma deaths.[3-5] It is believed that patients who have had a life threatening attack and those who die are from a similar demographic group. In a large study of patients admitted with a near fatal episode, two thirds of subsequent severe attacks or deaths had occurred within a year.[2 5] Interestingly, the association between asthma deaths and β agonist use is still debated and there has been concern that the use of long acting β agonists may increase asthma mortality.[6] This has not been confirmed in studies monitoring their use.[7 8] In contrast, there is a consensus that underuse of anti-inflammatory treatment in the period leading up to the acute severe attack worsens prognosis.[9]

Unfortunately, a proportion of asthmatic patients die despite reaching hospital alive. Such deaths can usually be attributed either to inadequate observation or treatment. Sadly, a number of patients suffer unobserved respiratory failure that progresses to cardiac arrest and anoxic brain damage.[10] A small number of patients are resistant to the most aggressive treatments and interventions.

Necroscopic studies of patients dying of acute severe asthma have found extensive mucus plugging of bronchi that has been termed "endobronchial mucus suffocation" (fig 13.1).[11] Microscopic examination reveals extensive inflammatory changes that involve all airway wall components and the pulmonary arterioles.[12 13] The degree of bronchial occlusion is much greater than in control asthmatic subjects, with mucus, desquamated epithelium, inflammatory cells and plasma exudate all contributing.[11] Sudden asphyxic asthma may be a distinct pathological subtype in which intense bronchoconstriction causes respiratory failure, often over the course of 1–2 hours.[14] Recovery appears to be rapid, which suggests that bronchoconstriction may be the predominant pathophysiological factor.[15]

INTENSIVE THERAPY AND MONITORING

Patients who fail to improve with optimal medical treatment in the emergency department should be considered for HDU or ICU admission to facilitate continuous monitoring of physiological parameters such as pulse oximetry, ECG, and arterial and central venous pressure. Equipment and experienced staff are also available for urgent procedures such as endotracheal intubation or the insertion of thoracostomy tubes.

Clinical, physiological and laboratory assessment

The immediate assessment of patients with asthma should include the degree of respiratory distress (ability to speak, respiratory rate, use of accessory muscles, air entry), degree of hypoxia (cyanosis, pulse oximetry, level of consciousness), and cardiovascular stability (arrhythmias, blood pressure). Accessory muscle use, wheeze, paradox, and tachypnoea may diminish as the patient tires.[16]

Forced expiratory volume in 1 second (FEV_1) and peak expiratory flow rate are the most used and convenient measures of airflow obstruction that support clinical findings and quantify the response to treatment.[17] Occasionally patients are too distressed to perform forced expiratory manoeuvres or there is a risk of precipitating further bronchoconstriction.[18] Expiratory airflow limitation results in a dynamic increase in end expiratory lung volume which interferes with inspiratory muscle function, both of the diaphragm and the chest wall. The positive alveolar pressure at end expiration (PEEP) due to residual elastic recoil has been termed intrinsic (PEEPi) and its presence is suggested by residual expiratory flow at the onset of inspiration. In spontaneously breathing patients the magnitude of PEEPi can be estimated by the change in intrapleural pressure (usually measured by an oesophageal pressure probe) between the onset of inspiratory effort and the onset of inspiratory flow (fig 13.2). The work of breathing is increased in the presence of PEEPi because the residual alveolar pressure must be overcome by muscle effort before inspiratory flow commences. Many patients also use expiratory muscles to aid expiration, which may paradoxically worsen dynamic airway collapse and PEEPi. Inspiratory muscle activity may also persist during expiration,[19-21] which contributes to increased expiratory work of breathing. In mechanically ventilated paralysed patients the magnitude of PEEPi is estimated by performing an end expiratory breath hold and measuring the airway pressure with reference to that of the atmosphere. In the presence of PEEPi a short expiratory time may lead to "breath stacking" and progressive hyperinflation as the next breath is initiated before the previous tidal volume has been completely exhaled. The pathological effects of PEEPi include hypotension due to reduced venous return and an increased risk of pneumothorax.[22]

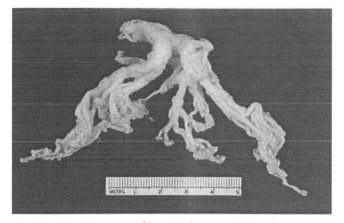

Figure 13.1 Mucus cast of bronchial tree coughed up by an asthmatic patient during an exacerbation. Reproduced with permission of E Klatt, Utah.

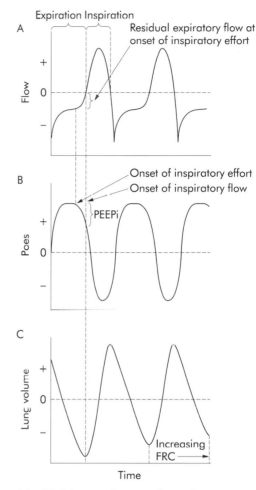

Figure 13.2 (A) Schematic diagram of an asthmatic patient exhibiting significant residual flow at end expiration. (B) The oesophageal pressure (Poes), an estimate of intrapleural pressure, shows the degree of pressure change required to overcome intrinsic pressure (PEEPi) and initiate inspiratory flow. (C) A progressive increase in lung volume (breath stacking) occurs if expiratory time is insufficient to allow complete exhalation of the tidal volume.

Pulse oximetry is an invaluable adjunct to monitoring since the avoidance or abolition of hypoxia is a prime goal of treatment. Regular arterial blood gas measurements provide a measure of gas exchange and facilitate the monitoring of serum potassium levels. The arterial carbon dioxide tension ($Paco_2$) and acid-base status help to identify the presence of pre-existing respiratory or metabolic acidosis, and the trend in $Paco_2$ is helpful when assessing the response to treatment. The degree of hypokalaemia and lactic acidosis may also guide treatment.[23] A chest radiograph is indicated to identify pneumothorax, areas of segmental or lobar collapse, or infiltrates that may suggest pneumonia. However, the yield is low.[24 25] An ECG may detect myocardial ischaemia or identify arrhythmias, especially in older patients.[26] Right axis deviation and right heart strain are common findings. Potassium, magnesium, calcium and phosphate deficiencies should be corrected to reduce the risk of arrhythmia and respiratory muscle weakness.

There are other causes of wheeze and respiratory distress that must be considered in the differential diagnosis. These include left ventricular failure, upper airway obstruction, inhaled foreign body, and aspiration of stomach contents.

Treatment

Intensive care treatment of the poorly responsive asthmatic patient should include high concentrations of inspired oxygen, continuous nebulisation of β agonists, intravenous corticosteroids, and respiratory support.[27–29] Clinicians must be aware of the need to optimise oxygenation and avoid dehydration and hypokalaemia. Unrestricted high concentrations of oxygen (60–100%) must be administered to abolish hypoxaemia,[27 30] unlike the patient with chronic obstructive lung disease where controlled limited oxygen is indicated.

Hypokalaemia is common and may be exaggerated by fluid resuscitation and the administration of β agonist bronchodilators. Repeated infusions of potassium chloride may be required with careful monitoring of serum levels and continuous ECG monitoring.

Specific asthma drug treatment

On admission to the ICU there should be a rapid review of earlier asthma treatment to identify elements that can be intensified or deficiencies remedied. Drugs contraindicated in asthma include β blockers, aspirin, non-steroidal anti-inflammatory drugs, and adenosine.

Corticosteroids

Evidence continues to accumulate that early treatment with adequate doses of corticosteroid improves outcome in severe acute asthma. There does not appear to be any benefit from high doses of hydrocortisone exceeding 400 mg/day, and no particular advantage of the intravenous over the oral route provided there is reliable gastrointestinal absorption.[31] Inhaled corticosteroids have not been fully evaluated in this setting.

β agonists

Salbutamol (albuterol in North America) is the most commonly prescribed β agonist for the treatment of acute asthma.[29] It appears to be more effective and induces less hypokalaemia when delivered by the inhaled route, although there is a theoretical rationale for administering salbutamol intravenously to bypass obstructed airways.[32] Concerns over blood levels and potential cardiotoxicity may inhibit more aggressive use of nebulised salbutamol.[33] However, continuous administration of nebulised salbutamol in doses approaching 20 mg/h can achieve bronchodilation without toxicity; indeed, the patient's heart rate may fall with alleviation of airway obstruction.[34]

Interpretation of the literature on continuous nebulised salbutamol is hampered by differences in the definitions of "continuous" (length of time) and the delivered doses used in individual studies. One study compared 27.5 mg salbutamol by either continuous or intermittent nebulisation over 6 hours[35] and, not surprisingly, showed little difference between intermittent and continuous regimens. Another study suggested benefit from prolonged continuous aerosol use only in severe asthma.[36] Doses of 0.3 mg/kg/h nebulised salbutamol have been safely used in children without significant toxicity.[37] Higher inhaled doses may be required in mechanically ventilated patients due to aerosol losses in the ventilator circuit.

Salbutamol delivered by metered dose inhaler (MDI) with a spacer device is at least as effective as nebulised drug in the management of acute asthma in the emergency department.[38] In patients with hypoxia and respiratory distress, however, nebulised drugs may be easier to administer. Even intranasal and intratracheal instillation of β agonists may be effective in an emergency situation.[39 40] Salbutamol is currently a racemic mixture of R and L forms. The S-enantiomer does not have β agonist effects and competes for the binding sites of the R form, levosalbutamol.[41] Formulations of levosalbutamol have fewer side effects and greater efficacy than the racemic mixture, suggesting that it may be preferable in acute severe asthma.[42] Terbutaline is an alternative β agonist that has been less widely studied but is effective by the inhaled, intravenous, and subcutaneous routes. Long acting β agonists such as salmeterol and eformoterol are not recommended because of their slow onset of action.

Both nebulised and intravenous adrenaline (epinephrine) are effective in the treatment of acute asthma. The putative benefits of the α-adrenergic component of adrenaline include reduced microvascular permeability and airway wall oedema, and less impairment of ventilation/perfusion matching than with more selective β agonists.[43] However, there does not appear to be any clinical benefit over β agonists such as salbutamol.[44]

Some of the metabolic and cardiovascular complications of acute severe asthma may be exacerbated by high dose β agonist therapy. Lactic acidosis as a result of parenteral β agonist use, anaerobic metabolism due to high work of breathing, tissue hypoxia, intracellular alkalosis, and reduced lactate clearance due to liver congestion all contribute to the complex metabolic disturbances of acute severe asthma. Haemodynamically significant arrhythmias are relatively infrequent, even with the combination of methylxanthines and β receptor agonists[45]; however, β agonist induced hypokalaemia heightens the risk.

Ipratropium
Ipratropium bromide has a mild additional bronchodilating effect when added to β agonists that may only be significant in severe asthma.[46] The safety profile and the fact that individual patients may obtain benefit have resulted in aerosolised ipratropium (500 μg 6 hourly) being recommended for the treatment of acute severe asthma.[47]

Aminophylline
The addition of aminophylline does not add to the bronchodilating effect of optimal doses of β agonists.[48] Other reported benefits of aminophylline such as improving diaphragmatic endurance, stimulating ventilatory drive, and anti-inflammatory effect do not seem to improve outcome in acute severe asthma.[49–53] Currently, aminophylline is not recommended as a first line drug in acute asthma management and its inclusion as a second line agent is still debated.[46] However, when other agents fail to achieve bronchodilation, aminophylline can be used providing dosing regimens are adhered to. Typically, a loading dose of 5 mg/kg by slow intravenous infusion over 20 minutes is followed by an infusion of 500 μg/kg/h. If prolonged administration is required, daily monitoring of blood theophylline levels is essential. The therapeutic range is 55–110 μmol/l (10–20 mg/l).

ASSISTED VENTILATION
If there is inadequate response to drug treatment or if the patient is in extremis at presentation, mechanical ventilation may be required.

> **Box 13.1   Contraindications to a trial of mask CPAP or NIV in acute severe asthma**
>
> - Need for immediate endotracheal intubation
> - Poor patient cooperation
> - Inability of the ventilator to supply high FiO_2
> - Hypercapnia (CPAP less likely to benefit than NIV)
> - Excess respiratory secretions
> - Lack of experienced staff and/or a high dependency area

Mask continuous positive airway pressure (CPAP) and non-invasive ventilation (NIV)
In spontaneously breathing patients the application of low levels of mask CPAP (3–8 cm H_2O) may improve respiratory rate, dyspnoea, and work of breathing in asthma, particularly if there is evidence of smoking related lung disease.[20 54 55] There is a danger that CPAP may worsen lung hyperinflation. If patients are intolerant of the mask or do not derive benefit, CPAP should be withdrawn. In hypercapnic patients CPAP alone may not improve ventilation.

Few studies have looked specifically at NIV in asthma. Low levels of CPAP and pressure support of 10–19 cm H_2O in acute severe asthma improved gas exchange and prevented endotracheal intubation in all but two of 17 hypercapnic patients.[56] However, the rate of intubation in patients with acute asthma, even in the presence of hypercapnia, is low at 3–8%.[28 57] It is reasonable to give asthmatic patients a trial of NIV over 1–2 hours in an HDU or ICU if there are no contraindications (box 13.1).[56] Deciding when to initiate NIV, when a trial of NIV has failed, and optimising NIV in this setting require considerable expertise. In our experience, high flow ventilators specifically designed for NIV (such as the BiPAP Vision; Respironics, Pittsburg, USA) that allow significant mask and mouth leaks are better tolerated than many conventional ICU ventilators.

Endotracheal intubation
Cardiopulmonary arrest and deteriorating consciousness are absolute indications for intubation and assisted ventilation. Hypercapnia, acidosis, and clinical signs of severe disease at presentation may not require immediate intubation before an aggressive trial of conventional bronchodilator therapy.[57 58] Conversely, progressive deterioration with increasing distress or physical exhaustion may warrant intubation and mechanical ventilation without the presence of hypercapnia.

Once it has been decided that mechanical ventilation is required, the necessary medications, suitable monitoring equipment, and expert help should be sought. An understanding of the pathophysiology and anticipation of difficulties can minimise the complications associated with endotracheal intubation and ventilation. The best technique for intubation is generally that most familiar to the clinician performing the procedure.

The process of intubation begins with explanation and reassurance for the patient, followed by pre-oxygenation. The asthmatic patient is often dehydrated and the combination of PEEPi, the loss of endogenous catecholamines, and the vasodilating properties of the anaesthetic agents can cause catastrophic hypotension.[59 60] Volume resuscitation before induction of anaesthesia can limit the degree of hypotension but vasoconstrictors such as ephedrine or metaraminol should be at hand.

Intubation is best performed by direct laryngoscopy after induction of general anaesthesia. Endoscopic methods have been advocated with either oral or nasal intubation,[16 58] but laryngeal spasm and further bronchoconstriction may occur. Satisfactory local anaesthesia of the oropharynx, nasopharynx, and larynx is therefore essential. Longer term sedation is required once the airway has been secured. Some recommendations for successful and safe endotracheal intubation are summarised in box 13.2.

> **Box 13.2 Summary of recommendations for the process of intubation**
>
> - Performed/supervised by experienced anaesthetists or intensivists
> - Skilled assistants in an appropriate environment
> - Good preparation and understanding of the pathophysiology
> - Correct electrolyte disturbances and rehydrate
> - Obtain reliable large bore venous access
> - Continuous ECG and pulse oximetry
> - Continuous arterial monitoring not essential, but helpful
> - Pre-oxygenate
> - Use familiar method of intubation
> - Use familiar sedatives and muscle relaxants
> - Prepare for the rapid correction of hypotension, arrhythmias and barotrauma.
> - Ventilator set up and ready to monitor airway pressures early
> - Get aerosol delivery system for the ventilator connected or commence parenteral bronchodilator therapy
> - Plan ongoing sedation/paralysis before intubation

> **Box 13.3 Initial ventilator settings in paralysed patients (adapted from Finfer and Garrard[109])**
>
> - FiO_2 = 1.0 (initially)
> - Long expiratory time (I:E ratio >1:2)
> - Low tidal volume 5–7 ml/kg
> - Low ventilator rate (8–10 breaths/min)
> - Set inspiratory pressure 30–35 cm H_2O on pressure control ventilation or limit peak inspiratory pressure to <40 cm H_2O
> - Minimal PEEP <5 cm H_2O

Drug therapy for intubation and mechanical ventilation

Anaesthetic agents and sedatives

Etomidate and thiopentone are short acting imidazole and barbiturate drugs, respectively, that are commonly used for intubation although rarely bronchospasm and anaphylactoid reactions have been reported. Longer term sedation may be obtained by infusion of midazolam (2–10 mg/h); metabolites may accumulate in renal and hepatic impairment. Propofol is a useful drug for intubation and intermediate term sedation, mainly because of its rapid onset and offset of action. It is easily titratable for intubation, providing deep sedation rapidly, although it has no analgesic properties. However, vasodilatation and hypotension occur, especially in dehydrated patients. Relatively little literature regarding its specific use in asthma is available. The doses of all the above agents need to be adjusted for patient size and pre-existing level of consciousness.

Ketamine is a general anaesthetic agent that has been used before, during, and after intubation in patients with acute severe asthma.[61–63] It has sympathomimetic and bronchodilating properties. The usual dose for intubation is 1–2 mg/kg given intravenously over 2–4 minutes. It may increase blood pressure and heart rate, lower seizure threshold, alter mood, and cause delirium. Inhalational anaesthetics used for gas induction have the advantage of bronchodilation and may make muscle relaxation unnecessary. However, specialised anaesthetic equipment is required for this approach.

Opioids are a useful addition to sedatives and provide analgesia during intubation and mechanical ventilation. Morphine in large boluses causes histamine release, which may worsen bronchoconstriction and hypotension. Some intravenous preparations also contain metabisulphite, to which some asthmatics are sensitive. Fentanyl is a better choice of opioid for intubation as it inhibits airway reflexes and is short acting. It causes less histamine release than morphine but large boluses may cause bronchospasm and chest wall rigidity.

Neuromuscular blocking drugs

Rapid sequence induction with cricoid pressure should be used to prevent aspiration of gastric contents. Suxamethonium, a depolarising muscle relaxant, is widely used. It has a rapid onset and short duration of action but may cause hyperkalaemia and increased intracranial pressure. Rocuronium, a non-depolarising muscle relaxant with an acceptably rapid onset, offers an alternative. Allergic sensitivity may occur to any neuromuscular blocking agent and most may also cause histamine release and the potential for bronchospasm, particularly in bolus doses. Atracurium boluses should be avoided because of this possibility and vecuronium or pancuronium infusions used for longer term maintenance of muscle relaxation.

Myopathy and muscle weakness are well recognised complications of the long term administration of non-depolarising neuromuscular blocking agents in asthmatic patients with an incidence of about 30%.[64–66] In most cases the myopathy is reversible, but may take weeks to resolve. There is an association between neuromyopathy and the duration of muscle relaxant drug use that is independent of corticosteroid therapy.[65] The use of neuromuscular blocking agents should therefore be kept to a minimum.

Mechanical ventilation

Mechanical ventilation provides respiratory support while drug therapy reverses bronchospasm and airway inflammation.[28] Abolishing hypoxia is the most important aim.

Modes of ventilation

Commonly adopted ventilation modes include pressure limited and time cycled (pressure control or bilevel ventilation) or volume limited and time cycled modes (synchronised intermittent mandatory ventilation, SIMV).[28] In pressure limited modes, maximum airway pressure is set and the tidal volume delivered depends on respiratory system compliance. Volume cycled modes, however, deliver a set tidal volume and can be successfully and safely used provided an airway pressure limit is set appropriately. As the patient improves and begins to breathe, spontaneously triggered modes of ventilation such as pressure support ventilation (PSV) can be introduced.

Ventilator settings

The major variables that need to be set when placing a patient on mechanical ventilation include the oxygen concentration of inspired gas (FiO_2), tidal volume (V_T) or inspiratory pressure, ventilator rate, inspiratory to expiratory time ratio (I:E ratio), and PEEP. The aims are to minimise airway pressure, allowing sufficient time for completion of expiration while achieving adequate alveolar ventilation. Suggested initial ventilator settings are shown in box 13.3.

Outcome is improved in mechanically ventilated asthmatics by limiting airway pressure using a low respiratory rate and tidal volume while permitting a moderate degree of hypercarbia and respiratory acidosis.[67] Hypercarbia has not been found to be detrimental except in patients with raised intracranial pressure or severe myocardial depression. Moderate degrees of hypercarbia with an associated acidosis (pH 7.2–7.15) are generally well tolerated. Reducing the respiratory rate to 8 or 10 breaths/min prolongs expiratory time so that I:E ratios of greater than 1:2 can be achieved. An attempt to increase minute ventilation (to reduce $PaCO_2$) by increasing the ventilator respiratory rate invariably reduces the expiratory time and I:E ratio, increases air trapping, and may paradoxically cause an increased $PaCO_2$. This has resulted in perceived failure of mechanical ventilation.[60]

Humidification of inspired gas is particularly important in asthmatic patients to prevent thickening of secretions and drying of airway mucosa, a stimulus for bronchospasm in itself.[69]

Ventilator alarms

These include peak pressure and low tidal volume/low minute ventilation alarms. If exceptionally high airway pressures occur or there is a sudden fall in V_T, blockage of the endotracheal tube, pneumothorax, or lobar collapse should be excluded. Plateau rather than peak airway pressure may provide the best measure of alveolar pressure and provide the best predictor of barotrauma, together with measures of hyperinflation such as PEEPi.[70]

Extrinsic PEEP

Low level CPAP may be beneficial in spontaneously breathing, mechanically ventilated patients, especially if expiratory muscle activity is contributing to dynamic airways collapse. However, in mechanically ventilated paralysed patients extrinsic PEEP was of no benefit at low levels and was detrimental at high levels because the fall in gas trapping was outweighed by the rise in functional residual capacity (FRC).[22] However, in this study large V_T were used (up to 18 ml/kg); furthermore PEEPi and arterial blood gases were not measured. Changes in FRC and gas trapping may guide the level of PEEP. Applied extrinsic PEEP should not exceed PEEPi.

Topical drug delivery to the ventilated patient

Mechanical ventilation, whether invasive or non-invasive, may compromise the delivery of bronchodilator aerosols. The amount of nebulised drug reaching the airways depends on the nebuliser design, driving gas flow, characteristics of the ventilator tubing, and the size of the endotracheal tube.[47 71] Drug delivery may vary from 0% to 42% in ventilated patients.[72] The presence of humidification alone may reduce drug deposition by as much as 40%, but may be reversed by the addition of a spacer device.[73 74] Both ultrasonic and jet nebulisers are effective in ventilated patients.[75] Nebulisers may, however, be a source of bacterial contamination.[76]

Metered dose inhalers have been widely used and may provide at least as good drug delivery as nebulisers, depending on actuator design and the presence of humidification and spacer devices.[77 78] The recommended characteristics of aerosol delivery systems used in ventilated patients are shown in box 13.4. Ideally, each aerosol delivery system should be evaluated for each type of ventilator circuit used.[73]

THERAPEUTIC OPTIONS IN THE NON-RESPONDING PATIENT

A proportion of patients improve rapidly following the introduction of mechanical ventilation, and weaning should occur in line with this improvement. Unfortunately, for some there is difficulty in achieving adequate ventilation or there is persistent hypoxia. Difficulty in ventilation may be due to refractory bronchospasm, extreme hyperinflation, or mucus plugging.

Manual compression

This technique was first described anecdotally by Watts in 1984.[79] Hyperinflation is relieved by manual compression of the chest wall during expiration.[80] The technique has been advocated and used with success in both intubated and non-intubated patients, although it has not been fully evaluated by a controlled clinical study in humans.[81 80]

Mucolytics

There is often a striking degree of mucus impaction in both large and small airways that contributes to hyperinflation, segmental and lobar collapse with shunting, increased airway

---

Box 13.4 Recommendations for aerosol delivery to mechanically ventilated patients

Metered dose inhaler (MDI) system
- Spacer or holding chamber
- Location in inspiratory limb rather than Y piece
- No humidification (briefly discontinue)
- Actuate during lung inflation
- Large endotracheal tube internal diameter
- Prolonged inspiratory time

Jet nebuliser system
- Mount nebuliser in inspiratory limb
- Delivery may be improved by inspiratory triggering
- Increase inspiratory time and decrease respiratory rate
- Use a spacer
- High flow to generate aerosol
- High volume fill
- Stop humidification
- Consider continuous nebulisation

Ultrasonic nebulisers
- Position in inspiratory limb prior to a spacer device
- Use high power setting
- Use a high volume fill
- Maximise inspiratory time
- Drugs must be stable during ultrasonic nebulisation

---

pressure, and barotrauma. Chest physiotherapy and mucolytics have no proven benefit. Bronchoscopic lavage with locally applied acetylcysteine may be used to help clear impacted secretions in selected refractory patients but its routine use is not advocated.[82] Recently, recombinant DNase, a mucolytic prescribed for sputum liquefaction in cystic fibrosis, has been used to treat mucus impaction in asthma but there are no clinical trials.[83]

Inhalational anaesthetic agents

Halothane, isoflurane, and sevoflurane are potent bronchodilators in asthmatic patients receiving mechanical ventilation who have failed to respond to conventional β adrenergic agents.[84] Experimental evidence indicates a direct effect on bronchial smooth muscle mediated via calcium dependent channels as well as by modulating vagal, histamine, allergen, and hypoxia induced bronchoconstrictor mechanisms.[85 86] Furthermore, these agents reduce pulmonary vascular tone resulting in lower pulmonary artery pressures in acute asthma.[87] Bronchodilator responses are seen in the form of reduced peak airway pressures within minutes, associated with improved ventilation distribution (lower $Paco_2$) and reduced air trapping.[88] Although bronchodilator effects are seen at sub-anaesthetic concentrations, these agents also offer a relatively expensive method of sedation. A few ICU ventilators, such as the Seimens Servo 900 series, can be fitted with a vaporiser allowing anaesthetic gases to be administered. Effective exhaled gas scavenging systems are required when using inhalational anaesthetics in the ICU. If this facility is not available a Cardiff canister can be added to the expiratory port of the ventilator to remove effluent anaesthetic gases. Significant side effects such as hypotension and myocardial irritability exist, and prolonged administration of some agents may result in bromide or fluoride toxicity.[89] Sevoflurane, a halogenated ether, is largely devoid of cardiorespiratory side effects and may be the preferred agent. Administration of sub-anaesthetic concentrations of these agents via face mask may relieve bronchospasm refractory to conventional treatment.[90]

One of the difficult aspects of mechanical ventilation of the acute asthmatic patient is the weaning and extubation process. The presence of the endotracheal tube within the larynx and trachea induces bronchoconstriction which becomes troublesome as the sedation is withdrawn in preparation for extubation.[91 92] Use of an inhalational anaesthetic agent allows the endotracheal tube to be removed under anaesthesia with the confident expectation of rapid recovery once the anaesthetic is discontinued.

Helium

A mixture of helium and oxygen (heliox) may reduce the work of breathing and improve gas exchange because of its low density that reduces airway resistance and hyperinflation. However, the benefits are marginal and the concentration of inspired oxygen is consequently decreased. Flow meters and nebuliser generator systems must be adapted for heliox use in ventilated patients.[93] The use of heliox to prevent intubation has not been studied, but dyspnoea scores were improved in one study, possibly by reducing the work of breathing.[94]

Magnesium sulphate

Early anecdotal reports suggested benefit from intravenous magnesium sulphate, which has been inconsistently supported by randomised studies.[95–99] A significant benefit was recently observed in children receiving intravenous magnesium sulphate (40 mg/kg) during acute asthma attacks.[100] Overall, the case for magnesium sulphate in acute asthma requires further evaluation in both adults and children.

Leukotriene inhibitors

Leukotrienes are inflammatory mediators known to be active in the airway inflammation of asthma. Leukotriene receptor antagonists (zafirlukast, montelukast) and synthesis blockers (zilueton) currently have a relatively minor role in the management of poorly controlled and aspirin sensitive asthma.[101] However, recent work has suggested a role for leukotriene antagonists in acute asthma.[102–105]

Platelet activating factor (PAF) inhibitors

PAF inhibitors attenuate the late response in asthma but have limited clinical efficacy.[106]

Nitric oxide (NO)

NO exerts a weak bronchodilator effect.[107] It dilates pulmonary arteries and, when inhaled, may improve ventilation/perfusion matching.

OUTCOME AND FOLLOW UP

ICU admission identifies an asthmatic patient as a member of a poor prognostic group.[3 5 108] Follow up should include a focus on anti-inflammatory therapy and a written management plan that may include the emergency use of intramuscular adrenaline. Issues such as access to health care services, compliance with treatment, avoidance of triggers, socioeconomic and psychosocial factors also need to be addressed.

ACKNOWLEDGEMENT

The authors would like to thank Dr Duncan Young for his review of the manuscript and helpful suggestions.

REFERENCES

1 **Kearney SE**, Graham DR, Atherton ST. Acute severe asthma treated by mechanical ventilation: a comparison of the changing characteristics over a 17 yr period. *Respir Med* 1998;**92**:716–21.

2 **Richards GN**, Kolbe J, Fenwick J, *et al*. Demographic characteristics of patients with severe life threatening asthma: comparison with asthma deaths. *Thorax* 1993;**48**:1105–9.

3 **Turner MO**, Noertjojo K, Vedal S, *et al*. Risk factors for near-fatal asthma. A case-control study in hospitalized patients with asthma. *Am J Respir Crit Care Med* 1998;**157**:1804–9.

4 **Sandford AJ**, Pare PD. The genetics of asthma. The important questions. *Am J Respir Crit Care Med* 2000;**161**:S202–6.

5 **Marquette CH**, Saulnier F, Leroy O, *et al*. Long-term prognosis of near-fatal asthma. A 6-year follow-up study of 145 asthmatic patients who underwent mechanical ventilation for a near fatal attack of asthma. *Am Rev Respir Dis* 1992;**146**:76–81.

6 **Abramson MJ**, Bailey MJ, Couper FJ, *et al*. Are asthma medications and management related to deaths from asthma? *Am J Respir Crit Care Med* 2001;**163**:12–8.

7 **Castle W**, Fuller R, Hall J, *et al*. Serevent nationwide surveillance study: comparison of salmeterol with salbutamol in asthmatic patients who require regular bronchodilator treatment. *BMJ* 1993;**306**:1034–7.

8 **Donohue JF**. The expanding role of long-acting beta-agonists. *Chest* 2000;**118**:283–5.

9 **Kallenbach JM**, Frankel AH, Lapinsky SE, *et al*. Determinants of near fatality in acute severe asthma. *Am J Med* 1993;**95**:265–72.

10 **Shugg AW**, Kerr S, Butt WW. Mechanical ventilation of paediatric patients with asthma: short and long term outcome. *J Paediatr Child Health* 1990;**26**:343–6.

11 **Saetta M**, Di Stefano A, Rosina C, *et al*. Quantitative structural analysis of peripheral airways and arteries in sudden fatal asthma. *Am Rev Respir Dis* 1991;**143**:138–43.

12 **Carroll N**, Elliot J, Morton A, *et al*. The structure of large and small airways in nonfatal and fatal asthma. *Am Rev Respir Dis* 1993;**147**:405–10.

13 **Faul JL**, Tormey VJ, Leonard C, *et al*. Lung immunopathology in cases of sudden asthma death. *Eur Respir J* 1997;**10**:301–7.

14 **Reid LM**. The presence or absence of bronchial mucus in fatal asthma. *J Allergy Clin Immunol* 1987;**80**:415–6.

15 **Wasserfallen JB**, Schaller MD, Feihl F, *et al*. Sudden asphyxic asthma: a distinct entity? *Am Rev Respir Dis* 1990;**142**:108–11.

16 **Corbridge TC**, Hall JB. The assessment and management of adults with status asthmaticus. *Am J Respir Crit Care Med* 1995;**151**:1296–316.

17 **Rodrigo G**, Rodrigo C. Assessment of the patient with acute asthma in the emergency department. A factor analytic study. *Chest* 1993;**104**:1325–8.

18 **Lim TK**. Status asthmaticus in a medical intensive care. *Singapore Med J* 1989;**30**:334–8.

19 **Hill AR**. Respiratory muscle function in asthma. *J Assoc Acad Minor Phys* 1991;**2**:100–8.

20 **Lougheed DM**, Webb KA, O'Donnell DE. Breathlessness during induced lung hyperinflation in asthma: the role of the inspiratory threshold load. *Am J Respir Crit Care Med* 1995;**152**:911–20.

21 **De Troyer A**, Pride NB. The chest wall and respiratory muscles. In: Roussos C, ed. *The thorax*. New York: Dekker, 1995: 1975–2006.

22 **Tuxen DV**. Detrimental effects of positive end-expiratory pressure during controlled mechanical ventilation of patients with severe airflow obstruction. *Am Rev Respir Dis* 1989;**140**:5–9.

23 **Appel D**, Rubenstein R, Schrager K, *et al*. Lactic acidosis in severe asthma. *Am J Med* 1983;**75**:580–4.

24 **Findley LJ**, Sahn SA. The value of chest roentgenograms in acute asthma in adults. *Chest* 1981;**80**:535–6.

25 **White CS**, Cole RP, Lubetsky HW, *et al*. Acute asthma. Admission chest radiography in hospitalized adult patients. *Chest* 1991;**100**:14–6.

26 **Myrianthefs MM**, Nicolaides EP, Pitiris D, *et al*. False positive ST-segment depression during exercise in subjects with short PR segment and angiographically normal coronaries: correlation with exercise-induced ST depression in subjects with normal PR and normal coronaries. *J Electrocardiol* 1998;**31**:203–8.

27 **British Thoracic Society**, British Paediatric Association, Research Unit of the Royal College of Physicians of London, *et al*. Guidelines on the management of asthma. *Thorax* 1993;**48**(Suppl):S1–24.

28 **Garrard CS**, Nolan K. Intensive care management of asthma. In: Webb AR, Shapiro MJ, Singer M, *et al*, eds. *Oxford textbook of intensive care*. Oxford: Oxford University Press, 1999:90–5.

29 **Garrard CS**, Benham S. Bronchodilators in intensive care. In: Webb AR, Shapiro MJ, Singer M, *et al*, eds. *Oxford textbook of intensive care*. Oxford: Oxford University Press, 1999:1241–4.

30 **Lipworth BJ**, Jackson CM, Ziyaie D, *et al*. An audit of acute asthma admissions to a respiratory unit. *Health Bull (Edinb)* 1992;**50**:389–98.

31 **Manser R**, Reid D, Abramson M. Corticosteroids for acute severe asthma in hospitalised patients. *Cochrane Database Syst Rev* 2000;2.

32 **Salmeron S**, Brochard L, Mal H, *et al*. Nebulized versus intravenous albuterol in hypercapnic acute asthma. A multicenter, double-blind, randomized study. *Am J Respir Crit Care Med* 1994;**149**:1466–70.

33 **Lin RY**, Smith AJ, Hergenroeder P. High serum albuterol levels and tachycardia in adult asthmatics treated with high-dose continuously aerosolized albuterol. *Chest* 1993;**103**:221–5.

34 **Lin RY**, Sauter D, Newman T, *et al*. Continuous versus intermittent albuterol nebulization in the treatment of acute asthma. *Ann Emerg Med* 1993;**22**:1847–53.

35 **Besbes-Ouanes L**, Nouira S, Elatrous S, *et al*. Continuous versus intermittent nebulization of salbutamol in acute severe asthma: a randomized, controlled trial. *Ann Emerg Med* 2000;**36**:198–203.

36 **Rudnitsky GS**, Eberlein RS, Schoffstall JM, *et al*. Comparison of intermittent and continuously nebulized albuterol for treatment of asthma in an urban emergency department. *Ann Emerg Med* 1993;**22**:1842–6.

37 **Papo MC**, Frank J, Thompson AE. A prospective, randomized study of continuous versus intermittent nebulized albuterol for severe status asthmaticus in children. *Crit Care Med* 1993;**21**:1479–86.

38 **Idris AH**, McDermott MF, Raucci JC, *et al*. Emergency department treatment of severe asthma. Metered-dose inhaler plus holding chamber is equivalent in effectiveness to nebulizer. *Chest* 1993;**103**:665–72.

39 **Weksler N**, Brill S, Tarnapolski A, *et al*. Intranasal salbutamol instillation in asthma attack. *Am J Emerg Med* 1999;**17**:686–8.

40 **Steedman DJ**, Robertson CE. Emergency endotracheal drug administration using aerosol. *Resuscitation* 1987;**15**:135–9.

41 **Boulton DW**, Fawcett JP. The pharmacokinetics of levosalbutamol: what are the clinical implications? *Clin Pharmacokinet* 2001;**40**:23–40.

42 **Handley DA**. Single-isomer beta-agonists. *Pharmacotherapy* 2001;**21**:21–7S.

43 **Baldwin DR**, Sivardeen Z, Pavord ID *et al*. Comparison of the effects of salbutamol and adrenaline on airway smooth muscle contractility in vitro and on bronchial reactivity in vivo. *Thorax* 1994;**49**:1103–8.

44 **Abroug F**, Nouira S, Bchir A, *et al*. A controlled trial of nebulized salbutamol and adrenaline in acute severe asthma. *Intensive Care Med* 1995;**21**:18–23.

45 **Molfino NA**, Nannini LJ, Martelli AN, *et al*. Respiratory arrest in near-fatal asthma. *N Engl J Med* 1991;**324**:285–8.

46 **Silverman R**. Treatment of acute asthma. A new look at the old and at the new. *Clin Chest Med* 2000;**21**:361–79.

47 **The COPD Guidelines Group of the Standards of Care Committee of the BTS**. BTS guidelines for the management of chronic obstructive pulmonary disease. *Thorax* 1997;**52**(Suppl 5):S1–28.

48 **Parameswaran K**, Belda J, Rowe BH. Addition of intravenous aminophylline to beta2-agonists in adults with acute asthma (Cochrane Review). *Cochrane Database Syst Rev* 2000;4.

49 **Murciano D**, Auclair MH, Pariente R, *et al*. A randomized, controlled trial of theophylline in patients with severe chronic obstructive pulmonary disease. *N Engl J Med* 1989;**320**:1521–5.

50 **Lakshminarayan S**, Sahn SA, Weil JV. Effect of aminophylline on ventilatory responses in normal man. *Am Rev Respir Dis* 1978;**117**:33–8.

51 **Ward AJ**, McKenniff M, Evans JM, *et al*. Theophylline: an immunomodulatory role in asthma? *Am Rev Respir Dis* 1993;**147**:518–23.

52 **Rodrigo C**, Rodrigo G. Treatment of acute asthma. Lack of therapeutic benefit and increase of the toxicity from aminophylline given in addition to high doses of salbutamol delivered by metered-dose inhaler with a spacer. *Chest* 1994;**106**:1071–6.

53 **Zainudin BM**, Ismail O, Yusoff K. Effect of adding aminophylline infusion to nebulised salbutamol in severe acute asthma. *Thorax* 1994;**49**:267–9.

54 **Mansel JK**, Stogner SW, Norman JR. Face-mask CPAP and sodium bicarbonate infusion in acute, severe asthma and metabolic acidosis. *Chest* 1989;**96**:943–4.

55 **Shivaram U**, Miro AM, Cash ME, *et al*. Cardiopulmonary responses to continuous positive airway pressure in acute asthma. *J Crit Care* 1993;**8**:87–92.

56 **Meduri GU**, Turner RE, Abou-Shala N, *et al*. Noninvasive positive pressure ventilation via face mask. First-line intervention in patients with acute hypercapnic and hypoxemic respiratory failure. *Chest* 1996;**109**:179–93.

57 **Mountain RD**, Sahn SA. Clinical features and outcome in patients with acute asthma presenting with hypercapnia. *Am Rev Respir Dis* 1988;**138**:535–9.

58 **Leatherman J**. Life-threatening asthma. *Clin Chest Med* 1994;**15**:453–79.

59 **Mansel JK**, Stogner SW, Petrini MF, *et al*. Mechanical ventilation in patients with acute severe asthma. *Am J Med* 1990;**89**:42–8.

60 **Zimmerman JL**, Dellinger RP, Shah AN, *et al*. Endotracheal intubation and mechanical ventilation in severe asthma. *Crit Care Med* 1993;**21**:1727–30.

61 **L'Hommedieu CS**, Arens JJ. The use of ketamine for the emergency intubation of patients with status asthmaticus. *Ann Emerg Med* 1987;**16**:568–71.

62 **Hemming A**, MacKenzie I, Finfer S. Response to ketamine in status asthmaticus resistant to maximal medical treatment. *Thorax* 1994;**49**:90–1.

63 **Howton JC**, Rose J, Duffy S, *et al*. Randomized, double-blind, placebo-controlled trial of intravenous ketamine in acute asthma. *Ann Emerg Med* 1996;**27**:170–5.

64 **Griffin D**, Fairman N, Coursin D, *et al*. Acute myopathy during treatment of status asthmaticus with corticosteroids and steroidal muscle relaxants. *Chest* 1992;**102**:510–4.

65 **Leatherman JW**, Fluegel WL, David WS, *et al*. Muscle weakness in mechanically ventilated patients with severe asthma. *Am J Respir Crit Care Med* 1996;**153**:1686–90.

66 **Margolis BD**, Khachikian D, Friedman Y, *et al*. Prolonged reversible quadriparesis in mechanically ventilated patients who received long-term infusions of vecuronium. *Chest* 1991;**100**:877–8.

67 **Darioli R**, Perret C. Mechanical controlled hypoventilation in status asthmaticus. *Am Rev Respir Dis* 1984;**129**:385–7.

68 **Shapiro MB**, Kleaveland AC, Bartlett RH. Extracorporeal life support for status asthmaticus. *Chest* 1993;**103**:1651–4.

69 **Scharf SM**, Heimer D, Walters M. Bronchial challenge with room temperature isocapnic hyperventilation. A comparison with histamine challenge. *Chest* 1985;**88**:586–93.

70 **Tuxen DV**, Williams TJ, Scheinkestel CD, *et al*. Use of a measurement of pulmonary hyperinflation to control the level of mechanical ventilation in patients with acute severe asthma. *Am Rev Respir Dis* 1992;**146**:1136–42.

71 **Thomas SH**, O'Doherty MJ, Fidler HM, *et al*. Pulmonary deposition of a nebulised aerosol during mechanical ventilation. *Thorax* 1993;**48**:154–9.

72 **Dhand R**, Tobin MJ. Inhaled bronchodilator therapy in mechanically ventilated patients. *Am J Respir Crit Care Med* 1997;**156**:3–10.

73 **Lange CF**, Finlay WH. Overcoming the adverse effect of humidity in aerosol delivery via pressurized metered-dose inhalers during mechanical ventilation. *Am J Respir Crit Care Med* 2000;**161**:1614–8.

74 **Harvey CJ**, O'Doherty MJ, Page CJ, *et al*. Effect of a spacer on pulmonary aerosol deposition from a jet nebuliser during mechanical ventilation. *Thorax* 1995;**50**:50–3.

75 **Harvey CJ**, O'Doherty MJ, Page CJ, *et al*. Comparison of jet and ultrasonic nebulizer pulmonary aerosol deposition during mechanical ventilation. *Eur Respir J* 1997;**10**:905–9.

76 **Craven DE**, Lichtenberg DA, Goularte TA, *et al*. Contaminated medication nebulizers in mechanical ventilator circuits. Source of bacterial aerosols. *Am J Med* 1984;**77**:834–8.

77 **Gay PC**, Patel HG, Nelson SB, *et al*. Metered dose inhalers for bronchodilator delivery in intubated, mechanically ventilated patients. *Chest* 1991;**99**:66–71.

78 **Duarte AG**, Momii K, Bidani A. Bronchodilator therapy with metered-dose inhaler and spacer versus nebulizer in mechanically ventilated patients: comparison of magnitude and duration of response. *Respir Care* 2000;**45**:817–23.

79 **Watts JI**. Thoracic compression for asthma. *Chest* 1984;**86**:505.

80 **Fisher MM**, Bowey CJ, Ladd-Hudson K. External chest compression in acute asthma: a preliminary study. *Crit Care Med* 1989;**17**:686–7.

81 **Eason J**, Tayler D, Cottam S, *et al*. Manual chest compression for total bronchospasm. *Lancet* 1991;**337**:366.

82 **Lang DM**, Simon RA, Mathison DA, *et al*. Safety and possible efficacy of fiberoptic bronchoscopy with lavage in the management of refractory asthma with mucous impaction. *Ann Allergy* 1991;**67**:324–30.

83 **Patel A**, Harrison E, Durward A, *et al*. Intratracheal recombinant human deoxyribonuclease in acute life-threatening asthma refractory to conventional treatment. *Br J Anaesth* 2000;**84**:505–7.

84 **Eger EI**. The pharmacology of isoflurane. *Br J Anaesth* 1984;**56**:71–99S.

85 **Hirshman CA**, Edelstein G, Peetz S, *et al*. Mechanism of action of inhalational anesthesia on airways. *Anesthesiology* 1982;**56**:107–11.

86 **Korenaga S**, Takeda K, Ito Y. Differential effects of halothane on airway nerves and muscle. *Anesthesiology* 1984;**60**:309–18.

87 **Saulnier FF**, Durocher AV, Deturck RA, *et al*. Respiratory and hemodynamic effects of halothane in status asthmaticus. *Intensive Care Med* 1990;**16**:104–7.

88 **Maltais F**, Reissmann H, Navalesi P, *et al*. Comparison of static and dynamic measurements of intrinsic PEEP in mechanically ventilated patients. *Am J Respir Crit Care Med* 1994;**150**:1318–24.

89 **Echeverria M**, Gelb AW, Wexler HR, *et al*. Enflurane and halothane in status asthmaticus. *Chest* 1986;**89**:152–4.

90 **Padkin AJ**, Baigel G, Morgan GA. Halothane treatment of severe asthma to avoid mechanical ventilation. *Anaesthesia* 1997;**52**:994–7.

91 **Gal TJ**. Pulmonary mechanics in normal subjects following endotracheal intubation. *Anesthesiology* 1980;**52**:27–35.

92 **Habre W**, Scalfaro P, Sims C, *et al*. Respiratory mechanics during sevoflurane anesthesia in children with and without asthma. *Anesth Analg* 1999;**89**:1177–81.

93 **Gluck EH**, Onorato DJ, Castriotta R. Helium-oxygen mixtures in intubated patients with status asthmaticus and respiratory acidosis. *Chest* 1990;**98**:693–8.

94 **Kass JE**, Terregino CA. The effect of heliox in acute severe asthma: a randomized controlled trial. *Chest* 1999;**116**:296–300.

95 **McNamara RM**, Spivey WH, Skobeloff E, *et al*. Intravenous magnesium sulfate in the management of acute respiratory failure complicating asthma. *Ann Emerg Med* 1989;**18**:197–9.

96 **Green SM**, Rothrock SG. Intravenous magnesium for acute asthma: failure to decrease emergency treatment duration or need for hospitalization. *Ann Emerg Med* 1992;**21**:260–5.

97 **Bloch H**, Silverman R, Mancherje N, *et al*. Intravenous magnesium sulfate as an adjunct in the treatment of acute asthma. *Chest* 1995;**107**:1576–81.

98 **Rowe BH**, Bretzlaff JA, Bourdon C, *et al*. Magnesium sulfate for treating exacerbations of acute asthma in the emergency department. *Cochrane Database Syst Rev* 2000;2.

99 **Chande VT**, Skoner DP. A trial of nebulized magnesium sulfate to reverse bronchospasm in asthmatic patients. *Ann Emerg Med* 1992;**21**:1111–5.

100 **Ciarallo L**, Brousseau D, Reinert S. Higher-dose intravenous magnesium therapy for children with moderate to severe acute asthma. *Arch Pediatr Adolescent Med* 2000;**154**:979–83.

101 **Drazen JM**, Israel E, O'Byrne PM. Treatment of asthma with drugs modifying the leukotriene pathway. *N Engl J Med* 1999;**340**:197–206.

102 **Kuitert LM**, Barnes NC. Leukotriene receptor antagonists: useful in acute asthma? *Thorax* 2000;**55**:255–6.

103 **Drazen JM**, O'Brien J, Sparrow D, *et al*. Recovery of leukotriene E4 from the urine of patients with airway obstruction. *Am Rev Respir Dis* 1992;**146**:104–8.

104 **Dworski R**, Fitzgerald GA, Oates JA, *et al*. Effect of oral prednisone on airway inflammatory mediators in atopic asthma. *Am J Respir Crit Care Med* 1994;**149**:953–9.

105 **Dockhorn RJ**, Baumgartner RA, Leff JA, *et al*. Comparison of the effects of intravenous and oral montelukast on airway function: a double blind, placebo controlled, three period, crossover study in asthmatic patients. *Thorax* 2000;**55**:260–5.

106 **Evans DJ**, Barnes PJ, Cluzel M, *et al*. Effects of a potent platelet-activating factor antagonist, SR27417A, on allergen-induced asthmatic responses. *Am J Respir Crit Care Med* 1997;**156**:11–6.

107 **Hogman M**, Frostell CG, Hedenstrom H, *et al*. Inhalation of nitric oxide modulates adult human bronchial tone. *Am Rev Respir Dis* 1993;**148**:1474–8.

108 **Molfino NA**, Nannini LJ, Rebuck AS, *et al*. The fatality-prone asthmatic patient. Follow-up study after near-fatal attacks. *Chest* 1992;**101**:621–3.

109 **Finfer SR**, Garrard CS. Ventilatory support in asthma. *Br J Hosp Med* 1993;**49**:357–60.

14 The pulmonary circulation and right ventricular failure

K McNeil, J Dunning, N W Morrell

The lungs are the only organs that receive the entire cardiac output which is delivered at a mean resting pulmonary arterial pressure of 15 mm Hg. The capacitance pulmonary arteries are larger in calibre and have thinner walls than their systemic counterparts. Moreover, the pulmonary circulation possesses little resting vascular tone and has a large reserve for recruitment of vascular segments that are normally non-perfused.[1] Thus, the pulmonary circulation is a low pressure, low resistance circuit capable of handling large increases in pulmonary blood flow (up to sixfold with strenuous exercise) with only small changes in pressure. The maintenance of a low pulmonary capillary pressure is vital in preserving the function of the blood-gas barrier.[2] In accordance with this low pressure circuit, the right ventricle (RV) is a thin muscle with limited contractile reserve, which has significant implications for both the prognosis associated with severe pulmonary hypertension (PHT) and for the principles underlying the clinical management of PHT and RV failure.

Both PHT and RV dysfunction are common complications of the complex medical disorders experienced in the intensive care unit. In most circumstances the PHT is mild or moderate in degree and associated with RV dysfunction rather than frank right heart failure. Occasionally, however, patients do present with life threatening PHT and associated RV failure requiring prompt and appropriate intervention.

Right heart dysfunction and PHT of varying severity are commonly encountered in patients with chronic lung disease and left ventricular failure, but these specific entities will not be considered further. This chapter will rather concentrate on the management of severe PHT in the setting of RV failure. In addition, we will discuss the relevance and treatment of PHT in the context of acute respiratory distress syndrome (ARDS) in adults. Definitions of PHT and calculations for mean pulmonary artery pressure (PAP) are shown in table 14.1.

In the intensive care unit haemodynamics are usually measured using a flow directed, balloon tipped pulmonary artery catheter. Cardiac output is most commonly and conveniently determined by thermodilution techniques. It can also be derived via the Fick principle but this is not used frequently in clinical practice. Transoesophageal echocardiography can also be used to estimate cardiac output using Doppler imaging. The procedure requires sedation, however, and is not therefore usually performed in cases with severe PHT unless the patient is intubated (or undergoing another essential procedure).

AETIOLOGY OF PULMONARY HYPERTENSION

The WHO consensus conference in 1998[3] reclassified PHT according to clinicopathological criteria. Both the site of pathology (arterial or venous) and causative factors (association with respiratory disease/hypoxia, thromboembolic disease, or primary vascular pathology) were included. This classification adds to our understanding of the mechanisms involved and provides a good starting point in developing a rational clinical approach to the management of severe PHT.

By this classification, the cause of PHT is divided into either an intrinsic disease of the pulmonary vessels or a vascular response to another disease process. In general, treatment for this second group should be directed at the underlying disease rather than at the pulmonary vasculature per se. Probably the commonest causes of PHT in the ITU are raised left atrial pressure and hypoxaemia. Treatment should be directed at the underlying cardiac or respiratory disease, respectively.

THE PULMONARY CIRCULATION IN ARDS

The acute respiratory distress syndrome (ARDS) is characterised by non-hydrostatic pulmonary oedema and refractory hypoxaemia, and complicates up to 25% of cases of the systemic inflammatory response syndrome The consensus definitions of ARDS and acute lung injury (ALI) are shown in table 14.2. PHT with increased pulmonary vascular resistance is common, even when systemic vascular resistance is low. The degree of pulmonary arterial hypertension is usually mild to moderate but promotes the accumulation of extravascular lung water and can cause right ventricular dysfunction, reducing ejection fraction and cardiac output. The presence of PHT has been shown to be an adverse prognostic indicator in patients with ARDS.[4][5]

Initially, a number of factors may contribute to the increase in PAP in ARDS.[6] Increased circulating levels of vasoactive mediators such as serotonin, endothelin-1, thromboxane and leukotrienes may contribute to the increase in pulmonary vascular tone. There may also be an important contribution from increased discharge from the sympathetic nervous system. Although hypoxic pulmonary vasoconstriction may play

---

Table 14.1 Definitions of pulmonary hypertension (PHT) and calculations for mean pulmonary artery pressure (PAP)

PHT definitions	Mean PAP
Rest	>25 mm Hg
Exercise	>30 mm Hg
Mild	<30 mm Hg
Moderate	30–45 mm Hg
Severe	>45 mm Hg

Calculation of mean PAP: (1) mPAP = dPAP + (sPAP − dPAP)/3; (2) mPAP = (2 × dPAP + sPAP)/3 (these are the same equation expressed in two commonly used forms); d – diastolic, s – systolic.

Table 14.2 Recommended criteria for definition of acute lung injury (ALI) and acute respiratory distress syndrome (ARDS). Modified from Bernard et al[42]

	Timing	Oxygenation	Chest radiograph	Pulmonary artery wedge pressure
ALI	Acute onset	PaO_2/FiO_2 ≤40 kPa (regardless of PEEP level)	Bilateral infiltrates on frontal chest radiograph	≤18 mm Hg or no clinical evidence of left atrial hypertension
ARDS	Acute onset	PaO_2/FiO_2 ≤26.7 kPa (regardless of PEEP level)	Bilateral infiltrates on frontal chest radiograph	≤18 mm Hg or no clinical evidence of left atrial hypertension

some role in increasing pulmonary vascular resistance locally, generally the pulmonary vascular response to hypoxia is reduced in patients with ARDS.[7] Indeed, administration of 100% oxygen to patients with ALI does not significantly alter pulmonary haemodynamics.[8] Structural changes in small pulmonary arteries (pulmonary vascular remodelling) develop in patients with ARDS of more than a few days duration, with the severity of the changes correlating with the duration of lung injury. Initially, acute endothelial injury and thromboemboli are visible on histopathological examination.[9] Fibrocellular intimal obliteration of arteries, veins, and lymphatic vessels occurs in those surviving more than 10 days.

Manipulation of the pulmonary circulation in patients with ARDS is aimed at improving systemic oxygen availability and improving right ventricular dysfunction.[10] Reducing pulmonary vascular resistance using vasodilators such as prostacyclin[11] or nitrates improves cardiac output in ARDS, but concurrent vasodilation occurring in poorly ventilated lung regions can worsen ventilation/perfusion (V/Q) matching, increasing shunt fraction and exacerbating hypoxaemia. The aim of inhaled vasodilator treatment is to confine vasodilation to those areas of the pulmonary circulation receiving the most ventilation, optimising V/Q matching. Thus, inhaled nitric oxide (NO) reduces pulmonary vascular resistance, improves right ventricular function, and improves arterial oxygenation in patients with ARDS.[12 13] The current recommendation is that NO treatment in ARDS should be limited to patients who are optimally ventilated and have an arterial oxygen tension (PaO_2) of <12 kPa with a fractional inspired oxygen (FiO_2) of 1.0.[14] Similar improvements have been reported with the use of nebulised prostacyclin in ARDS. However, large randomised trials have not shown that selective pulmonary vasodilators alter the outcome in ARDS in terms of a reduction in either the duration of mechanical ventilation or mortality.[15]

SEVERE PULMONARY HYPERTENSION

In general, the clinical presentation of severe PHT reflects the degree of resulting right heart dysfunction or failure. The structure and geometry of the RV dictates its ability to cope with increased PAP.

If the pressure increase occurs over a long period of time (months to years), the RV has a limited capacity to cope via hypertrophy. By contrast, after severe acute rises in pulmonary vascular resistance—for example, following a massive central pulmonary embolism—the ability of the RV to adapt is severely limited. Usually it simply dilates and can rarely generate, nor less sustain, a systolic pressure of 50 mm Hg.[16] This results in a low output and haemodynamic shock. Occasionally in this acute setting the venous pulses, especially the femoral pulse, will become "arterialised" due to marked

tricuspid regurgitation and, with the accompanying systemic hypotension, can be mistaken for its arterial counterpart.

Right ventricular failure is also manifest as systemic venous hypertension. This results in the classical clinical signs of jugular venous engorgement (with "cV" waves due to tricuspid regurgitation), pulsatile hepatomegaly, lower limb oedema, and occasionally anasarca. In addition to these clinically obvious effects there is also a concomitant congestion of the splanchnic circulation in general, with resulting gut oedema. In these circumstances patients often become refractory to oral diuretics, presumably due to poor absorption.

Other less usual presentations may develop in patients with severe primary pulmonary hypertension (PPH) attributable to the effects of venous hypertension. Renal dysfunction is common, resulting from both arterial hypotension and the high renal venous pressure. This reduces the filtration pressure across the glomerulus and may result in nephrotic syndrome as the presenting clinical manifestation of PHT. Similarly, visual disturbances associated with papilloedema and delirium due to severe cerebral venous hypertension mimicking cavernous sinus thrombosis may occur. In all cases effective treatment of the PHT leading to improvement in RV function and reduction in systemic venous pressures can lead to resolution.

Investigation of severe PHT

In most cases severe PHT can be readily diagnosed on clinical grounds. Where right heart failure dominates the clinical picture, severe PHT is usually evident. However, it is imperative to elucidate the underlying cause in order to administer appropriate treatment.

Patients with severe PHT and RV failure are frequently too unwell or too unstable to undergo definitive investigations. Where feasible, spiral CT angiography is the investigation of choice for the diagnosis of acute central pulmonary embolism. This examination will identify large central clots with positive and negative predictive values of over 90% compared with pulmonary angiography.[17] Radiological signs of severe PHT such as enlargement of the pulmonary arteries and right sided chambers are also evident. Conversely, the left sided chambers are normal or reduced (compressed) in size.

Echocardiography at the bedside may show signs of RV pressure overload as well as excluding other causes of haemodynamic collapse such as pericardial tamponade.[18] With severe RV dilation and dysfunction, left ventricular function as assessed by echocardiography is usually reduced due to paradoxical movement of the septum and distortion of normal left/right heart dynamics. It is vitally important in this setting to attribute correctly the low cardiac output state to the right sided problems as there are important differences in the principles of treating a failing RV and those used to support the left side.

Pulmonary artery catheterisation will confirm a low cardiac index in association with a raised pulmonary vascular resistance. A low pulmonary artery capillary occlusion pressure (<15 mm Hg), reflecting reduced left atrial pressure, effectively excludes left heart dysfunction as the cause of PHT and the low output state. However, in patients with severely deranged haemodynamics, accurate placement of a pulmonary artery catheter can be difficult and the data obtained need to be interpreted with caution.

TREATMENT
General principles
Pulmonary hypertension (PHT)

The principles of treating PHT are based upon reducing RV afterload and preventing or treating the complications of RV dysfunction. Attempted correction of hypoxaemia is mandatory in the treatment of any patient with severe PHT. In the presence of a right to left shunt this may not be possible, but in these situations it is usually possible at least to ameliorate the added oxygen desaturation associated with sleep and exercise. As in any low cardiac output state, anticoagulation is desirable.

With intrinsic disease of the pulmonary arteries, several vasodilator strategies can be considered. For patients requiring mechanical ventilation inhaled NO can be used to maximise V/Q matching, as vasodilation only occurs in ventilated areas.[19] Prostacyclin (PGI$_2$) is also an effective pulmonary vasodilator but, when administered intravenously, can result in worsening of V/Q matching.[20] The short biological half life of inhaled NO (seconds) leads to a greater effect on the pulmonary than the systemic circulation, its biological effects being rapidly eliminated by reaction with haemoglobin. Prostacyclin has a rather longer half life in the circulation (1–2 minutes) and usually lowers pulmonary and systemic vascular resistance, although the systemic effects can be minimised by inhaled treatment. Calcium channel blockers should not be used in patients with significant cardiac dysfunction as their negative inotropic effects may further impair RV performance.[21] Nitric oxide donors such as nitroprusside or nitrates are rarely effective in this setting, and usually exacerbate the systemic hypotension associated with the low cardiac output syndrome.

Right heart dysfunction

The RV is designed to work with a low pressure circuit and, as such, has limited contractile reserve. For this reason RV support is aimed at reducing afterload. Severe acute RV dysfunction associated with PHT may present during heart or lung transplantation or surgery for pulmonary embolus or severe mitral valve disease. Inhaled NO may be useful in this setting to decrease pulmonary vascular resistance without reducing systemic arterial pressure, which is essential for the maintenance of coronary perfusion to the right ventricle. Inhaled NO in the dose range 20–40 ppm may benefit these patients.[14] Unless the pulmonary vascular resistance can be reduced, inotropes are ineffective, imposing more work on a struggling RV. Inotropes can transiently improve cardiac output for 6–12 hours but inevitably the RV fails, resulting in a lethal downward spiral of increasing inotrope requirements but diminishing effect. Inotropes are, however, useful for supporting or augmenting RV contractility in situations where the pulmonary vascular resistance can be reduced through concomitant administration of vasodilator therapy. In this respect, a phosphodiesterase inhibitor such as enoximone[22] is our preferred choice as its vasodilator properties contrast with the pulmonary vasoconstrictor effects characteristic of catecholamines.

Intra-aortic balloon counterpulsation is useful for short term RV support,[23] augmenting coronary blood flow and increasing central systemic blood pressure, thereby reducing the need for pressor agents such as noradrenaline which are potent pulmonary vasoconstrictors. Most devices used in the context of RV support are modified from those used to support the failing left heart. When the lung function remains adequate to allow sufficient oxygenation and carbon dioxide removal, mechanical assist devices alone may be used to support the RV. When severe lung injury accompanies RV failure, mechanical RV support can be incorporated into either extracorporeal membrane oxygenation (ECMO) or extracorporeal carbon dioxide removal (ECCOR) circuits.

Paracorporeal devices such as the Abiomed are implanted through a sternotomy using right atrial or ventricular cannulation for drainage to the pump chamber, with return to the pulmonary artery through a vascular conduit sutured to the pulmonary trunk. Such a procedure is highly invasive and the subsequent management of the pump is complex. In particular, maintaining a balance between vasodilator agents, inotropes, and filling pressures may be difficult to achieve.

Overflowing the pump can result in gross pulmonary oedema, compounding an already difficult situation. A further source of difficulty may be experienced with the management of anticoagulation. While it is important to achieve adequate anticoagulation, intracranial haemorrhage may result if tight control is not maintained. Success is most likely in centres where there is familiarity with the management of these devices and their complications.

Although the use of ECMO is more complex, cannulation and the establishment of the ECMO circuit is less invasive than that required for most paracorporeal pulsatile ventricular assist devices. This technique is only of value when the insult necessitating its use is reversible. Although well established in children, its adoption in adult practice has been less widespread. Key components to successful intervention include early institution (ventilated less than 5 days), a flexible approach to cannulation (established percutaneously via femoral and jugular routes), and readiness to support other systems including the kidneys and liver.

Any attempt to support the RV with a mechanical device in the face of PHT is complicated. A multidisciplinary approach must be adopted, and there is no simple unifying technique. The advent of small axial and rotary blood pumps currently undergoing trials in left ventricular dysfunction may improve the outlook in this area in years to come.

Atrial septostomy has been used in the treatment of patients with severe PHT and RV compromise.[24] This treatment evolved from the observation that patients with PPH and a patent foramen ovale lived longer than those with no septal defect.[25] Creating a shunt at the atrial level decompresses the right sided chambers and augments left atrial filling with a concomitant increase in cardiac output and systemic oxygen transport. The resulting reduction in RV end diastolic pressure and wall tension are postulated to improve Starling haemodynamics and RV contractility. Although the resulting right to left shunt causes systemic oxygen desaturation (which is especially marked with exercise when PAP rises), this can usually be controlled with supplemental oxygen.

The clinical benefits reported following septostomy include resolution of syncopal and pre-syncopal episodes, decreased cough, decreased systemic venous congestion, and improved exercise tolerance. Our own experience of this procedure suggests it is most effective before the onset of severe RV dysfunction and, conversely, as reported by others,[26] it has not been effective in patients with end stage right heart failure or acute right heart failure severe enough to require admission to the ITU. Atrial septostomy has been used primarily in advanced PPH as a bridge to heart-lung transplantation,[24] although its exact role (in particular the optimal timing of the procedure) is not known. As our own experience with this procedure has developed, it is being used earlier in the course of disease. Experience of the procedure in any form of severe PHT is very limited and at present there are no controlled clinical studies in any disease group.

Thromboembolic disease

The most common cause of acute severe PHT is massive central pulmonary thromboembolism. Some of the mechanisms involved in the development of shock in the setting of acute massive pulmonary embolism (PE) are shown in fig 14.1. The overall mortality from massive PE is 6–8%, increasing to 30% if complicated by systemic hypotension.[27] Of those patients who fail to survive, 67% die within 1 hour of the onset of symptoms.[28]

The diagnosis of massive PE is suggested by the clinical presentation of right ventricular failure, a normal or oligaemic chest radiograph, and a suggestive ECG (right ventricular strain).[29] In more stable patients there may be time to organise spiral CT pulmonary angiography.[17 30] Echocardiography (either transthoracic or transoesophageal) may reveal thrombus in the pulmonary outflow tract or show signs of right ventricular dysfunction/hypokinesis.[18 31]

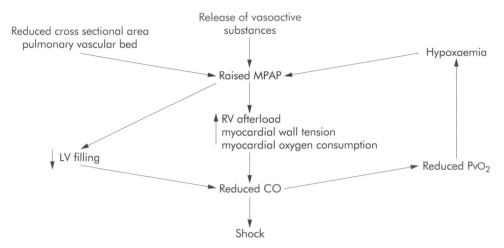

Figure 14.1 Factors involved in the generation of acute right ventricular failure following massive pulmonary embolism. MPAP=mean pulmonary artery pressure; CO=cardiac output; LV=left ventricle; PvO₂=ventricular oxygen tension.

Oxygen and analgesia should be given to all patients immediately. Invasive monitoring of the central venous pressure will guide cautious fluid and colloid replacement to optimise right sided filling pressures. The central venous pressure should be maintained at 15–20 cm H₂O. Overfilling worsens right ventricular function, but inadequate filling (or indeed overly aggressive diuresis) also compromises RV haemodynamics. If haemodynamic compromise is present and there are no contraindications (shown in box 14.1), thrombolysis should be considered for acute massive PE.[32][33] The rationale for this is the greater mortality in patients with right ventricular dysfunction following acute PE.[34] Thrombolysis leads to more rapid restoration of RV function than heparin alone.[28] However, the potential benefits must justify the 1% risk of cerebral and fatal bleeding,[35] and the effects of thrombolysis on mortality still need to be confirmed by a prospective randomised trial. Two hour infusion regimens of streptokinase (1.5 million units), urokinase and recombinant tissue plasminogen activator (rt-PA; 100 mg) followed by a heparin infusion have similar efficacy and safety profiles.[36] Thrombolysis may be considered in all age groups and in postoperative patients. The risk of major haemorrhage with these agents increases with increasing age and body mass index. Bolus and front loaded regimens (administered over <2 hours) are simpler to use and are as effective as longer duration infusions. Streptokinase should not be used if patients have been previously treated with this agent. There is no benefit of direct central versus peripheral administration of thrombolytic agents.

Patients may require inotropic treatment as the RV afterload is reduced and RV function recovers.[37] It is important to maintain systemic arterial pressure and to ensure adequate perfusion of the right coronary artery.

Studies have now shown that echocardiography can also provide important prognostic information in acute PE. Although cardiogenic shock occurs in less than 5% of patients with PE, RV dysfunction or hypokinesis occurs in up to 40% of patients with a normal systemic blood pressure. The finding of RV dysfunction increases the mortality from PE at 14 days and 3 months. In a Swedish study[34] mortality at 1 year was 45% in patients presenting with RV dysfunction compared with 15% in those with normal echocardiography. The benefits of thrombolysis may therefore extend to patients without overt shock but with RV dysfunction of any degree. This was borne out by the results from a multicentre registry showing a favourable clinical outcome in haemodynamically stable patients with major PE following thrombolysis.[38] Again, these promising results await confirmation in a prospective randomised trial.

If thrombolysis is contraindicated (see box 14.1) in acute massive PE, other treatment options include mechanical clot

---

Box 14.1 Indications and contraindications for thrombolytic treatment of acute PE

Indications

- Massive PE: first line treatment
- Haemodynamic compromise
- Failure to respond to anticoagulants

Contraindications

Absolute

- Recent major trauma or operation (within 10 days)
- Recent cerebrovascular accident (within 2 months)
- Bleeding diathesis
- Active internal bleeding

Relative

- Prolonged cardiopulmonary resuscitation
- Pregnancy
- Diabetic proliferative retinopathy

---

fragmentation, transvenous catheter embolectomy, or surgical embolectomy.[33] Insertion of an inferior vena caval filter should be considered in the presence of active haemorrhage to prevent further potentially fatal embolism. Surgical embolectomy may be appropriate in the setting of an experienced cardiovascular surgical unit. It should be reserved for severely compromised patients in refractory cardiogenic shock or patients requiring intermittent resuscitation.[39] To be effective it must be performed as soon as possible. Total perioperative mortality is approximately 30%, with the highest mortality rates (~60%) in those patients who require preoperative cardiopulmonary resuscitation.[40][41] An approach to the treatment of a patient with massive PE is shown in fig 14.2. In this setting, it is vitally important that chronic thromboembolic disease is excluded as the treatment of these two conditions is vastly different. Attempted surgical embolectomy (as opposed to pulmonary endarterectomy) in a patient with chronic thromboembolic PHT is fraught with disaster.

For patients with chronic thromboembolic PHT, the treatment of choice is pulmonary endarterectomy. In experienced hands this procedure results in a sustained reduction in pulmonary pressures and RV remodelling.[43] Within the UK, Papworth Hospital is the National Specialist Commissioning Advisory Group (NSCAG) designated centre for pulmonary endarterectomy.

CONCLUSION

Unrecognised or untreated severe PHT has a poor prognosis related directly to the limited contractile reserves of the RV.

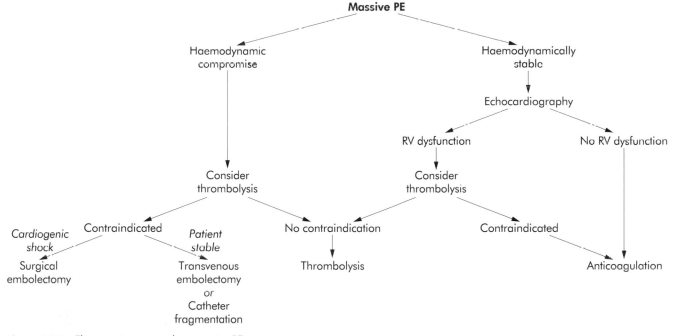

Figure 14.2 Therapeutic approach to massive PE.

Appropriate treatment hinges on identification of the underlying cause and effective reduction in RV afterload. The commonest cause of acute severe PHT is massive pulmonary thromboembolism and, if no contraindications exist, thrombolytic therapy is the treatment of choice. Pulmonary vasodilators such as intravenous prostacyclin or inhaled NO are often effective in other cases where increased pulmonary vascular tone is present. Whatever the underlying cause, without effective afterload reduction the RV will inevitably fail and it is thus of the utmost importance that inotropes are not relied on to support the RV without effective treatment of the underlying problem.

REFERENCES

1 **Rodman DM**, Voelkel NF. Regulation of vascular tone. In: Crystal RG, West JB, et al, eds. *The lung*. Scientific Foundations. Philadelphia: Lippincott-Raven, 1997: 1473–92.

2 **West JB**. Pulmonary capillary stress failure. *J Appl Physiol* 2000;**89**:2483–9.

3 **Rich S**, ed. *Primary pulmonary hypertension: executive summary of a WHO meeting*. Geneva: World Health Organisation, 1998.

4 **Villar J**, Blazquez MA, Lubillo S, et al. Pulmonary hypertension in acute respiratory failure. *Crit Care Med* 1989;**17**:523–6.

5 **Leeman M**. Pulmonary hypertension in acute respiratory distress syndrome. *Monaldi Arch Chest Dis* 1999;**54**:146–9.

6 **Wort SJ**, Evans TW. The role of the endothelium in modulating vascular control in sepsis and related conditions. *Br Med Bull* 1999;**55**:30–48.

7 **Leeman M**. The pulmonary circulation in acute lung injury: a review of some recent advances. *Intensive Care Med* 1991;**17**:254–60.

8 **Santos C**, Ferrer M, Roca J, et al. Pulmonary gas exchange response to oxygen breathing in acute lung injury. *Am J Respir Crit Care Med* 2000;**161**:26–31.

9 **Tomashefski JF**, Davies P, Boggis C, et al. The pulmonary vascular lesions of the adult respiratory distress syndrome. *Am J Pathol* 1983;**112**:112–26.

10 **Naeije R**. Medical treatment of pulmonary hypertension in acute lung disease. *Eur Respir J* 1993;**6**:1521–8.

11 **Radermacher P**, Santak B, Wust HJ, et al. Prostacyclin and right ventricular function in patients with pulmonary hypertension associated with ARDS. *Intensive Care Med* 1990;**16**:227–32.

12 **Rossaint R**, Falke KJ, Lopez F, et al. Inhaled nitric oxide for the adult respiratory distress syndrome. *N Engl J Med* 1993;**328**:399–405.

13 **Fierobe L**, Brunet F, Dhainaut JF, et al. Effect of inhaled nitric oxide on right ventricular function in adult respiratory distress syndrome. *Am J Respir Crit Care Med* 1995;**151**:1414–9.

14 **Cuthbertson BH**, Dellinger P, Dyar OJ, et al. UK guidelines for the use of inhaled nitric oxide therapy in adult ICUs. *Intensive Care Med* 1997;**23**:1212–8.

15 **Lundin S**, Mang H, Smithies M, et al. Inhalation of nitric oxide in acute lung injury: results of a European multicentre study. The European Study Group of inhaled nitric oxide. *Intensive Care Med* 1999;**25**:911–9.

16 **McIntyre KM**, Sasahara AA. Determinants of right ventricular function and haemodynamics after pulmonary embolism. *Chest* 1974;**65**:534–43.

17 **Remy-Jardin M**, Remy J, Deschildre F, et al. Diagnosis of pulmonary embolism with spiral CT: comparison with pulmonary angiography and scintigraphy. *Radiology* 1996;**200**:699–706.

18 **Jardin F**, Dubourg O, Bourdarias JP. Echocardiographic pattern of acute cor pulmonale. *Chest* 1997;**111**:209–17.

19 **Hayward CS**, Kelly RP, MacDonald PS. Inhaled nitric oxide in cardiology practice. *Cardiovasc Res* 1999;**43**:628–38.

20 **Otulana B**, Higenbottam T. The role of physiological deadspace and shunt in the gas exchange of patients with pulmonary hypertension: a study of exercise and prostacyclin infusion. *Eur Respir J* 1988;**1**:732–7.

21 **Gaine SP**, Rubin LJ. Primary pulmonary hypertension. *Lancet* 1998;**352**:719–25.

22 **Bauer J**, Dapper F, Demirakca S, et al. Perioperative management of pulmonary hypertension after heart transplantation in childhood. *J Heart Lung Transplant* 1997;**16**:1238–47.

23 **Arafa OE**, Geiran OR, Andersen K, et al. Intraaortic balloon pumping for predominantly right ventricular failure after heart transplantation. *Ann Thorac Surg* 2000;**70**:1587–93.

24 **Rothman A**, Sklansky MS, Lucas VW, et al. Atrial septostomy as a bridge to lung transplantation in patients with severe pulmonary hypertension. *Am J Cardiol* 1999;**84**:682–6.

25 **Rozkovec A**, Montanes P, Oakley CM. Factors that influence the outcome of primary pulmonary hypertension. *Br Heart J* 1986;**55**:449–58.

26 **Rich S**, Dodin E, McLaughlin VV. Usefulness of atrial septostomy as a treatment for primary pulmonary hypertension and guidelines for its application. *Am J Cardiol* 1997;**80**:369–71.

27 **Alpert JS**, Smith R, Carlson CJ, et al. Mortality in patients treated for pulmonary embolism. *JAMA* 1976;**236**:1477–80.

28 **Dalen JE**, Alpert JS. Natural history of pulmonary embolism. *Prog Cardiovasc Dis* 1975;**17**:259–70.

29 **British Thoracic Society Standards of Care Committee**. Suspected pulmonary embolism: a practical approach. *Thorax* 1997;**52**(Suppl 4):S1–24.

30 **Blum AG**, Delfau F, Grignon B, et al. Spiral-computed tomography versus pulmonary angiography in the diagnosis of acute massive pulmonary embolism. *Am J Cardiol* 1994;**74**:96–8.

31 **McConnell MV**, Solomon SD, Rayan ME, et al. Regional right ventricular dysfunction detected by echocardiography in acute pulmonary embolism. *Am J Cardiol* 1996;**78**:469–73.

32 **Jerjes-Sanchez C**, Ramirez-Rivera A, Garcia ML, et al. Streptokinase and heparin versus heparin alone in massive pulmonary embolism: a randomised controlled trial. *J Thromb Thrombolysis* 1995;**2**:227–9.

33 **Goldhaber SZ**. Pulmonary embolism. *N Engl J Med* 1998;**339**:93–104.

34 **Ribeiro A**, Lindmarker P, Juhlin-Dannfelt A, et al. Echocardiography Doppler in pulmonary embolism: right ventricular dysfunction as a predictor of mortality rate. *Am Heart J* 1997;**134**:479–87.

35 **Konstantinides S**, Geibel A, Kasper W. Submassive and massive pulmonary embolism: a target for thrombolytic therapy. *Thromb Haemost* 1999;**82**(Suppl 1):104–8.

36 **Meneveau N**, Schiele F, Metz D, *et al.* Comparative efficacy of a two-hour regimen of streptokinase versus alteplase in acute massive pulmonary embolism: immediate clinical and hemodynamic outcome and one-year follow up. *J Am Coll Cardiol* 1998;**31**:1057–63.

37 **Layish DT**, Tapson VF. Pharmacologic hemodynamic support in massive pulmonary embolism. *Chest* 1997;**111**:218–24.

38 **Konstantinides S**, Geibel A, Olschewski M, *et al.* Association between thrombolytic treatment and the prognosis of hemodynamically stable patients with major pulmonary embolism: results of a multicentre registry. *Circulation* 1997;**96**:882–8.

39 **Elliott CG**. Embolectomy, catheter extraction, or disruption of pulmonary emboli: editorial review. *Curr Opin Pulm Med* 1995;**1**:298–302.

40 **Doerge H**, Schoendube FA, Voss M, *et al.* Surgical therapy of fulminant pulmonary embolism: early and late results. *Thorac Cardiovasc Surg* 1999;**47**:9–13.

41 **Gulba DC**, Schmid C, Borst HG, *et al.* Medical compared with surgical treatment for massive pulmonary embolism. *Lancet* 1994;**343**:576–7.

42 **Bernard GR**, Artigas A, Brigham KL, *et al.* The American-European consensus conference on ARDS. *Am J Respir Crit Care Med* 1994;**149**:818–24.

43 **Archibald CJ**, Auger WR, Fedullo PF, *et al.* Long-term outcome after pulmonary thromboendarterectomy. *Am J Respir Crit Care Med* 1999;**160**:523–8.

15 Thoracic trauma, inhalation injury and post-pulmonary resection lung injury in intensive care

E D Moloney, M J D Griffiths, P Goldstraw

Trauma to the respiratory tract may cause respiratory failure and critical illness by several mechanisms. In this article we discuss three such conditions that are best managed by a multidisciplinary approach between physicians and surgeons. Thoracic trauma and inhalation injury are common causes of respiratory failure and critical illness often in young patients who have a good prognosis if the original insult is survivable. The pathogenesis of post-pulmonary resection lung injury is discussed as a well defined human model of the acute respiratory distress syndrome (ARDS) whose management is discussed in detail elsewhere in this book.

Despite the disparate nature of these conditions, common themes emerge in the supportive management of such patients while they recover (fig 15.1). For example, atelectasis and sputum retention follow all major pulmonary insults, including surgery, as a consequence of impaired cough and shallow respiration caused by pain and weakness. The tendency to develop respiratory failure and pneumonia may be minimised by adequate pain relief, mobilisation, and physiotherapy. Intermittent non-invasive ventilatory support and tracheal aspiration facilitated by a nasopharyngeal airway or a mini-tracheostomy help a patient with an inadequate cough.

THORACIC TRAUMA
Epidemiology
Thoracic trauma accounts for 20–25% of deaths following trauma and contributes to another 25% of trauma-related deaths. Blunt thoracic injuries have a higher mortality than penetrating injuries because of a higher incidence of injury to other organs. However, in both adults and children the predominant cause of death in patients with blunt thoracic trauma is head injury.[1][2] Approximately one third of all patients admitted to trauma centres have sustained serious injuries to the chest and the lung parenchyma is injured in a high proportion of these.[3] The leading causes of blunt and penetrating thoracic trauma are road traffic accidents, and stabbings and gun shot wounds, respectively.

Blunt thoracic trauma can produce a spectrum of injuries—including rib fractures, pneumothorax, flail segments and pulmonary contusion (fig 15.2)—all of which can impair pulmonary function.[4] Mortality for patients with three or more rib fractures is double that of patients without rib fractures (1.8% versus 3.9%),[2] and the presence of thoracic trauma increases the overall risk of death from 27% to 33%.[1] The presence of three or more rib fractures in an injured adult identifies a small group with an increased risk of splenic and liver injury.[1] Similarly, the presence of pneumothorax, haemothorax, pulmonary contusion, and a flail segment are each associated with an increased risk of death.[1]

Thoracic trauma is a significant aetiological factor in up to 20% of the 1 500 000 cases per year of ARDS in the United States.[5] ARDS may occur as a result of direct lung injury or from the systemic sequelae of extrathoracic injury.[6][7] In mechanically ventilated trauma patients, 18% developed ARDS when pulmonary contusion was their only risk factor. However, the incidence rose to 35% when other risk factors were present.[8] Pulmonary contusion is the most common injury seen in association with thoracic trauma, occurring in 30–75% of patients suffering major thoracic injury.[9] Contusion occurs more frequently following blunt thoracic injury and is an important factor leading to respiratory failure. It causes disruption of the alveolar-capillary membrane and increased pulmonary shunting, which may be exacerbated by a reduction in compliance caused by rib fracture or by attendant pain and muscle spasm. In one series 11% of patients with serious isolated pulmonary contusions died, whereas the mortality was much higher (22%) in patients with associated injuries.[10]

Management
The first priorities in managing thoracic trauma are securing an adequate airway and ventilation, controlling bleeding, and restoring adequate tissue perfusion. Mechanical ventilation is indicated when gas exchange is inadequate, despite aggressive pain management and pulmonary toilet.[11][12] The cervical spine should be stabilised during tracheal intubation in cases of severe blunt trauma. If an arrhythmia, hypotension, and/or changes in the central nervous system occur during or immediately after endotracheal intubation, air embolism should be suspected. Air embolism is a rare cause of intractable shock and cardiac arrest following thoracic trauma.[13]

Decreased breath sounds on one side, hypotension, neck vein distension, and deviation of the trachea suggest the presence of a tension pneumothorax warranting immediate needle decompression or tube thoracostomy.[11] A small well tolerated pneumothorax in a spontaneously breathing patient may suddenly be converted into a tension pneumothorax after positive pressure is applied to the airway. Nearly all air leaks will eventually seal if the lung is fully expanded and the chest tube is placed on suction. Generally, surgical intervention is considered if an air leak persists for 14 days. The exception to this rule is the patient with a major bronchial injury, which is suggested by a very large air leak, an inability to re-expand the lung with closed tube thoracostomy, and usually confirmed by bronchoscopy. In general, injuries to the trachea or major bronchi require operative repair.[14]

Hypotension without neck vein distension, tracheal deviation and dullness to percussion

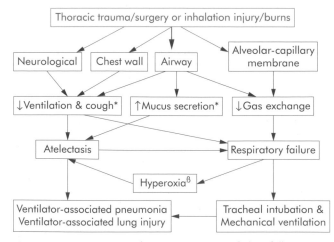

Figure 15.1   Common pathways to respiratory failure following thoracic trauma or inhalation injury. *Optimising pain relief, sputum clearance and respiratory mechanics are crucial in preventing respiratory failure at an early stage in the recovery period. §Hyperoxia causes reabsorption atelectasis.

suggests a significant haemothorax. In most cases bleeding will stop once the lung has been re-expanded using tube thoracostomy. Indications for thoracotomy are an initial loss of at least 1500 ml of blood upon placement of the chest tube, or continued bleeding of 200–300 ml/h.[14] Haemorrhage is the major preventable cause of trauma deaths in hospital, and hypotension following injury should be considered to be due to hypovolaemia until proved otherwise. Patients who have a retained haemothorax are at risk of empyema or a fibrothorax with lung entrapment. Non-operative management using closed tube thoracostomy has a lower likelihood of success when there is a significant amount of retained clot, if the fluid is viscous, or if it has a low pH. A larger empyema generally requires thoracotomy with decortication and drainage, particularly if an extensive pleural peel has developed.[14]

Sternal fracture may be associated with cardiac injury and is an indication for a 12 lead electrocardiogram (ECG) and cardiac monitoring for 12 hours. Acute cardiac tamponade should be suspected in patients who have refractory shock and evidence of raised central venous pressure. Pericardiocentesis and emergency thoracotomy may be life saving in this group of patients.[14] Echocardiography can be used as a non-invasive means of evaluating stable patients with a possible myocardial contusion or tamponade. Disruption of the aorta and great vessels, suggested by fracture of the first and second ribs, requires operative management that needs to be performed immediately if the patient is haemodynamically unstable. Aortography or chest CT scanning are definitive tests for blunt aortic injury and should be obtained in patients who have a wide mediastinum. Transoesophageal echocardiography can be performed instead of aortography in selected patients, allowing good views of the descending aorta but not the upper ascending aorta or aortic arch.[14] Penetrating injuries to the oesophagus are relatively uncommon, and blunt injuries to the oesophagus are rare. In patients not undergoing surgical exploration of a penetrating wound, the diagnosis of oesophageal injury can be made from radiographic studies. In general, oesophageal injuries are managed operatively. If the injury is more than 24 hours old, mediastinal inflammation may make it impossible to close the perforation; in this case, drainage with or without diversion may be the only option.[14]

Patients with rib fractures are more likely to require thoracotomy and their length of stay in the ICU is also significantly increased. Multiple rib fractures and flail chest (at least three contiguous ribs, each fractured in two places) suggest associated intrathoracic injury[15] and pneumothorax or haemothorax.[16] The mortality rate for patients with flail chest

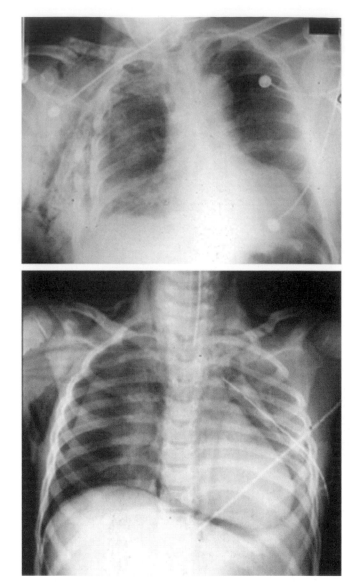

Figure 15.2   Radiographic features of thoracic trauma. (A) Right sided flail segment associated with ipsilateral pulmonary contusion, surgical emphysema and fractured clavicle. (B) The result of blunt thoracic trauma in a child causing bilateral pneumothoraces, pulmonary contusion and pneumopericardium; note the absence of rib fractures. The possible mediastinal displacement to the left suggests that the undrained right sided pneumothorax is under tension.

injuries is 30–33%,[16 17] with 30% of deaths related to intrathoracic injury, 30% to extrathoracic injury (most commonly closed head injury), and 30% related to multiple organ failure and ARDS.[16] In a study of 144 consecutive patients with blunt chest trauma, the mortality rate for pulmonary contusion alone or flail chest alone was 16%, whereas the combination of pulmonary contusion and flail chest resulted in a mortality rate of 42%.[17] Flail chest can lead to paradoxical ventilation, generating inefficient ventilation with progressive respiratory distress and failure. Respiratory failure in flail chest may also result from the increased work of breathing, pain, compromised cough, and atelectasis. A flail chest alone is not an indication for mechanical ventilation if the patient has adequate gas exchange. Thus, not all patients require tracheal intubation but rather alleviation of pain so that effective tidal volumes and vital capacities can be generated.[18] However, patients with flail chest require mechanical ventilation more frequently than those without flail segment.[16 17] The use of non-invasive positive pressure ventilation (NIPPV) in patients with a flail segment and lesser degrees of pulmonary contusion has also been described.[19] The decision to stabilise the chest wall surgically in flail chest is based on the experience and judgement of the surgeon. To date, the goal of minimising intubation time by internal fixation of rib fractures has not been proven to be effective in a randomised trial. However, a patient who either fails to wean or manifests a persistent chest wall deformity may benefit from surgical management. In addition, if thoracotomy is indicated for other reasons in a patient with a flail segment, it would appear reasonable to take the opportunity to stabilise the rib fractures.

Traditionally, the effect of the flail segment on pulmonary mechanics was thought to be the most significant aspect of the injury. However, pain is now recognised as the primary factor affecting pulmonary function.[20] By enabling the patient to take adequate tidal volumes and cough effectively, relief of pain from rib fractures can prevent the development of atelectasis, pneumonia, and sepsis, and obviate the need for mechanical ventilation in patients with severe chest trauma.[20 21] The standard of care has evolved from intubation and mechanical ventilation for all patients to optimisation of pain control combined with chest physiotherapy.[21] Systemic analgesics may be helpful in relieving pain but detrimental to the patient with marginal pulmonary mechanics in whom any reduction in respiratory drive may lead to hypoxia, atelectasis, and the need for mechanical ventilation.[22] The development of regional techniques has revolutionised the management of blunt thoracic trauma, providing a range of options for analgesia that should be tailored to individual needs.[23] The use of epidural catheters for continuous administration of opiates or local anaesthetics is the preferred technique for pain control in severe thoracic trauma and rarely produces any clinically significant alteration in pulmonary function.[24–27] Useful alternatives are intercostal nerve blocks and intrapleural local anaesthetic infusions.[28] The primary disadvantage of intercostal nerve blocks, however, is their relatively short duration of action (12.3 hours in one study[29]), requiring repeated injections for adequate pain control after trauma. The mechanism of action of intrapleural analgesia is unclear, but may be the simultaneous blockade of multiple intercostal nerves or nerve endings in the pleura.[30] A retrospective review of outcome factors among elderly patients after thoracic trauma showed clear improvement when an epidural catheter was used for analgesia compared with systemic narcotic alone.[31] There was a decreased incidence of pulmonary complications in the epidural group, and the incidence of pneumonia, ARDS, and death was significantly lower in these patients.[31] In a further study in which the efficacy of epidural and intrapleural catheters for pain relief and improvements in pulmonary function was compared, continuous epidural analgesia was clearly superior.[32] The only negative effect of epidural analgesia consistently found in this study was hypotension that was easily corrected.[32]

Most patients with penetrating chest injuries can be treated non-operatively, with only 10–15% requiring surgery.[33 34] In a series of 373 patients with penetrating lung injuries, chest tube insertion was found to be the only treatment required in 76% of patients and, of the remaining 24% who underwent exploratory thoracotomy, half required pulmonary repair or resection.[35] The majority of patients with mild to moderate chest wall injury who survive the acute phase recover with little or no pulmonary disability.[36]

INHALATION INJURY
Epidemiology
Inhalation injury can be thermal and/or chemical. It accompanies severe burns in up to 35% of those admitted to burn centres and accounts for 50–70% of burn related deaths.[37–39] The first comprehensive description of inhalation injury resulted from the 1942 Boston Coconut Grove fire in which 491 people died.[40] Furthermore, in the aftermath of the

2001 World Trade Center terrorist attack in New York, inhalation injury was the most frequent reason that survivors sought medical attention.[41] Inhalation injury predisposes burn patients to pneumonia, respiratory failure, and death.[42] Most burn patients who die have multiple organ failure[43]; in one study mortality was 67% in patients with isolated pulmonary failure but 92% when pulmonary failure was complicated by failure of at least one other system.[44] The incidence of ARDS complicating burns is 2–7%,[45] but is significantly higher in patients with inhalation injury.[42] In a review of 529 burn patients admitted over a 4 year period, patients with inhalation injury had a 73% incidence of respiratory failure and a 20% incidence of ARDS.[42] Advances in the treatment of burn victims have reduced mortality to 2–3% in those without respiratory complications compared with 46% in those with concomitant inhalation injury.[46]

Burn size is an important predictor of the development of pulmonary complications.[47] Smoke inhalation with minimal or no cutaneous burn is associated with chemical tracheobronchitis that does not add significantly to the morbidity and mortality of thermal injury. Patients with an inhalation injury and a medium sized burn often develop significant sequelae of their pulmonary injury which can add up to 20% to the expected mortality.[47] The importance of inhalation injury without pulmonary complications is controversial. While some have found that this does not add to mortality,[42] others have reported that inhalation injury increased mortality by 60% when complicated by pneumonia, and by as much as 20% even in the absence of infection.[47] It is possible, however, that in some patients without proven pneumonia, inhalation injury produced other complications that adversely affected outcome such as prolonged ventilator dependence, confinement to bed, and atelectasis.

Pathogenesis
Inhalation injuries can produce a wide spectrum of clinical effects. Smoke inhalation is a particularly challenging clinical problem because, apart from thermal injury, patients are often exposed to a large number of inhaled toxins such as pyrolysis products of plastics and other chemicals.[48] Death from smoke inhalation may be caused by direct pulmonary injury or asphyxia caused by oxygen deprivation or carbon monoxide exposure. Simple asphyxia may occur during a fire because the ambient oxygen level in a burning room may fall to less than 10%. Older individuals and those with pre-existing lung diseases may be more susceptible to the effects of inhalation injury.[49] In individuals with no past history of airway disease, the emergence of significant bronchial hyperreactivity after inhalation injury from irritating agents such as chlorine gas[50] is known as reactive airways disease syndrome (RADS).[51 52]

Irritant gases may produce a variety of clinical problems, including upper airway mucosal irritation and inflammation, laryngospasm, bronchoconstriction, atelectasis, and ARDS. Water solubility plays a key role in determining where inhaled gases deposit in the respiratory tract. Because the respiratory tract is lined with mucus, gases that are highly water soluble such as ammonia, sulphur dioxide, and hydrogen chloride generally cause acute irritant injury to mucous membranes, including the eyes and the lining of the nose and upper airway, and spare the lower respiratory tract. However, high solubility gases are also capable of causing lower tract injury at sufficiently high doses. Less soluble gases such as phosgene, ozone, and nitrogen oxides often have no effect on the upper airway, but they penetrate into the lower airway and irritate the small airways and gas exchange surface.[53] Gases of intermediate solubility such as chlorine may exert irritant effects widely throughout the respiratory tract. Furthermore, the particle size of inhaled substances determines the site and nature of the injury. Most particles that are smaller than $100\ \mu m$ can enter the airway. Particles with a diameter of

<10 µm can reach the lower respiratory tract, and those with a diameter of <5 µm can deposit in the terminal bronchi and alveoli. The effect of size is especially important for dusts and aerosols which can contain particles with diameters ranging from 50 µm to less than 1 µm.

Thermal injury is usually limited to the upper airway because of its efficiency as a heat exchanger and the low thermal capacity of air. However, thermal injury to the trachea and bronchi can result following exposure to steam. Chemical injury of the airway can be caused by irritants or cytotoxic chemicals that either adhere to fine particles in smoke or become aerosolised. Injury can occur at all levels of the airway and is typically patchy; even a short exposure to highly reactive irritants can result in loss of cilia and superficial epithelial erosions. Depletion of the free radical scavenger glutathione in the lungs of smoke exposed animals suggests a role for reactive oxygen species (ROS) mediated injury.[54] The damage from inhaled irritants can disrupt epithelial cell tight junctions, the influx of inflammatory cells, and leakage of interstitial fluid. Injury to the alveolar-capillary membrane caused by smoke inhalation is primarily mediated by neutrophils.[55–57] Cast formation may occur in small airways causing obstruction and atelectasis which decreases compliance and impairs gas exchange. Diffuse pneumonitis is the most common acute manifestation of injury to the pulmonary parenchyma, with clinical features that include dyspnoea, cough, and hypoxaemia. Although this is usually a self-limited process, more severe injury can lead to ARDS. Chronic sequelae of lower respiratory tract injury include bronchiolitis obliterans, cryptogenic organising pneumonia, and pulmonary fibrosis.[58]

Management

Clinical findings (facial burns, singed nasal vibrissae, or burned eyelashes) and chest radiography, which is often normal initially, are poor predictors of inhalation injury.[47] Vital signs and oxygen saturation may also be normal, even after significant inhalation injury. It is prudent to hospitalise patients with a history of significant smoke inhalation for at least 24 hours of observation because complications may not be immediately apparent. Importantly, the presence of stridor indicates significant upper airway oedema and warrants immediate tracheal intubation, since oedema and upper airway narrowing are typically progressive, usually peaking 12–24 hours after injury. Nebulised adrenaline may provide temporary relief but is not a definite treatment and frequent monitoring for evidence of progressive airway compromise must be continued.

Fibreoptic bronchoscopy may help in identifying incipient upper airway obstruction caused by oedema, providing it is carried out in circumstances that allow for securing the airway should the procedure lead to further deterioration.[59] Pulmonary toilet may be beneficial if there is significant endobronchial cast formation or if there is excessive carbonaceous material in the lungs.[60] However, a normal appearance of the upper airway on bronchoscopic examination does not exclude inhalation injury as distal injury caused by fine particulates which do not precipitate in the large calibre airways can be missed. Combining bronchoscopy with xenon-133 ventilation-perfusion lung scintiphotography, when the bronchoscopic findings are negative or equivocal, provides a highly sensitive means of diagnosing inhalation injury.[61]

Carbon monoxide poisoning is responsible for approximately 80% of the deaths associated with smoke inhalation.[62] The diagnosis is confirmed and the severity of poisoning estimated by measuring the percentage of haemoglobin saturated as carboxyhaemoglobin. Any patient suspected of inhalation injury should therefore receive 100% oxygen via a tight fitting non-rebreathing mask until carbon monoxide poisoning is excluded and the carboxyhaemoglobin level is less than 10%.

Physical examination of patients suffering from carbon monoxide poisoning typically shows cyanosis, although a cherry red skin colour may be encountered in well ventilated patients. Although hyperbaric oxygen therapy has some proponents, the accompanying risks and the lack of data confirming long term benefit provide no support for its use outside prospective randomised trials.[63]

Severe airway damage can denude the epithelium and lead to the formation of bloody casts consisting of inspissated mucus and blood clots. Aerosolised heparin (10 000 IU every 6 hours) can reduce the likelihood of endobronchial clot formation and respiratory decompensation.[64] In animal models, treatment with heparin alone did not attenuate pulmonary dysfunction after severe smoke injury, but combined treatment with nebulised heparin and systemic lisophylline had beneficial effects on pulmonary function in association with a decrease in blood flow to poorly ventilated areas and less lipid peroxidation.[65] Several other new experimental treatments for inhalation injury have shown promise in animal studies or limited human trials. For example, ascorbic acid infusions reduced the severity of respiratory dysfunction in burns patients with inhalation injury.[66] Neither prophylactic corticosteroids nor antibiotics are of benefit for smoke inhalation.[67] Nevertheless, patients with significant mucosal injury are at high risk for developing pneumonia, in which case antibiotic therapy should be instituted promptly. Corticosteroids should be given to patients with airflow obstruction unresponsive to inhaled bronchodilators. A chest wall eschar can limit gas exchange by restricting chest wall expansion and result in the need for relatively high airway pressures. Chest wall escharotomy which releases this constricting band can be lifesaving.

LUNG INJURY FOLLOWING LUNG RESECTION
Epidemiology

ARDS is defined as the acute onset of respiratory failure with refractory hypoxaemia (arterial oxygen tension (Pao_2)/inspiratory oxygen fraction (Fio_2) ratio <200 mm Hg) and bilateral infiltrates on frontal chest radiography that cannot be explained by, but may co-exist with, increased left atrial pressure (occluded pulmonary artery pressure (Ppa) <18 mm Hg).[68] ARDS is the extreme manifestation of a spectrum of acute lung injury (ALI) defined identically except for the presence of less severe refractory hypoxaemia (Pao_2/Fio_2 <300 mm Hg). The extent to which lung resection fulfils this requirement remains controversial as pneumonectomy, by definition, precludes the development of bilateral pulmonary infiltrates. However, most authorities now accept that many patients with what has been termed "post-pneumonectomy pulmonary oedema (PPO)" display the physiological and radiological defining criteria for ALI/ARDS.[69]

The reported mortality rate for ALI/ARDS associated with thoracotomy and pulmonary resection varies from 2% to 12%.[70 71] ALI/ARDS is the commonest cause of death following pulmonary resection,[72 73] and the majority die as a result of multiple organ failure.[74] The mortality rate remains high despite advances in supportive techniques. Before a consensus definition of ALI/ARDS was agreed, the incidence was reported to vary from 4% to 7% following pneumonectomy and from 1% to 7% after lobectomy, with an associated mortality of 50–100%.[75–77] A retrospective study using the consensus definition[68] found an incidence of 2.2%/5.2% for ALI/ARDS following lobectomy and 1.9%/4.9% after pneumonectomy.[78] A further study showed an incidence of 6%, 3.7%, and 1% for ALI/ARDS following pneumonectomy, lobectomy, and minor resections, respectively.[73] In this latter study ALI/ARDS contributed to 72% of all postoperative deaths.

No correlation has been found between age, preoperative lung function, arterial blood gas analysis, or duration of

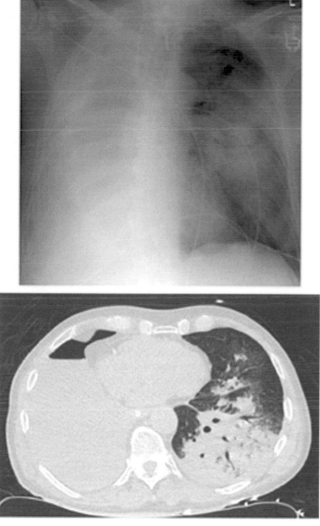

Figure 15.3 Radiographic features of acute lung injury following a right sided pneumonectomy. The CT scan shows dense dependent collapse and consolidation with overlying patchy consolidation and ground glass opacification.

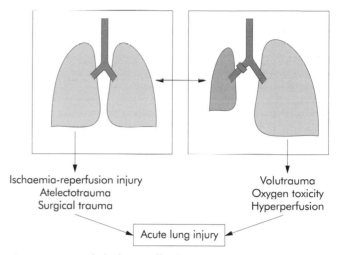

Figure 15.4 Both the lungs suffer damage that may contribute to acute lung injury during one lung ventilation and resection.

surgery and the development of ALI/ARDS.[72 78] However, men over the age of 60 years, especially when undergoing lung resection for lung cancer, form a high risk group.[73] Furthermore, no correlation has been found between the side of resection and the development of ALI/ARDS, but the risk increases progressively with more extensive resections.[73 75 79] ALI may present up to 7 days after surgery,[73 77] but most patients present between 1 and 3 days postoperatively.[75 76] Excessive perioperative administration of crystalloid may precipitate respiratory failure,[74 77] although recently the perceived role of fluid overload has diminished.[75 76] The high protein content of the alveolar oedema fluid and the frequent delay in presentation suggest that perioperative fluid overload is not the primary cause of post-pulmonary resection lung injury. The differential diagnosis includes lower respiratory tract infection and cardiogenic pulmonary oedema (fig 15.3]). Both can be investigated in the intubated patient by tracheal aspiration or bronchoscope guided sampling and pulmonary arterial catheterisation.

Pathogenesis
During pulmonary resection one lung is mechanically ventilated while clamping one lumen of a double lumen endotracheal tube collapses the lung being operated on. Repeated collapse and reinflation occur during the course of thoracotomy as the surgeon carries out the many steps in the operation. These cycles cause ischaemia-reperfusion (IR)

injury that are likely to resemble the insult suffered by a transplanted lung.[80 81] IR injury combined with the oxygen toxicity required to counterbalance the effects of shunt in the deflated lung induce the formation of reactive oxygen species (ROS) and reactive nitrogen species (RNS). Similarly, the gas exchange surface in the ventilated lung may be damaged by hyperperfusion, hyperoxia, and overdistension. Clinical observations suggest that injury to the non-operated side may be more important, as shown by a significant increase in density on the CT scan of the non-operated lung in eight out of nine patients following pulmonary resection.[82] Conversely, when the other lung that has been subjected to surgical trauma is re-expanded, IR leads to neutrophil recruitment and activation[80 83 84] and the formation of ROS,[85–87] and may cause systemic effects through the return of toxic metabolites to the circulation (fig 15.4).[88]

Under normal circumstances endogenous antioxidants closely regulate redox balance. However, if these defence mechanisms become overwhelmed, high levels of ROS/RNS may directly damage lipids, proteins and DNA, while lower levels affect signal transduction causing a change in cell behaviour without necessarily damaging or killing the cell. ROS have been implicated in the onset and progression of ARDS, both in animal models and clinical studies, in which markers of oxidative damage have been identified.[89 90] Iron is a catalyst for hydroxyl radical formation, and in patients with ARDS aberrant iron metabolism has been identified. Levels of chelatable redox active iron in bronchoalveolar lavage (BAL) fluid are greater in survivors of ARDS than in non-survivors.[91] Paradoxically, non-survivors had increased levels of transferrin and iron binding antioxidant activity.[92] After lobectomy the increase in hydrogen peroxide in exhaled breath condensate was greater than in breath from patients following pneumonectomy.[93] This may be explained by the increased tissue handling and dissection involved in doing a lobectomy compared with a pneumonectomy. Others have reported changes in several markers in the plasma indicating oxidative stress following lung resection (protein thiol, protein carbonyl, and myeloperoxidase levels), but no differences were observed between patients undergoing lobectomy and those undergoing pneumonectomy.[94]

Activated neutrophils in the lungs of patients with ALI produce ROS.[95 97] However, neutrophil depletion does not attenuate experimental IR mediated lung injury.[80] Following IR in the isolated perfused rat lung model, non-leucocyte derived ROS appear before neutrophil-endothelial cell adhesion and activation occur.[98] In humans an increase in pulmonary vascular permeability persists throughout the course of ARDS and correlates with the severity of lung injury and the neutrophil content of the BAL fluid.[99] Studies in rodents have looked at the effects of IR on hypoxic pulmonary vasoconstriction using albumin escape as a marker of endothelial integrity.[100] The integrity of the endothelium was maintained for up to 30 minutes of ischaemia alone. If, however, a shorter period of ischaemia was followed by reperfusion, the tendency for oedema formation was dramatically increased.[100] This suggests that short periods of ischaemia followed by reperfusion may cause as much damage as much longer periods of ischaemia alone.

CONCLUSION

Thoracic trauma and inhalation injury are common causes of respiratory failure and critical illness often in young patients who have a good prognosis if the original insult is survivable. Blunt thoracic trauma can produce a spectrum of injuries including rib fractures, pneumothorax, flail segments and pulmonary contusion, all of which can impair pulmonary function. Inhalation injury can be both thermal and/or chemical, and predisposes burn patients to pneumonia, respiratory failure, and death. ALI/ARDS is the most common cause of death following pulmonary resection, the pathogenesis of which results from IR injury. The mortality rate remains high despite advances in supportive techniques.

Despite the disparate nature of these conditions, common themes emerge in the supportive management of such patients. For example, atelectasis and sputum retention follow all major pulmonary trauma, including surgery, as a consequence of impaired cough and shallow respiration caused by pain and weakness. The tendency to develop respiratory failure and pneumonia may be minimised by adequate pain relief, mobilisation, and physiotherapy. Intermittent non-invasive ventilatory support and tracheal aspiration facilitated by a nasopharyngeal airway or a mini-tracheostomy may be required to help a patient with an inadequate cough. These conditions are best managed by a multidisciplinary approach.

REFERENCES

1 **Gaillard M**, Herve C, Mandin L, *et al*. Mortality prognostic factors in chest injury. *J Trauma* 1990;**30**:93–6.
2 **Lee RB**, Bass SM, Morris JA Jr, *et al*. Three or more rib fractures as an indicator for transfer to a level I trauma center: a population-based study. *J Trauma* 1990;**30**:689–94.
3 **Tominaga GT**, Waxman K, Scannell G, *et al*. Emergency thoracotomy with lung resection following trauma. *Am Surg* 1993;**59**:834–7.
4 **Webb WR**. Thoracic trauma. *Surg Clin North Am* 1974;**54**:1179–92.
5 **Bass TL**, Miller PK, Campbell DB, *et al*. Traumatic adult respiratory distress syndrome. *Surg Clin North Am* 1997;**7**:429–42.
6 **Ashbaugh DG**, Bigelow DB, Petty TL, Levine BE. Acute respiratory distress in adults. *Lancet* 1967;ii:319–23.
7 **Russell GB**, Campbell DB. Thoracic trauma and the adult respiratory distress syndrome. *Semin Thorac Cardiovasc Surg* 1992;**4**:241–6.
8 **Maunder RJ**, Hudson LD. *Adult respiratory distress syndrome*. New York: Marcel Dekker 1991: 1–21.
9 **Chopra PS**, Kroncke GM, Berkoff HA, *et al*. Pulmonary contusion a problem in blunt chest trauma. *Wisconsin Med J* 1977;**76**:S1–3.
10 **DeMuth WE**, Smith JM. Pulmonary contusion. *Am J Surg* 1965;**109**:819.
11 **Richardson JD**, Adams L, Flint LM. Selective management of flail chest and pulmonary contusion. *Ann Surg* 1982;**196**:481–7.
12 **Majeski JA**. Management of flail chest after blunt trauma. *South Med J* 1981;**74**:848–9.
13 **Saada M**, Goarin JP, Riou B, *et al*. Systemic gas embolism complicating pulmonary contusion. Diagnosis and management using transesophageal echocardiography. *Am J Respir Crit Care Med* 1995;**152**:812–5.
14 **American College of Surgeons**. *Advanced trauma life support program for doctors*. Chicago, IL: American College of Surgeons, 1997.
15 **Freedland M**, Wilson RF, Bender JS, *et al*. The management of flail chest injury: factors affecting outcome. *J Trauma* 1990;**30**:1460–8.
16 **Ciraulo DL**, Elliott D, Mitchell KA, *et al*. Flail chest as a marker for significant injuries. *J Am Coll Surg* 1994;**178**:466–70.
17 **Clark GC**, Schecter WP, Trunkey DD. Variables affecting outcome in blunt chest trauma: flail chest vs. pulmonary contusion. *J Trauma* 1988;**28**:298–304.
18 **Cicala RS**, Voeller GR, Fox T, *et al*. Epidural analgesia in thoracic trauma: effects of lumbar morphine and thoracic bupivacaine on pulmonary function. *Crit Care Med* 1990;**18**:229–31.
19 **Garfield MJ**, Howard-Griffin RM. Non-invasive positive pressure ventilation for severe thoracic trauma. *Br J Anaesth* 2000;**85**:788–90.

20 **Rankin AP**, Comber RE. Management of fifty cases of chest injury with a regimen of epidural bupivacaine and morphine. *Anaesth Intensive Care* 1984;**12**:311–4.
21 **Trinkle JK**, Richardson JD, Franz JL, *et al*. Management of flail chest without mechanical ventilation. *Ann Thorac Surg* 1975;**19**:355–63.
22 **Egbert LD**, Bendixen HH. Effect of morphine on breathing pattern: a possible factor in atelectasis. *JAMA* 1964;**188**:485–8.
23 **Karmakar MK**, Ho AM. Acute pain management of patients with multiple fractured ribs. *J Trauma* 2003;**54**:615–25.
24 **Dittmann M**, Steenblock U, Kranzlin M, *et al*. Epidural analgesia or mechanical ventilation for multiple rib fractures? *Intensive Care Med* 1982;**8**:89–92.
25 **Johnston JR**, McCaughey W. Epidural morphine. A method of management of multiple fractured ribs. *Anaesthesia* 1980;**35**:155–7.
26 **Ullman DA**, Fortune JB, Greenhouse BB, *et al*. The treatment of patients with multiple rib fractures using continuous thoracic epidural narcotic infusion. *Reg Anesth* 1989;**14**:43–7.
27 **Rawal N**, Sjostrand UH, Dahlstrom B, *et al*. Epidural morphine for postoperative pain relief: a comparative study with intramuscular narcotic and intercostal nerve block. *Anesth Analg* 1982;**61**:93–8.
28 **Haenel JB**, Moore FA, Moore EE, *et al*. Extrapleural bupivacaine for amelioration of multiple rib fracture pain. *J Trauma* 1995;**38**:22–7.
29 **Nunn JF**, Slavin G. Posterior intercostal nerve block for pain relief after cholecystectomy. Anatomical basis and efficacy. *Br J Anaesth* 1980;**52**:253–60.
30 **Shafei H**, Chamberlain M, Natrajan KN, *et al*. Intrapleural bupivacaine for early post-thoracotomy analgesia: comparison with bupivacaine intercostal block and cryofreezing. *Thorac Cardiovasc Surg* 1990;**38**:38–41.
31 **Wisner DH**. A stepwise logistic regression analysis of factors affecting morbidity and mortality after thoracic trauma: effect of epidural analgesia. *J Trauma* 1990;**30**:799–804.
32 **Luchette FA**, Radafshar SM, Kaiser R, *et al*. Prospective evaluation of epidural versus intrapleural catheters for analgesia in chest wall trauma. *J Trauma* 1994;**36**:865–9.
33 **Siemens R**, Polk HC Jr, Gray LA Jr, *et al*. Indications for thoracotomy following penetrating thoracic injury. *J Trauma* 1977;**17**:493–500.
34 **McSwain NE Jr**. Blunt and penetrating chest injuries. *World J Surg* 1992;**16**:924–9.
35 **Graham JM**, Mattox KL, Beall AC Jr. Penetrating trauma of the lung. *J Trauma* 1979;**19**:665–9.
36 **Landercasper J**, Cogbill TH, Lindesmith LA. Long-term disability after flail chest injury. *J Trauma* 1984;**24**:410–4.
37 **Herndon DN**, Langner F, Thompson P, *et al*. Pulmonary injury in burned patients. *Surg Clin North Am* 1987;**67**:31–46.
38 **Herndon DN**, Barrow RE, Linares HA, *et al*. Inhalation injury in burned patients: effects and treatment. *Burns Incl Therm Inj* 1988;**14**:349–56.
39 **Zawacki BE**, Jung RC, Joyce J, *et al*. Smoke, burns, and the natural history of inhalation injury in fire victims: a correlation of experimental and clinical data. *Ann Surg* 1977;**185**:100–10.
40 **Saffle JR**. The 1942 fire at Boston's Coconut Grove nightclub. *Am J Surg* 1993;**166**:581–91.
41 **Centers for Disease Control and Prevention**. Rapid assessment of injuries among survivors of the terrorist attack on the World Trade Center—New York City, September 2001. *JAMA* 2002;**287**:835–8.
42 **Hollingsed TC**, Saffle JR, Barton RG, *et al*. Etiology and consequences of respiratory failure in thermally injured patients. *Am J Surg* 1993;**166**:592–6.
43 **Hamit HF**. Factors associated with deaths of burned patients in a community hospital. *J Trauma* 1978;**18**:405–18.
44 **Marshall WG Jr**, Dimick AR. The natural history of major burns with multiple subsystem failure. *J Trauma* 1983;**23**:102–5.
45 **Fowler AA**, Hamman RF, Zerbe GO, *et al*. Adult respiratory distress syndrome. Prognosis after onset. *Am Rev Respir Dis* 1985;**132**:472–8.
46 **Haponik EF**, Crapo RO, Herndon DN, *et al*. Smoke inhalation. *Am Rev Respir Dis* 1988;**138**:1060–3.
47 **Shirani KZ**, Pruitt BA Jr, Mason AD Jr. The influence of inhalation injury and pneumonia on burn mortality. *Ann Surg* 1987;**205**:82–7.
48 **Kimmel EC**, Still KR. Acute lung injury, acute respiratory distress syndrome and inhalation injury: an overview. *Drug Chem Toxicol* 1999;**22**:91–128.
49 **Rajpura A**. The epidemiology of burns and smoke inhalation in secondary care: a population-based study covering Lancashire and South Cumbria. *Burns* 2002;**28**:121–30.
50 **Leroyer C**, Malo JL, Girard D, *et al*. Chronic rhinitis in workers at risk of reactive airways dysfunction syndrome due to exposure to chlorine. *Occup Environ Med* 1999;**56**:334–8.
51 **Alberts WM**, Brooks SM. Reactive airways dysfunction syndrome. *Curr Opin Pulm Med* 1996;**2**:104–10.
52 **Bardana EJ Jr**. Reactive airways dysfunction syndrome (RADS): guidelines for diagnosis and treatment and insight into likely prognosis. *Ann Allergy Asthma Immunol* 1999;**83**:583–6.
53 **Schwartz DA**. Acute inhalational injury. *Occup Med* 1987;**2**:297–318.
54 **LaLonde C**, Nayak U, Hennigan J, *et al*. Plasma catalase and glutathione levels are decreased in response to inhalation injury. *J Burn Care Rehabil* 1997;**18**:515–9.
55 **Guha SC**, Herndon DN, Evans MJ, *et al*. Is the CD18 adhesion complex of polymorphonuclear leukocytes involved in smoke-induced lung damage? A morphometric study. *J Burn Care Rehabil* 1993;**14**:503–11.
56 **Isago T**, Noshima S, Traber LD, *et al*. Analysis of pulmonary microvascular permeability after smoke inhalation. *J Appl Physiol* 1991;**71**:1403–8.

57 **Ischiropoulos H**, Mendiguren I, Fisher D, *et al.* Role of neutrophils and nitric oxide in lung alveolar injury from smoke inhalation. *Am J Respir Crit Care Med* 1994;**150**:337–41.

58 **Wright JL**. Inhalational lung injury causing bronchiolitis. *Clin Chest Med* 1993;**14**:635–44.

59 **Hunt JL**, Agee RN, Pruitt BA Jr. Fiberoptic bronchoscopy in acute inhalation injury. *J Trauma* 1975;**15**:641–49.

60 **Nakae H**, Tanaka H, Inaba H. Failure to clear casts and secretions following inhalation injury can be dangerous: report of a case. *Burns* 2001;**27**:189–91.

61 **Agee RN**, Long JM 3rd, Hunt JL, *et al.* Use of 133-xenon in early diagnosis of inhalation injury. *J Trauma* 1976;**16**:218–24.

62 **Zikria BA**, Weston GC, Chodoff M, *et al.* Smoke and carbon monoxide poisoning in fire victims. *J Trauma* 1972;**12**:641–5.

63 **Grube BJ**, Marvin JA, Heimbach DM. Therapeutic hyperbaric oxygen: help or hindrance in burn patients with carbon monoxide poisoning? *J Burn Care Rehabil* 1988;**9**:249–52.

64 **Cox CS Jr**, Zwischenberger JB, Traber DL, *et al.* Heparin improves oxygenation and minimizes barotrauma after severe smoke inhalation in an ovine model. *Surg Gynecol Obstet* 1993;**176**:339–49.

65 **Tasaki O**, Mozingo DW, Dubick MA, *et al.* Effects of heparin and lisofylline on pulmonary function after smoke inhalation injury in an ovine model. *Crit Care Med* 2002;**30**:637–43.

66 **Tanaka H**, Matsuda T, Miyagantani Y, *et al.* Reduction of resuscitation fluid volumes in severely burned patients using ascorbic acid administration: a randomized, prospective study. *Arch Surg* 2000;**135**:326–31.

67 **Nieman GF**, Clark WR, Hakim T. Methylprednisolone does not protect the lung from inhalation injury. *Burns* 1991;**17**:384–90.

68 **Bernard GR**, Artigas A, Brigham KL, *et al.* The American-European Consensus Conference on ARDS. Definitions, mechanisms, relevant outcomes, and clinical trial coordination. *Am J Respir Crit Care Med* 1994;**149**:818–24.

69 **Williams EA**, Evans TW, Goldstraw P. Acute lung injury following lung resection: is one lung anaesthesia to blame? *Thorax* 1996;**51**:114–6.

70 **Romano PS**, Mark DH. Patient and hospital characteristics related to in-hospital mortality after lung cancer resection. *Chest* 1992;**101**:1332–7.

71 **Wada H**, Nakamura T, Nakamoto K, *et al.* Thirty-day operative mortality for thoracotomy in lung cancer. *J Thorac Cardiovasc Surg* 1998;**115**:70–3.

72 **Ruffini E**, Parola A, Papalia E, *et al.* Frequency and mortality of acute lung injury and acute respiratory distress syndrome after pulmonary resection for bronchogenic carcinoma. *Eur J Cardiothorac Surg* 2001;**20**:30–6.

73 **Kutlu CA**, Williams EA, Evans TW, *et al.* Acute lung injury and acute respiratory distress syndrome after pulmonary resection. *Ann Thorac Surg* 2000;**69**:376–80.

74 **Zeldin RA**, Normandin D, Landtwing D, *et al.* Postpneumonectomy pulmonary edema. *J Thorac Cardiovasc Surg* 1984;**87**:359–65.

75 **Turnage WS**, Lunn JJ. Postpneumonectomy pulmonary edema. A retrospective analysis of associated variables. *Chest* 1993;**103**:1646–50.

76 **Waller DA**, Gebitekin C, Saunders NR, *et al.* Noncardiogenic pulmonary edema complicating lung resection. *Ann Thorac Surg* 1993;**55**:140–3.

77 **Mathru M**, Blakeman B, Dries DJ, *et al.* Permeability pulmonary edema following lung resection. *Chest* 1990;**98**:1216–8.

78 **Hayes JP**, Williams EA, Goldstraw P, *et al.* Lung injury in patients following thoracotomy. *Thorax* 1995;**50**:990–1.

79 **Keagy BA**, Lores ME, Starek PJ, *et al.* Elective pulmonary lobectomy: factors associated with morbidity and operative mortality. *Ann Thorac Surg* 1985;**40**:349–52.

80 **Lu YT**, Hellewell PG, Evans TW. Ischemia-reperfusion lung injury: contribution of ischemia, neutrophils, and hydrostatic pressure. *Am J Physiol* 1997;**273**:L46–54.

81 **De Perrot M**, Liu M, Waddell TK, *et al.* Ischaemia-reperfusion-induced lung injury. *Am J Respir Crit Care Med* 2003;**167**:490–511.

82 **Padley SP**, Jordan SJ, Goldstraw P, *et al.* Asymmetric ARDS following pulmonary resection: CT findings initial observations. *Radiology* 2002;**223**:468–73.

83 **Anderson BO**, Moore EE, Moore FA, *et al.* Hypovolemic shock promotes neutrophil sequestration in lungs by a xanthine oxidase-related mechanism. *J Appl Physiol* 1991;**71**:1862–5.

84 **Terada LS**, Dormish JJ, Shanley PF, *et al.* Circulating xanthine oxidase mediates lung neutrophil sequestration after intestinal ischemia-reperfusion. *Am J Physiol* 1992;**263**:L394–401.

85 **McCord JM**. Oxygen-derived radicals: a link between reperfusion injury and inflammation. *Fed Proc* 1987;**46**:2402–6.

86 **Adkison D**, Hollwarth ME, Benoit JN, *et al.* Role of free radicals in ischemia-reperfusion injury to the liver. *Acta Physiol Scand Suppl* 1986;**548**:101–7.

87 **Williams EA**, Quinlan GJ, Anning PB, *et al.* Lung injury following pulmonary resection in the isolated, blood-perfused rat lung. *Eur Respir J* 1999;**14**:745–50.

88 **Parks DA**, Granger DN. Contributions of ischemia and reperfusion to mucosal lesion formation. *Am J Physiol* 1986;**250**:G749–53.

89 **Pittet JF**, Mackersie RC, Martin TR, *et al.* Biological markers of acute lung injury: prognostic and pathogenetic significance. *Am J Respir Crit Care Med* 1997;**155**:1187–205.

90 **Metnitz PG**, Bartens C, Fischer M, *et al.* Antioxidant status in patients with acute respiratory distress syndrome. *Intensive Care Med* 1999;**25**:180–5.

91 **Gutteridge JM**, Mumby S, Quinlan GJ, *et al.* Pro-oxidant iron is present in human pulmonary epithelial lining fluid: implications for oxidative stress in the lung. *Biochem Biophys Res Commun* 1996;**220**:1024–7.

92 **Gutteridge GMC**, Quinlan G, Evans TW. Primary plasma antioxidants are secreted in patients with adult respiratory distress syndrome. *J Lab Clin Med* 1994;**124**:263–73.

93 **Lases EC**, Duurkens VA, Gerritsen WB, *et al.* Oxidative stress after lung resection therapy: a pilot study. *Chest* 2000;**117**:999–1003.

94 **Williams EA**, Quinlan GJ, Goldstraw P, *et al.* Postoperative lung injury and oxidative damage in patients undergoing pulmonary resection. *Eur Respir J* 1998;**11**:1028–34.

95 **Tate RM**, Repine JE. Neutrophils and the adult respiratory distress syndrome. *Am Rev Respir Dis* 1983;**128**:552–9.

96 **Lamb NJ**, Gutteridge JM, Baker C, *et al.* Oxidative damage to proteins of bronchoalveolar lavage fluid in patients with acute respiratory distress syndrome: evidence for neutrophil-mediated hydroxylation, nitration, and chlorination. *Crit Care Med* 1999;**27**:1738–44.

97 **Grace PA**. Ischaemia-reperfusion injury. *Br J Surg* 1994;**81**:637–47.

98 **Seibert AF**, Haynes J, Taylor A. Ischemia-reperfusion injury in the isolated rat lung. Role of flow and endogenous leukocytes. *Am Rev Respir Dis* 1993;**147**:270–5.

99 **Sinclair DG**, Braude S, Haslam PL, *et al.* Pulmonary endothelial permeability in patients with severe lung injury. Clinical correlates and natural history. *Chest* 1994;**106**:535–9.

100 **Messent M**, Griffiths MJ, Evans TW. Pulmonary vascular reactivity and ischaemia-reperfusion injury in the rat. *Clin Sci* 1993;**85**:71–5.

16 Illustrative case 1: cystic fibrosis

S R Thomas

CASE REPORT

A 26 year old man was admitted to the intensive care unit (ICU) on two occasions. Cystic fibrosis (CF) had been diagnosed at 2 months when he was failing to thrive and he was subsequently found to be homozygous for the ΔF508 mutation. At 19 years of age his respiratory tract secretions were colonised by *Burkholderia cepacia*. He had recurrent pneumothoraces requiring two surgical pleurodeses. Immediately before his ICU admissions his forced expiratory volume in 1 second (FEV_1) was 31% predicted. He had pancreatic insufficiency at the time of diagnosis and developed diabetes at the age of 23. He also had CF related liver disease, portal hypertension, and oesophageal varices.

He was admitted to the CF centre with a history of increased breathlessness and sputum production with haemoptysis. Intravenous antibiotics were commenced. *Staphylococcus aureus* and *B cepacia* were cultured in the sputum. On the night after admission he had a massive haematemesis requiring resuscitation, endotracheal intubation, and transfer to the ICU. An emergency endoscopy identified bleeding oesophageal varices that were banded. Bronchoscopic examination showed aspirated blood throughout the bronchial tree. He was successfully weaned from mechanical ventilation and transferred back to a high dependency area. The subsequent inpatient stay was complicated by decompensation of his liver disease and ascites. He also developed *B cepacia* septicaemia and was eventually allowed to go home almost 1 month after discharge from the ICU.

Three weeks after discharge from the CF centre he presented to his local hospital with haematemesis. After a further episode of haemorrhage, an endotracheal tube and subsequently a Sengstaken-Blakemore tube were inserted. Endoscopy the following day did not suggest variceal haemorrhage, but a bronchoscopy showed blood predominantly in the right bronchial tree. He required a massive blood transfusion and was transferred back to the ICU at the CF centre. Bronchial angiography demonstrated abnormal bronchial arteries in the right upper lobe and some abnormal vessels in the left lower lobe, which were embolised. After a failed extubation, a percutaneous tracheostomy was inserted. He continued to have episodes of haemoptysis and developed worsening ascites that compromised diaphragmatic function. The ascites did not improve with conservative management and was drained on two occasions. Hypernatraemia developed probably as a result of a sodium containing elemental feed, intravenous antibiotics, and hyperaldosteronism associated with liver disease. A change to a low sodium non-elemental feed in combination with pancreatic enzymes corrected the hypernatraemia. He subsequently developed *B cepacia* septicaemia and the intravenous antibiotics were changed based on new sensitivities. Gradual weaning from pressure support ventilation was achieved and he was breathing spontaneously via a tracheostomy 25 days after admission. He was transferred to the respiratory ward on day 28 and discharged home 18 days later. He died suddenly after only 12 days at home following what was thought to be a massive haematemesis.

MANAGEMENT OF CF PATIENTS IN THE ICU

Most critically ill patients with CF have end stage disease and intensive care is not considered; however, when the possibility of intensive care arises for individual patients it is often difficult to determine whether this is appropriate. When a patient with CF is admitted to the ICU a number of specialist issues arise—such as the management of haemoptysis, the treatment of infective exacerbations, and nutritional support—which will be discussed below. Close liaison between the CF and ICU teams is required. Non-invasive ventilation of patients with CF has been found to be highly effective, but does not usually occur in the ICU in the UK and will not be discussed extensively here.

Selecting CF patients for ICU care

The selection of patients with CF who are suitable for admission to the ICU is not easy, partly because there are relatively few published data on which to base the decision. One retrospective multicentre study published in 1978 examined the outcomes of 46 patients who developed respiratory failure between the ages of 1 month and 32 years[1]; 21 were aged over 15 years. In 35 episodes (69%) the patients died while receiving mechanical ventilation, and only eight patients (16%) survived for more than 6 weeks after discharge. In this small study age did not appear to influence the probability of survival. Another study examined the outcomes of five mechanically ventilated patients under 1 year of age.[2] All were successfully weaned from mechanical ventilation and discharged home, and were alive 2–6 years later.

Two more recent studies, one in the USA[3] and one in the UK,[4] have reached somewhat different conclusions. This is partly related to differences in approach and differences in the definition of "survivors".

The US study[3] examined the outcomes of 76 adult patients with CF admitted to an ICU at a CF and transplant centre. The difference between UK and USA practice is exemplified by the observation that, of a total of 136 admissions, only 32 episodes required endotracheal intubation and 30 were admitted for antibiotic desensitisation. Thirty three episodes were precipitated by massive haemoptysis and 11 of these patients (73%) were alive 1 year after discharge from the ICU. The authors did not state whether any of these patients required endotracheal intubation, but this seems unlikely as all of the intubation episodes appear to be accounted for by infective exacerbations. There were a total of 65 admissions for infective exacerbations, 32 of which required endotracheal intubation. A total of 71% of the respiratory failure episodes resulted in survival to ICU discharge. This included 15 episodes that did not require any ventilatory support and 18 episodes that required non-invasive ventilation only. Twenty (62%) of the patients who received endotracheal intubation survived to be discharged from the ICU. Two patients were alive without transplantation 1 year after discharge and 10 had successful transplants. Although 17 subjects who were admitted with respiratory failure received transplants and 14 were alive 1 year later, the proportion of the patients who were transplanted from the ventilator and were alive 1 year later was not stated.

The UK study[4] examined the outcomes of 31 patients with CF admitted over 8 years to the ICU who required endotracheal intubation. In the UK most patients in the ICU require endotracheal intubation, and restrictions on bed availability mean that other patients are cared for in high dependency units or elsewhere. The patients were divided into two groups. The first group included 12 patients admitted on 13 occasions for respiratory failure, either due to aspiration of blood (three episodes) or infective exacerbations. Five subjects (38%) survived to hospital discharge, a figure similar to the American study described above, but only two patients (16%) survived beyond 6 months. The second group included 16 patients admitted to the ICU after surgical procedures on 18 occasions, 16 of which followed surgical pleurodesis. Fourteen of the subjects survived to hospital discharge and 11 (65%) survived beyond 6 months.

What conclusions can be drawn from these studies? It would appear that outcomes are good in infants requiring mechanical ventilation because of respiratory failure and in patients requiring ventilation after surgical pleurodesis. The outcome in patients admitted to the ICU after massive haemoptysis and haematemesis also appears relatively good. The outcome in the patients in the US study[3] also appeared favourable with the majority alive at 1 year, although (as mentioned above) it appears that these subjects did not require endotracheal intubation. Although the outcomes of patients with infective exacerbations in the US study appeared favourable, the population studied was different from that in the UK study in that only a minority required endotracheal intubation. In addition, many of the patients receiving mechanical ventilation subsequently had lung transplants, whereas none of the UK patients who were intubated were transplanted. Both the recent UK and US studies found that FEV$_1$ was not predictive of survival.

The role of transplantation for endotracheally intubated patients remains controversial. Although one study[5] has documented a 1 year survival rate of 50% in 10 patients who received mechanical ventilation for up to 42 days, many centres do not consider these patients for transplantation. At the Royal Brompton and Harefield Hospitals[6] only two of five patients who had been intubated and mechanically ventilated survived transplantation, and both survivors were ventilated for less than 24 hours preoperatively. The poorer outcome of ventilated patients receiving transplants coupled with severely restricted organ availability discourages transplantation in this group. The different ways in which centres prioritise patients for transplantation will also influence whether organs will become available within a reasonable time scale for ventilated patients. In contrast, non-invasive ventilation is well established as a bridging technique to transplantation.

There are probably many reasons for the poor outcome from invasive ventilation in these patients. They usually have severe pre-existing pulmonary disease and may also have associated liver disease. Even with optimal physiotherapy, sputum clearance will be less effective than in a conscious patient who is able to cough effectively and cooperate with physiotherapy.

Reversible factors need to be identified before deciding to intubate and ventilate a patient with CF, and those with end

stage disease should not normally receive this form of support. The relative lack of published evidence makes it difficult to make decisions for individual patients and, where possible, both the patient and the family need to be involved in the decision making process. It is only rarely appropriate to ventilate patients with CF who develop respiratory failure, and this is well illustrated by the experience at the Royal Brompton Hospital where only 16 such episodes have occurred over an 8 year period.[4]

Management of massive haemoptysis

Guidelines have been published for the management of massive haemoptysis (>240 ml/day).[7 8] Medical treatment includes the correction of coagulation defects with vitamin K and fresh frozen plasma. An infective exacerbation is often a precipitant and intravenous antibiotics should be commenced. The affected lung should be kept dependent in an attempt to avoid contamination of the other lung. There is case report evidence for the use of tranexamic acid.[9] An attempt should be made to localise the site of bleeding. This can be achieved in a number of ways. Many patients experience a sensation of gurgling in a particular part of the chest[8 10 11] and a recent study has shown that this is a reliable guide.[8] The chest radiograph may also show unilateral air space shadowing. If doubt remains, bronchoscopy should be performed. Bronchial embolisation is effective[8] and carries a low risk of complications that include chest pain, dysphagia, bronchial necrosis, bowel ischaemia, and, very rarely, paraplegia.[10 12 13]

Management of infective exacerbations

Antibiotics should be selected based on the most recent sputum culture. *Pseudomonas aeruginosa* is usually treated with an aminoglycoside in combination with another antipseudomonal antibiotic. Combination therapy is thought to reduce the risk of emergence of resistance. Although a recent study has suggested that monotherapy with tobramycin is effective,[14] it cannot be recommended in the ICU setting. The choice of antipseudomonal antibiotic includes carbapenems such as meropenem, carboxypenicillins such as ticarcillin, ureidopenicillins such as azlocillin, or third generation cephalosporins such as ceftazidime. Piperacillin appears to be associated with febrile reactions in patients with CF[15] and should be avoided. Once daily tobramycin does appear to be effective in patients with CF,[16] but this conclusion is based on a small study and confirmation is required. *Burkholderia cepacia* is usually multiresistant but may be sensitive to chloramphenicol, cotrimoxazole, ceftazidime, temocillin, or meropenem.[17] If the pulmonary pathogen is unknown, antipseudomonal antibiotics should always be given in conjunction with an antistaphylococcal antibiotic such as flucloxacillin. Aminoglycosides have a higher volume of distribution in CF patients than in non-CF individuals so a higher dose is usually required. Monitoring of aminoglycoside drug levels is essential.

Regular physiotherapy is crucial in these patients as they are unable to clear their secretions spontaneously. Whether toilet bronchoscopy is better than blind endobronchial suction is unknown, but inspection of the bronchi and suction is used when ventilatory problems arise and sputum plugging is suspected.

The role of recombinant human deoxyribonuclease (DNase) is uncertain in ventilated patients. In patients with CF it reduces the frequency of infective exacerbations[18 19] and has been shown to be safe and effective in those with severe disease.[20] However, efficacy is thought to be dependent upon effective sputum clearance which is more difficult in the ventilated patient. The effect of DNase on sputum clearance in ventilated patients has not been studied directly but, when a patient has been receiving DNase before admission to the ICU, it is generally continued.

Table 16.1 Common cystic fibrosis related pathologies, complications and principal elements of management in intensive care (for details see text)

CF related pathology	Complication	Management
Lung disease		
Bacterial colonisation of airways	Infective exacerbations	• Antibiotics • Physiotherapy • DNase
	Multiresistant pathogens	• Antibiotics selected according to sensitivities
	Sputum plugging	• Endobronchial suction • Bronchoscopy • DNase
Obstructive lung disease	Difficult ventilation Prolonged weaning	• Bronchodilators • Tracheostomy • NIV
Other	Haemoptysis	• Tranexamic acid • Bronchial artery embolisation
Gastrointestinal disease	Pancreatic insufficiency	• Pancreatic enzymes • Elemental feed
	Distal intestinal obstruction syndrome	• Maintain good hydration • Lactulose • N-acetyl cysteine • Gastrografin enema
Liver disease	Coagulopathy	• Vitamin K • Fresh frozen plasma
	Thrombocytopenia Altered drug metabolism	• Platelet transfusion • Careful drug prescribing practice
	Variceal haemorrhage	• Variceal banding
Diabetes	Hyperglycaemia	• Intravenous insulin
Other		
CF upper airway disease	Sinusitis	• Avoid nasal intubation • Antibiotics

Tracheostomies and weaning

Weaning patients with CF from mechanical ventilation is frequently prolonged and tracheostomies are often used to facilitate this process. A percutaneous rather than a surgical technique may be preferred for convenience and a lower incidence of complications.[21] There is limited experience in the use of percutaneous tracheostomies in patients with CF, and it is unknown whether the infected bronchial secretions in these patients predispose to a higher incidence of postoperative infections.

Non-invasive ventilation

As described above, invasive ventilation is associated with poor outcomes. Non-invasive ventilation has therefore been investigated as an alternative and has been shown to be effective in selected cases.[22 23] It may also be used to facilitate weaning from mechanical ventilation.

Gastrointestinal pathology and liver disease

Early nutritional support should be commenced. An elemental feed may be used or, alternatively, a standard feed with pancreatic enzyme supplementation. In those with liver disease a feed with a low sodium content should be used to avoid hypernatraemia.

Patients with CF who are acutely unwell, especially after surgery,[24] are at risk of developing the distal intestinal obstruction syndrome (DIOS); fever, dehydration,[25] and opioid analgesia may all contribute. Preventative strategies include the avoidance of dehydration, continuation of pancreatic enzyme supplementation, use of lactulose, and a carefully considered approach to the use of opioids. Treatment options include nasogastric or rectal N-acetyl cysteine, Gastrografin enemas, and intestinal lavage with a balanced electrolyte solution containing polyethylene glycol. Surgery can usually be avoided.

The incidence of liver disease in patients with CF depends on how it is defined, but it may occur in 25% of subjects[26] and symptomatic liver disease occurs in less than 5% of cases. Many patients with CF have a small increase in the liver isoenzyme of alkaline phosphatase and γ-glutamyl-transpeptidase but, if these enzymes are raised to more than four times normal, then liver disease is usually present. The presence of liver disease undoubtedly increases the risk of complications occurring during an ICU admission because of an increased risk of bleeding due to thrombocytopenia and coagulopathy. Oesophageal varices may be present. Care should be taken with the use of drugs that are metabolised by the liver or excreted in the bile. Ascites may cause diaphragmatic splinting and may need to be drained to facilitate ventilation.

Diabetes

A significant proportion of patients have CF related diabetes (CFRD). The prevalence appears to increase with age and one study has reported a prevalence of about 15%.[27] Tight control of blood glucose levels is associated with improved survival in critically ill non-CF patients.[28]

CONCLUSION

Intensive care is only appropriate for a small number of patents with CF with reversible complications of their disease. Limited evidence is available to help in deciding which patients should be selected for support of organ failures in the ICU and how such patients should be managed. There is a need for more research in this area. A summary of some of the problems that may be experienced is given in table 16.1.

Where possible, severely ill CF patients should be transferred to their CF specialist centre and this will facilitate optimal treatment of their multisystem disease. It is also easier for decisions about continuation of treatment to be made where pre-existing trusting relationships have developed between patients, their relatives, and their clinicians.

REFERENCES

1 **Davis PB**, Di Sant'Agnese PA. Assisted ventilation for patients with cystic fibrosis. *JAMA* 1978;**239**:1851–4.

2 **Garland JS**, Chan YM, Kelly KJ, *et al*. Outcome of infants with cystic fibrosis requiring mechanical ventilation for respiratory failure. *Chest* 1989;**96**:136–8.

3 **Sood N**, Paradowski LJ, Yankaskas JR. Outcomes of intensive care unit care in adults with cystic fibrosis. *Am J Respir Crit Care Med* 200;**163**:335–8.

4 **Thomas SR**, Evans TW, Geddes TW, *et al*. CF in adults: outcome after admission to intensive care (abstract). *Pediatr Pulmonol* 2000;**20**(Suppl):292.

5 **Massard G**, Shennib H, Metras D, *et al*. Double-lung transplantation in mechanically ventilated patients with cystic fibrosis. *Ann Thorac Surg* 1993;**55**:1087–91.

6 **Swami A**, Evans TW, Morgan CJ, *et al*. Ventilation of patients with end stage cystic fibrosis (abstract). *J Cardiothorac Vasc Anaesth* 1992;**6**(Suppl I):47.

7 **Schidlow DV**, Taussig LM, Knowles MR. Cystic Fibrosis Foundation consensus conference report on pulmonary complications of cystic fibrosis. *Pediatr Pulmonol* 1993;**15**:187–98.

8 **Brinson GM**, Noone PG, Mauro MA, *et al*. Bronchial artery embolization for the treatment of hemoptysis in patients with cystic fibrosis. *Am J Respir Crit Care Med* 1998;**157**:1951–8.

9 **Graff GR**. Treatment of recurrent severe hemoptysis in cystic fibrosis with tranexamic acid. *Respiration* 2001;**68**:91–4.

10 **Tonkin IL**, Hanissian AS, Boulden TF, *et al*. Bronchial arteriography and embolotherapy for hemoptysis in patients with cystic fibrosis. *Cardiovasc Intervent Radiol* 1991;**14**:241–6.

11 **Cohen AM**, Doershuk CF, Stern RC. Bronchial artery embolization to control hemoptysis in cystic fibrosis. *Radiology* 1990;**175**:401–5.

12 **Ivanick, MJ**, Thorwarth W, Donohue J, *et al*. Infarction of the left main-stem bronchus: a complication of bronchial artery embolization. *Am J Roentgenol* 1983;**141**:535–7.

13 **Lemoigne F**, Rampal P, Petersen R. Fatal ischemic colitis after bronchial artery embolization. *Presse Med* 1983;**12**:2056–7.

14 **Master V**, Roberts GW, Coulthard KP, *et al*. Efficacy of once-daily tobramycin monotherapy for acute pulmonary exacerbations of cystic fibrosis: a preliminary study. *Pediatr Pulmonol* 2001;**31**:367–76.

15 **Stead RJ**, Kennedy HG, Hodson ME, *et al*. Adverse reactions to piperacillin in adults with cystic fibrosis. *Thorax* 1985;**40**:184–6.

16 **Whitehead A**, Conway SP, Etherington C, *et al*. Once-daily tobramycin in the treatment of adult patients with cystic fibrosis. *Eur Respir J* 2002;**19**:303–9.

17 **Ciofu O**, Jensen T, Pressler T, *et al*. Meropenem in cystic fibrosis patients infected with resistant Pseudomonas aeruginosa or Burkholderia cepacia and with hypersensitivity to beta-lactam antibiotics. *Clin Microbiol Infect* 1996; **2**:91–8.

18 **Fuchs HJ**, Borowitz DS, Christiansen DH, *et al*. Effect of aerosolized recombinant human DNase on exacerbations of respiratory symptoms and on pulmonary function in patients with cystic fibrosis. The Pulmozyme Study Group. *N Engl J Med* 1994;**331**:637–42.

19 **Quan JM**, Tiddens HA, Sy JP, *et al*. A two-year randomized, placebo-controlled trial of dornase alfa in young patients with cystic fibrosis with mild lung function abnormalities. *J Pediatr* 2001;**139**:813–20.

20 **Shah PI**, Bush A, Canny GJ, *et al*. Recombinant human DNase I in cystic fibrosis patients with severe pulmonary disease: a short-term, double-blind study followed by six months open-label treatment. *Eur Respir J* 1995;**8**:954–8.

21 **Freeman BD**, Isabella K, Lin N, *et al*. A meta-analysis of prospective trials comparing percutaneous and surgical tracheostomy in critically ill patients. *Chest* 2000;**118**:1412–8.

22 **Hodson ME**, Madden BP, Steven MH, *et al*. Non-invasive mechanical ventilation for cystic fibrosis patients: a potential bridge to transplantation. *Eur Respir J* 1991;**4**:524–7.

23 **Madden BP**, Kariyawasam H, Siddiqi AJ, *et al*. Noninvasive ventilation in cystic fibrosis patients with acute or chronic respiratory failure. *Eur Respir J* 2002;**19**:310–3.

24 **Minkes RK**, Langer JC, Skinner MA, *et al*. Intestinal obstruction after lung transplantation in children with cystic fibrosis. *J Pediatr Surg* 1999;**34**:1489–93.

25 **Hodson ME**, Mearns MB, Batten JC. Meconium ileus equivalent in adults with cystic fibrosis of pancreas: a report of six cases. *BMJ* 1976;**2**:790–1.

26 **Nagel RA**, Westaby D, Javaid A, *et al*. Liver disease and bile duct abnormalities in adults with cystic fibrosis. *Lancet* 1989;**ii**:1422–5.

27 **Lanng S**, Thorsteinsson B, Lund-Andersen C, *et al*. Diabetes mellitus in Danish cystic fibrosis patients: prevalence and late diabetic complications. *Acta Paediatr* 1994;**83**:72–7.

28 **Van den Berghe G**, Wouters P, Weekers F, *et al*. Intensive insulin therapy in the critically ill patients. *N Engl J Med* 2001;**345**:1359–67.

17 Illustrative case 2: interstitial lung disease

A T Jones, R M du Bois, A U Wells

CASE REPORT

A 31 year old man with a 5 month history of Jo-1 negative dermatomyositis was admitted to the intensive care unit (ICU) with respiratory failure. Five months previously he had developed severe myositis which responded to corticosteroid treatment (prednisolone 1 mg/kg) with symptomatic improvement and a fall in creatine kinase. Six weeks later he developed chest radiographic infiltrates, extensive ground glass opacification on high resolution computed tomographic (HRCT) scanning (fig 17.1), and hypoxaemic respiratory failure despite maintenance treatment with prednisolone 20 mg daily. He deteriorated despite antimicrobial and increased corticosteroid treatment, requiring mechanical ventilation. A thoracoscopic biopsy specimen taken while on the ventilator disclosed diffuse alveolar damage admixed with organising pneumonia. Intravenous methylprednisolone (750 mg daily for 3 days) allowed weaning from ventilatory support and eventual discharge from hospital on prednisolone (0.5 mg/kg) and azathioprine (200 mg once daily). One month later he was readmitted with increasing dyspnoea and was treated for cytomegalovirus (CMV) pneumonitis diagnosed on the basis of a positive urinary detection of early antigen fluorescent foci (DEAFF) test and bronchoalveolar lavage (BAL) immunofluorescence. After a good initial response, progression of interstitial lung disease became evident radiologically and a single dose of intravenous cyclophosphamide (1.4 g) was administered.

One week later he developed increasing dyspnoea associated with increasing oxygen requirements and a low grade fever, but there were no major changes in chest radiographic abnormalities or inflammatory indices which were only mildly increased. Broad spectrum antibiotic treatment was instituted with cotrimoxazole to cover pneumocystis pneumonia (PCP) and intravenous ganciclovir to cover recrudescence of CMV pneumonitis. However, all cultures, including specific testing for CMV antigen, were negative. Continued deterioration prompted transfer to the ICU 48 hours after admission.

Examination of bronchoalveolar lavage (BAL) samples revealed no evidence of infection. Having failed to identify an infective agent and in the presence of broad spectrum antimicrobial treatment, the patient's continued decline was treated with three further daily doses of intravenous methylprednisolone and a further dose of intravenous cyclophosphamide. The transplantation investigation protocol was initiated and cyclosporin was added in the hope of decreasing steroid requirements. However, intermittent noninvasive support was increasingly necessary and tracheal intubation and mechanical ventilation were required 7 days after admission to the ICU. Despite vasopressor support, adjustment of antimicrobial treatment (including the empirical addition of liposomal amphotericin), and the use of granulocyte colony stimulating factor to treat pancytopenia, he continued to deteriorate and died 30 days after admission to the ICU. No clear evidence of underlying infection was obtained. Overall, the balance of probability strongly favoured inexorable progression of underlying interstitial lung disease.

MANAGEMENT OF PATIENTS WITH DIFFUSE INTERSTITIAL LUNG DISEASE IN THE ICU

Use of diagnostic techniques

This case illustrates important management difficulties in patients with diffuse interstitial lung disease (DILD) who progress to respiratory failure. Clinically, the differential diagnosis usually consists of deterioration of the underlying disease demanding increased immunosuppression, and infection requiring antimicrobial treatment and a reduction in immunosuppressive treatment. The distinction is important, whatever the likely outcome. Young patients with connective tissue disease may have an excellent long term outcome if they survive an acute episode—be it infective or due to inflammatory DILD—and prolonged aggressive intervention is appropriate. By contrast, major progression of fibrotic disease generally denotes a very poor outcome once mechanical ventilation has been instituted in idiopathic and connective tissue disease alike; prolonged ventilation is inappropriate.

Unfortunately, in most connective tissue diseases and other forms of DILD no serological marker correlates closely with pulmonary disease activity. The distinction between the onset of infection and progression of disease is complicated by the marked similarities in clinical presentation (fever, cough, increased breathlessness, and increased radiographic shadowing). Similarly, laboratory indices of infection (white blood cell count, erythrocyte sedimentation rate, C reactive protein) lack sensitivity or specificity as all may be influenced by the underlying pulmonary inflammation or systemic disease activity. The development of organ dysfunction or nosocomial infection in patients requiring intensive care may add to the diagnostic difficulties. Ideal markers that distinguish between infection and inflammation in patients requiring critical care and in those with autoimmune disease are not yet available for routine clinical use.[1 2]

Chest radiography is often unhelpful in discriminating between infection and progression of DILD in patients requiring critical care.[3] HRCT scanning is central to the diagnosis and management of DILD[4] and is a safe means of obtaining clinical and physiological information in critically ill patients.[5] It may be diagnostic in advanced DILD,[6] obviating the need for invasive investigation. When it is inconclusive diagnostically, CT may define the optimal site for surgical biopsy. However, although fairly accurate in the exclusion of ventilator associated pneumonia in

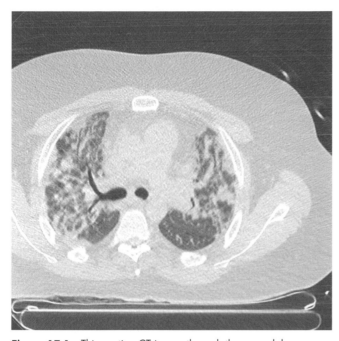

Figure 17.1 Thin section CT image through the upper lobes showing patchy consolidation, some of which is peribronchial. There is a generalised non-specific increase in attenuation of the lung parenchyma. The consolidation could represent autoimmune organising pneumonia associated with connective tissue disease (in view of its bronchocentric distribution), but an infective cause for the changes (or a coexisting infective component) cannot be excluded. Poor quality images are also a major constraint in the patient with severe dyspnoea at rest. Some of the ground glass attenuation may be technical.

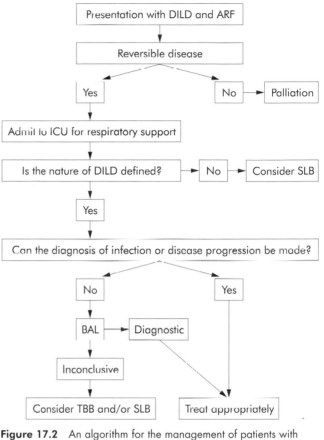

Figure 17.2 An algorithm for the management of patients with diffuse interstitial lung disease (DILD) and acute respiratory failure (ARF). BAL=bronchoalveolar lavage; TBB=transbronchial biopsy; SLB=surgical lung biopsy.

ARDS,[7] CT scanning has not been evaluated as a diagnostic test for opportunistic infection in the ventilated patient with DILD. As illustrated by the present case, the interpretation of ground glass opacification on the CT scan is not always straightforward, especially in connective tissue diseases where opportunistic infection may coexist with a number of primary pulmonary disease processes. In this setting, invasive or semi-invasive investigation is often required. In the present case there was a compelling need to define the underlying interstitial lung disease and an immediate diagnostic surgical lung biopsy (SLB) was performed, obviating semi-invasive less definitive procedures. However, in cases in which the underlying diagnosis is known and the problem is one of distinguishing between infection and disease progression, a more calibrated approach is usually appropriate including BAL and transbronchial biopsy (TBB) before SLB (fig 17.2).

In a case where pulmonary infiltrates are associated with immunosuppressive therapy, BAL makes a crucial contribution to the detection of opportunistic infection.[8 9] The spectrum of likely infective organisms depends on a variety of factors including the presence of neutropenia,[10] the nature of the underlying disease process and immunosuppressive therapy,[11 12] the prior administration of antimicrobial treatment,[13] and the timing of the BAL relative to hospital admission and the onset of ventilation.[14 15] Bacterial pathogens are isolated most commonly, but staining and cultures should be undertaken to exclude fungal, mycobacterial, and viral infections. In addition, non-infectious causes of diffuse radiographic shadowing including malignancy and alveolar haemorrhage may be identified. New diagnostic techniques applicable to BAL fluid include antigen detection (e.g. *Aspergillus* spp, *Cryptococcus neoformans*, *Legionella pneumophilia*), antibody detection (e.g. antipneumolysin for pneumococcal pneumonia), special methods for culture (BACTEC radiometric culture for mycobacteria), and techniques from molecular biology such as the polymerise chain reaction. However, the appropriate use of new diagnostic tests is often difficult to rationalise; their clinical usefulness is likely to be heavily dependent upon the quality of specimen, BAL technique, and population studied.[16] It is advisable for clinicians to seek microbiological advice before performing BAL if the use of novel diagnostic procedures is contemplated.

BAL is generally safe in immunosuppressed patients including those with haematological dysfunction[17] and in critically ill patients requiring mechanical ventilation.[18 19] However, deterioration in respiratory mechanics and gas exchange is well recognised and may be clinically significant.[20 21] Thus, BAL should be performed in the ICU in high risk patients; occasionally it is appropriate to institute mechanical ventilation before BAL is undertaken.

The diagnosis of CMV pneumonitis was unexpected but illustrates the diagnostic usefulness of BAL. CMV pneumonitis is probably rare outside transplant patients and those infected with HIV.[22–24] In patients infected with HIV the clinical significance of positive CMV serological testing is uncertain.[24] There are few data in other patient groups[25] but CMV pneumonitis is associated with a high rate of mortality (>80%) if treatment is delayed.[26 27] Serological evidence of previous CMV infection is common in adults, especially after the age of 40. As CMV pneumonitis typically presents with fever, dyspnoea and diffuse infiltrates on the chest radiograph, it may be very difficult to make the crucial distinction between infection and progression of disease.[28] Diagnostic viral cytopathic changes in TBB or open lung biopsy specimens tend to occur in advanced infection by which time antiviral treatment may be less efficacious, reinforcing continued interest in non-invasive techniques that promise rapid diagnosis.[24 25]

The added value of TBB in patients undergoing BAL remains contentious. In a retrospective study of immunosuppressed patients TBB was more sensitive than BAL (77% *v* 48%

in HIV disease, 55% v 20% in haematological malignancy, 57% v 27% in renal transplant recipients) and there were few serious complications.[29] In patients with HIV infection it has been argued that a negative BAL result should prompt a repeat BAL with TBB at the most abnormal site; this approach has a diagnostic yield of 90% for nodules or focal infiltrates.[30] In a retrospective study of mechanically ventilated patients, TBB was diagnostic in 35% of cases and led to a change in management in 60% of "medical" patients and in 25% of patients following lung transplantation.[31] The frequency of pneumothorax was higher (10.4%) than is generally reported in non-ventilated subjects (5%), but there were no serious complications. At subsequent open lung biopsy or necroscopic examination there was a concordance of 85% with TBB findings. The authors argue that TBB is safe in mechanically ventilated patients with undiagnosed pulmonary infiltrates and may obviate the need for SLB.

When BAL and TBB are non-diagnostic, SLB may be warranted. Although widely accepted in DILD in general,[4] the role of SLB has been questioned in ventilated subjects because of a perception of higher risk and reduced benefit in critically ill patients. However, it can be argued that diagnostic accuracy in this patient group (which is central to confident management) justifies the increased incidence of perioperative complications. The diagnostic yield of SLB in ventilated patients has varied from 46% to 100%,[32–35] but the influence of diagnosis on management is not always easy to quantify. In one study the attainment of a definitive diagnosis resulted in continuation of existing treatment in 33% of patients, increased immunosuppression in 26%, initiation of immunosuppression in 22%, and a change in antimicrobial treatment in 19%.[32] In ventilated patients the mortality rate with SLB may be as high as 10% and operative complications, occurring in approximately 20%, may influence survival.[32–35] However, mortality after the initial postoperative period is probably largely ascribable to progression of the underlying condition rather than to the surgical procedure, although controlled clinical data are lacking. Factors predicting mortality in ventilated patients with pulmonary infiltrates undergoing SLB have included an immunocompromised status at the onset of respiratory failure or current immunosuppressive treatment, severe hypoxia, multiorgan failure, and older age.[33–35]

In immunocompromised patients in the ICU, high inpatient and 1 year mortality rates (50% and 90%, respectively) are often cited to suggest that SLB adds little to the management provided that broad spectrum antibiotic cover (including cotrimoxazole to cover PCP) and a trial of corticosteroid treatment are instituted.[36 37] However, "patient benefit" is not always synonymous with eventual survival. Inappropriate immunosuppressive therapy may be associated with infective complications. SLB may identify irreversible disease, allowing inappropriate support to be minimised[33 34] and withdrawal of care issues to be discussed definitively with the relatives.[38 39] Finally, immunocompromised patients with underlying DILD can be viewed as "special cases" with regard to the performance of SLB because of the unique difficulties in distinguishing between infection and progression of the primary disease.

Role of lung transplantation

Mechanical ventilation is widely regarded as a strong relative contraindication to lung transplantation because of the high risk of pneumonia due to airway microbial colonisation, severe muscular deconditioning due to immobility, and other complications such as sepsis, deep venous thrombosis, gastrointestinal haemorrhage, altered gut motility, and nutritional problems.[40] The International Society of Heart Lung Transplantation/United Network for Organ Sharing has documented a threefold increase in 1 year mortality in mechanically ventilated patients compared with those who are nonventilated.[41] However, in small populations from selected

centres, outcomes have been similar to those in non-ventilated recipients. In a recent report of 21 patients who were transplanted while being mechanically ventilated, six developed acute allograft dysfunction and all died within a year with three not surviving the postoperative period.[42] However, there were no postoperative deaths among the remaining 15 patients and their long term survival (40%) did not differ from non-ventilated patients undergoing transplantation. Thus, mechanical ventilation should not be viewed as an absolute contraindication to transplantation. In our patient the factors favouring attempted transplantation included his age, relatively brief history (minimising severe muscular deconditioning), and the lack of evidence of relentless systemic disease activity.

Non-invasive ventilation decreases the need for tracheal intubation and increases the likelihood of successful weaning from mechanical ventilation, both resulting in a lower incidence of nosocomial infection.[43] The successful use of non-invasive ventilation as a bridge to transplantation in patients developing respiratory failure has been reported.[44 45] In view of the general scarcity of donor organs, the indications for transplantation in patients receiving mechanical ventilation are necessarily imprecise and controversial. Decisions should not be subject to generic guidelines but must be individualised, taking into account such factors as the presence of reversible superimposed processes (with a realistic chance of bridging to surgery with treatment) and the likelihood of expeditious transplantation. Immediate transplantation during an acute episode is seldom practicable.

CONCLUSION

In patients with interstitial lung disease who deteriorate to respiratory failure, the distinction between infection and progression of disease is often difficult and sometimes, as in the presented case, the two may coexist. Accurate management requires BAL which is best performed in the ICU in those with borderline respiratory failure; TBB may be a useful adjunct. In selected cases SLB may be invaluable both diagnostically and as an aid to confident management. Although seldom justifiable, transplantation of a ventilated patient is not absolutely contraindicated, especially in young non-deconditioned patients.

REFERENCES

1 **Brunkhorst R**, Eberhardt OK, Haubitz M, et al. Procalcitonin for discrimination of systemic autoimmune disease and systemic bacterial infection. Intensive Care Med 2000;**26**:S199–201.

2 **Reinhart K**, Karsai W, Meisner M. Procalcitonin as a marker of the systemic inflammatory response to infection. Intensive Care Med 2000;**26**:1193–200.

3 **Hansell DM**. Imaging the injured lung. In: Evans TW, Haslett C, eds. Acute respiratory distress in adults. London: Chapman and Hall, 1996: 361–79.

4 **British Thoracic Society**. BTS guidelines on the diagnosis, assessment and treatment of diffuse parenchymal lung disease in adults. Thorax 1999;**54**(Suppl 1):S4–14.

5 **Pesenti A**, Tagliabue P, Patroniti N, et al. Computerised tomography scan imaging in acute respiratory distress syndrome. Intensive Care Med 2001;**27**:631–9.

6 **Primack SL**, Hartman TE, Hansell DM, et al. End stage lung disease: findings in 61 patients. Radiology 1993;**189**:681–6.

7 **Winer-Muram HT**, Steiner RM, Gurney JW, et al. Ventilator-associated pneumonia in patients with adult respiratory distress syndrome: CT evaluation. Radiology 1998;**208**:193–9.

8 **Klech H**, Hutter C. Clinical guidelines for bronchoalveolar lavage (BAL): Report of the European Society of Pneumonology Task Force Group on BAL. Eur Respir J 1990;**3**:937–74.

9 **Stover DE**, Zaman MB, Hajdu SI, et al. Bronchoalveolar lavage in the diagnosis of diffuse pulmonary infiltrates in the immunocompromised host. Ann Intern Med 1984;**101**:1–7.

10 **Cordonnier C**, Escudier E, Verra F, et al. Bronchoalveolar lavage during neutropenic episodes: diagnostic yield and cellular pattern. Eur Respir J 1994;**7**:114–20.

11 **Ewig S**, Torres A, Riquelme R, et al. Pulmonary complications inpatients with haematological malignancies treated at a respiratory ICU. Eur Respir J 1998;**12**:116–22.

12 **Dunagan DP**, Baker AM, Hurd DD, *et al.* Bronchoscopic evaluation of pulmonary infiltrates following bone ,marrow transplantation. *Chest* 1997;**111**:135–41.

13 **Hohenadel IA**, Kiworr M, Genitsariotis R, *et al.* Role of bronchoalveolar lavage in immunocompromised patients with pneumonia treated with broad spectrum antibiotic and antifungal regimen. *Thorax* 2001;**56**:115–20.

14 **Fagon J**, Chastre J, Wolf M, *et al.* Invasive and noninvasive strategies for management of suspected ventilator-associated pneumonia. *Ann Intern Med* 2000;**132**:621–30.

15 **Mehta R**, Niederman MS. Adequate empirical therapy minimizes the impact of diagnostic methods in patients with ventilator-associated pneumonia. *Crit Care Med* 2000;**28**:3092–4.

16 **Mayaud C**, Cadranel J. A persistent challenge: the diagnosis of respiratory disease in the non-AIDS immunocompromised host. *Thorax* 2000;**55**:511–7.

17 **Saito H**, Anaissie EJ, Morice RC, *et al.* Bronchoalveolar lavage in the diagnosis of pulmonary infiltrates in patients with acute leukaemia. *Chest* 1988;**94**:745–9.

18 **Steinberg KP**, Mitchel DR, Maunder RJ, *et al.* Safety of bronchoalveolar lavage in patients with adult respiratory distress syndrome. *Am Rev Respir Dis* 1993;**148**:556–61.

19 **Montravers P**, Gauzit R, Dombret MC, *et al.* Cardiopulmonary effects of bronchoalveolar lavage in critically ill patients. *Chest* 1993;**106**:1541–7.

20 **Klein U**, Karzai W, Zimmermann P, *et al.* Changes in pulmonary mechanics after fibreoptic bronchoalveolar lavage in mechanically ventilated patients. *Intensive Care Med* 1998;**12**:1289–93.

21 **Verra F**, Hmouda H, Rauss A, *et al.* Bronchoalveolar lavage in immunocompromised patients. Clinical and functional consequences. *Chest* 1992;**101**:1215–20.

22 **Mann M**, Shelhamer JH, Masur H, *et al.* Lack of clinical utility of bronchoalveolar lavage cultures for cytomegalovirus in HIV infection. *Am J Respir Crit Care Med* 1997;**155**:1723–8.

23 **Mera JR**, Whimbey E, Elting L, *et al.* Cytomegalovirus pneumonia in adult nontransplantation patients with cancer: review of 20 cases occurring from 1964 through 1990. *Clin Infect Dis* 1996;**22**:1046–50.

24 **Baughman RP**. Cytomegalovirus: the monster in the closet. *Am J Respir Crit Care Med* 1997;**156**:1–2.

25 **Tamm M**, Traenkle P, Grilli B, *et al.* Pulmonary cytomegalovirus infection in immunocompromised patients. *Chest* 2001;**119**:838–43.

26 **Reed EC**, Bowden RA, Dandliker PS, *et al.* Treatment of cytomegalovirus with ganciclovir and intravenous cytomegalovirus immunoglobulin in patients with bone marrow transplants. *Ann Intern Med* 1988;**109**:783–8.

27 **Emmanuel D**, Cunningham I, Jules-Elysee K, *et al.* Cytomegalovirus pneumonia after bone marrow transplantation successfully treated with combination of ganciclovir and high-dose intravenous immune globulin. *Ann Intern Med* 1988;**109**:777–82.

28 **Smith CB**. Cytomegalovirus pneumonia: state of the art. *Chest* 1989;**95**:182–7S.

29 **Cazzadori A**, Di Perri G, Todeschini G, *et al.* Transbronchial biopsy in the diagnosis of pulmonary infiltrates in immunocompromised patients. *Chest* 1995;**107**:101–6.

30 **Cadranel J**, Gillet-Juvin K, Antoine M. Site directed bronchoalveolar lavage and transbronchial biopsy in HIV-infected patients with pneumonia. *Am J Respir Crit Care Med* 1995;**152**:1103–6.

31 **O'Brien JD**, Ettinger NA, Shevlin D, *et al.* Safety and yield of transbroncial biopsy in mechanically ventilated patients. *Crit Care Med* 1997;**25**:440–6.

32 **Canver CC**, Menttzer RM. The role of open lung biopsy in early and late survival of ventilator-dependent patients with diffuse idiopathic lung disease. *J Cardiovasc Surg* 1994;**35**:151–5.

33 **Flabouris A**, Myburgh J. The utility of open lung biopsy in patients requiring mechanical ventilation. *Chest* 1999;**115**:811–7.

34 **Warner DO**, Warner MA, Divertie MB. Open lung biopsy in patients with diffuse pulmonary infiltrates and acute respiratory failure. *Am Rev Respir Dis* 1988;**137**:90–4.

35 **Poe RH**, Wahl GW, Qazi R, *et al.* Predictors of mortality in the immunocompromised patient with pulmonary infiltrates. *Arch Intern Med* 1986;**146**:1304–8.

36 **Potter D**, Pass HI, Brower S, *et al.* Prospective randomized study of open lung biopsy versus empirical antibiotic therapy for acute pneumonitis in non-neutropenic cancer patients. *Ann Thorac Surg* 1985;**40**:422–8.

37 **McKenna RJ**, Mountain CF, McMurtrey MJ. Open lung biopsy in immunocompromised patients. *Chest* 1984;**86**:671–4.

38 **Ferrand E**, Robert R, Ingrand P, *et al.* Witholding and withdrawal of life support therapy in intensive care units in France: a prospective survey. *Lancet* 2001;**357**:9–14.

39 **Abbott KH**, Breen CM, Abernethy AP, *et al.* Families looking back: one year after discussion of withdraw or withholding life-sustaining therapy. *Crit Care Med* 2001;**29**:197–201.

40 **American Thoracic Society**. International giudelines for the selection of lung transplant candidates. *Am J Respir Crit Care Med* 1998;**158**:335–9.

41 **O'Brien GD**, Criner GJ. Mechanical ventilation as a bridge to lung transplantation. *J Heart Lung Transplant* 1999;**18**:255–65.

42 **Meyers BF**, Lynch JP, Battafarano RJ, *et al.* Lung transplant is warranted in stable, ventilator-dependent patients. *Ann Thorac Surg* 2000;**70**:1675–8.

43 **Evans TW**, Albert RK, Angus DC, *et al.* International Consensus Conferences in Intensive Care Medicine: Noninvasive positive pressure ventilation in acute respiratory failure. *Am J Respir Crit Care Med* 2001;**163**:283–91.

44 **Hodson ME**, Madden BP, Steven MH. Noninvasive mechanical ventilation for cystic fibrosis patients: a potential bridge to transplantation. *Eur Respir J* 1991;**4**:524–7.

45 **Quarata AJ**, Roy B, O'Brien GD, *et al.* Noninvasive positive pressure ventilation as bridge therapy to lung transplantation or volume reduction surgery. *Am J Respir Crit Care Med* 1996;**153**:A608.

18 Illustrative case 3: pulmonary vasculitis

ME Griffith, S Brett

CASE REPORT

A 28 year old man was admitted from a local hospital to the intensive care unit (ICU) at Hammersmith Hospital via the operating theatre. He had presented with a 3 month history of nasal stuffiness, epistaxis and haemoptysis, and had recently noticed increasing shortness of breath. He had lost 6 kg in weight and reported night sweats. His initial chest radiograph showed diffuse peripheral shadowing and a subsequent computed tomographic (CT) scan confirmed the presence of multiple infiltrative lesions (fig 18.1). Bronchoscopy showed evidence of recent diffuse haemorrhage; bronchoalveolar lavage cytology revealed an eosinophilia but was negative for acid fast bacilli, legionella, and fungi. Over the next few days he deteriorated, requiring endotracheal intubation and ventilation. He was transferred for an open lung biopsy. Lung histology was non-specific showing diffuse alveolar haemorrhage with fibrin deposition, fibroblastic proliferation, and a predominantly neutrophilic inflammatory infiltrate. Following the lung biopsy the patient was admitted to the ICU with severe hypoxaemic respiratory failure.

The patient had no significant past medical history. He was born in India and raised in the UK; his last visit abroad was to India 2 years before admission. He was a sales manager for a building company and did not smoke. On admission to ICU he was pyrexial at 38°C. He was paralysed and ventilated requiring 95% oxygen. There were no rashes, eyes and joints were normal, but he was noted to have a slight crusting of his nares. The blood pressure was 114/54 mm Hg supported by norepinephrine and dopexamine infusions. Clinical biochemistry results were: C reactive protein 99 mg/l, Na 135 mmol/l, K 4.3 mmol/l, urea 6.1 mmol/l, creatinine 52 µmol/l, albumin 16 g/l, ionised calcium 1.88 mmol/l, bilirubin 8 µmol/l, alkaline phosphatase 134 U/l (normal range 30–130), and alanine aminotransferase 76 U/l (0–31). The blood film showed a leucoerythroblastic picture; the counts were haemoglobin 7.5 g/dl, mean cell volume 89 fl, white cell count 15×10^9/l (neutrophil leucocytosis), platelets 324×10^9/l. Urine microscopy showed multiple red cell casts. Urgent ANCA (antineutrophil cytoplasmic antibodies) immunofluorescence was strongly positive for C-ANCA; anti-PR3 ELISA was also strongly positive at 89% (0–15%). This confirmed the clinical diagnosis of Wegener's granulomatosis and treatment was initiated with prednisolone and cyclophosphamide. In view of the severity of his lung haemorrhage he underwent five episodes of plasma exchange. His renal function deteriorated over 6 days and he required continuous renal replacement therapy for fluid balance and metabolic control. The aetiology of the renal failure was multifactorial with sepsis and nephritis contributing. As he was receiving heavy immunosuppression, he was given anti-infective prophylaxis with co-trimoxazole, fluconazole, and isoniazid. In order to minimise further lung haemorrhage, his intravascular volume was kept as low as possible by tightly controlling fluid balance. He sustained one episode of line sepsis treated with vancomycin. He required high concentrations of oxygen (Fio_2 >0.5) for 10 days and then his condition gradually improved; a tracheostomy was performed and his trachea was ultimately decannulated 15 days after ICU admission. His renal function recovered and he was discharged from hospital 46 days after admission with a creatinine level of 86 µmol/l. His pulmonary function was clinically good and was not assessed formally.

DISCUSSION
Presentation and diagnosis
This case illustrates the importance of the aggressive pursuit and treatment of the cause of acute respiratory failure. The history in this case provided important clues, but in some cases of acute severe respiratory failure a clinical picture of hypoxaemic respiratory failure with non-specific changes on the chest radiograph is all that is available on presentation to the ICU. The initial differential diagnosis is wide and includes most obviously infective agents, but also interstitial lung disease and vasculitis. High resolution CT scanning can be helpful but, unless it is performed in held static inspiration with arms out of the field, can be misleading. Serological tests are extremely valuable but may not be rapidly available.

Systemic vasculitis is characteristically a multifocal disease with a variety of clinical manifestations according to the size of the blood vessel involved and the organs affected. It is classified according to the size of the smallest vessel involved.[1] Alveolar haemorrhage results from small vessel vasculitides involving the lungs; these include Wegener's granulomatosis, microscopic polyangiitis and, rarely, Churg-Strauss syndrome. They can present at any age but occur most commonly in patients in their 50s and 60s and there is a slight male predominance.[2 3] There are reports of vasculitis occurring in families,[4–7] but most cases arise sporadically and, unlike most autoimmune diseases, so far no consistent HLA associations have been identified,[8] although there are associations with certain complement alleles and alleles of α_1-antitrypsin.[9–12] Environmental factors such as silica exposure,[13–15] drugs,[3 16] and infections[17–19] may play a part; however, although these may be important in elucidating the pathogenesis of vasculitis, in practice most cases have no obvious genetic or environmental precipitant. As can be seen from this case presentation, prompt diagnosis of vasculitis is vital, not only to instigate appropriate treatment but also to avoid unnecessary invasive diagnostic procedures. In retrospect, the previously arranged open lung biopsy in this case was probably not required and was precipitated by the deteriorating state of the patient and the need to secure a diagnosis. The

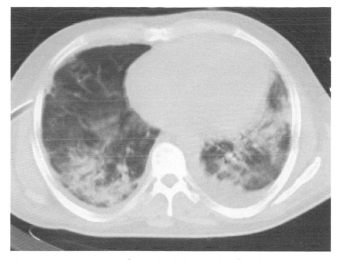

Figure 18.1 CT scan of a ventilated patient with pulmonary haemorrhage. Scattered dense airspace shadowing can be seen with some background ground glass shadowing. Small effusions are also visible. Courtesy of Dr Jeremy Levy.

ANCA result arrived on the ITU at the same time as the patient returned from theatre.

Small vessel vasculitis in the lung involves destruction of arterioles, capillaries and venules by an infiltration of activated neutrophils. This results in interstitial oedema and diffuse alveolar haemorrhage. Repeated episodes of lung haemorrhage may result in pulmonary fibrosis.[20] Haemoptysis is a common presenting feature, although it can be late or even absent even in the face of significant alveolar bleeding.[21] Other symptoms include dyspnoea, fever, and weight loss. Patients are anaemic, hypoxaemic, and have diffuse infiltrative shadowing on the chest radiograph. Alveolar haemorrhage can sometimes be confirmed on bronchoscopy, with haemosiderin-laden macrophages seen on cytological examination of lavage fluid. However, patients may be too hypoxic to undergo this procedure. Carbon monoxide transfer coefficient corrected for lung volume (Kco) will be raised. In the ITU patients are often ventilated, and methods of measuring Kco in ventilated patients have been reported and validated, although they are often only available in specialist centres where operators are familiar with their interpretation.[22 23] A CT scan of the chest is often unhelpful in determining the aetiology of alveolar haemorrhage, although it may reveal cavitating lesions typical of granulomatous infiltration. Lung biopsies frequently demonstrate necrotic tissue or show non-specific inflammation and haemorrhage, particularly if obtained via the transbronchial route, but the yield can be improved by open lung biopsy. If there is evidence of renal involvement a renal biopsy is more likely to be diagnostic and will usually show a focal necrotising glomerulonephritis.

Patients with vasculitis may present with isolated pulmonary haemorrhage, but usually there is also systemic involvement. Most patients with Wegener's granulomatosis have granulomatous lesions in the upper respiratory tract which result in chronic sinusitis, epistaxis, chronic otitis media, and deafness. Involvement of the trachea can present with life threatening stridor. Granulomas are also found in many sites outside the respiratory system including the kidney, central nervous system, prostate, parotid and orbit.[3] Patients with microscopic polyangiitis and Wegener's granulomatosis also present with systemic symptoms secondary to the small vessel vasculitis. Urine abnormalities include microscopic haematuria and proteinuria, with red cell casts on microscopy. The serum creatinine may initially be in the normal range, but acute renal failure tends to develop quite rapidly. Renal and respiratory involvement both have a significant effect on mortality.[3 24 25] Other organs in which vasculitis commonly occurs are skin, joints, muscles, gastrointestinal system, peripheral and central nervous system, and the eye.

Routine blood counts often show a normocytic or microcytic anaemia with a neutrophil leucocytosis, although there can also be eosinophilia (especially in Churg-Strauss syndrome) and thrombocythaemia. Thrombocytopenia suggests alternative causes of lung haemorrhage such as primary haematological abnormalities or systemic lupus erythematosus, in which case there will often be accompanying low complement levels and positive antinuclear antibodies. The erythrocyte sedimentation rate and C reactive protein level will both be raised. Biochemistry will often show a low serum albumin, raised alkaline phosphatase, and raised urea and creatinine. These results may point to a diagnosis of vasculitis but are relatively non-specific. The most important serological tests in the diagnosis of vasculitis are antineutrophil cytoplasmic antibodies (ANCA). ANCA were first described in 1982[26] and subsequently was found to be associated with both Wegener's granulomatosis and microscopic polyangiitis. There are two main patterns of ANCA—cytoplasmic (C) and perinuclear (P)—defined by their appearance on indirect immunofluorescence using ethanol fixed neutrophils. The main target antigen of C-ANCA is proteinase 3 (PR3).[27–30] P-ANCA have a wider range of specificities but, in systemic vasculitis, they are usually specific for myeloperoxidase (MPO).[31] Most patients with Wegener's granulomatosis have anti-PR3 specific ANCA, patients with Churg-Strauss syndrome and polyarteritis nodosa have anti-MPO ANCA, and patients with microscopic polyangiitis have either anti-PR3 or anti-MPO ANCA. If immunofluorescence is used alone, then C-ANCA is more specific than p-ANCA for vasculitis since perinuclear staining is not only produced by anti-myeloperoxidase antibodies but also by antinuclear antibodies and antibodies to neutrophil enzymes not associated with vasculitis. All serum that is ANCA positive should therefore be tested in PR3 and MPO ELISA as this greatly increases their specificity.[32] In a large European trial for the standardisation of ANCA assays, the specificity of immunofluorescence alone was found to be 97% for C-ANCA and 81% for a P-ANCA pattern. The combination of C-ANCA with anti-PR3 and P-ANCA with anti-MPO both had a specificity of 99%.[33] However, a negative ANCA assay does not exclude the possibility of vasculitis as there are a few cases of small vessel vasculitides that are ANCA negative.[34 35] In these cases a tissue diagnosis should be sought.

Management

Systemic vasculitis should be treated with cyclophosphamide (we use 3 mg/kg/day, reduced in the elderly to 2 mg/kg/day) combined with prednisolone. Historically, cyclophosphamide was continued for at least a year after remission.[36 37] However, in view of the side effect profile of cyclophosphamide, many clinicians now substitute azathioprine in stable patients at 3 months. The European Vasculitis Study Group has set up a series of multicentre randomised controlled trials to investigate the roles of different immunosuppressive regimes in vasculitis. The first of these trials to be completed has recently confirmed that azathioprine is as effective as cyclophosphamide for maintenance of remission after 3 months,[38] More recently mycophenylate mofetil, levamisole, and TNF directed treatment have also been used.[39] In patients with fulminant disease such as dialysis dependent renal failure and alveolar haemorrhage, there may be an additional benefit from plasma exchange or intravenous methylprednisolone[40 41] and the results of the current European trials should clarify this. In patients who fail to respond to this treatment or who cannot tolerate cyclophosphamide due to marrow suppression, there may also be a role for immunoabsorption,[42 43] pooled immunoglobulin,[44 45] or monoclonal antibodies,[46] although so far much of the evidence is anecdotal. Lung haemorrhage is a major cause of early mortality and aggressive supportive therapy is important. Patients should be kept relatively intravascularly depleted until the lung haemorrhage is controlled, and clearly exacerbating pulmonary oedema must be avoided. Although acute renal failure may be exacerbated by this regimen, this is of secondary importance as the patient can be supported with renal replacement therapy and acute tubular necrosis caused by initial volume depletion is likely to recover in the long term. However, care must be taken to avoid hypoperfusion of the splanchnic circulation with consequent gut and liver dysfunction that may result in multiple organ failure.

There is little evidence on which to base ventilatory strategies for adults. A rational approach is to limit excessive tidal volume excursions or pressure changes which are likely to damage further the fragile vasculature and exacerbate haemorrhage. Modest gas exchange targets should therefore be set. However, profound hypoxaemia and hypercapnia should be avoided as this may exacerbate pulmonary hypertension. A high inspired oxygen fraction may be harmful on theoretical grounds concerning oxidant stress, but a compromise needs to be found until the patient responds to specific treatment. Extracorporeal membrane oxygenation has been used successfully in a small number of cases[47] but cannot currently be recommended.

In summary, patients admitted to the ICU with suspected pulmonary vasculitis have a high mortality of around 25–50%, depending upon aetiology. These patients should be discussed early with a centre which has specialist expertise in this area to ensure prompt diagnosis and access to adjuvant therapies such as plasma exchange. ANCA assays are vital in the diagnosis, and patients with suspected lung haemorrhage should be tested within 24 hours of presentation. This will help to minimise morbidity and mortality from these diseases. Good long term survival can be achieved with prompt treatment with appropriate immunosuppressive agents. Continued low dose immunosuppression and follow up are required long term as there is a high incidence of relapse.

REFERENCES

1 **Jennette JC**, Falk RJ, Andrassy K, et al. Nomenclature of systemic vasculitides. Proposal of an international consensus conference. Arthritis Rheum 1994;**37**:187–92.
2 **Luqmani RA**, Bacon PA, Beaman M, et al. Classical versus non-renal Wegener's granulomatosis. Q J Med 1994;**87**:161–7.
3 **Gaskin G**, Pusey CD. Systemic vasculitis. In: Davison AM, Cameron JS, Grunfeld JP, et al, eds. Oxford textbook of clinical nephrology. Oxford: Oxford University Press, 1996: 877–911.
4 **Franssen CF**, ter Maaten JC, Hoorntje SJ. Brother and sister with myeloperoxidase associated autoimmune disease. Ann Rheum Dis 1994;**53**:213.
5 **Heuze-Claudot L**, Leroy B, Chevailler A, et al. A familial ANCA associated pulmonary renal syndrome. Clin Exp Immunol 1993;**93**(Suppl 1):40.
6 **Knudsen BB**, Joergensen T, Munch-Jensen B. Wegener's granulomatosis in a family. A short report. Scand J Rheumatol 1988;**17**:225–7.
7 **Muniain MA**, Moreno JC, Gonzalez Campora R. Wegener's granulomatosis in two sisters. Ann Rheum Dis 1986;**45**:417–21.
8 **Griffith ME**, Pusey CD. HLA genes in ANCA-associated vasculitides. Exp Clin Immunogenet 1997;**14**:196–205.
9 **Finn JE**, Zhang L, Agrawal S, et al. Molecular analysis of C3 allotypes in patients with systemic vasculitis. Nephrol Dial Transplant 1994;**9**:1564–7.
10 **Esnault VL**, Testa A, Audrain M, et al. Alpha 1-antitrypsin genetic polymorphism in ANCA-positive systemic vasculitis. Kidney Int 1993;**43**:1329–32.
11 **Elzouki AN**, Segelmark M, Wieslander J, et al. Strong link between the alpha 1-antitrypsin PiZ allele and Wegener's granulomatosis. J Intern Med 1994;**236**:543–8.
12 **Griffith ME**, Lovegrove JU, Gaskin G, et al. C-antineutrophil cytoplasmic antibody positivity in vasculitis patients is associated with the Z allele of alpha-1-antitrypsin, and P- antineutrophil cytoplasmic antibody positivity with the S allele. Nephrol Dial Transplant 1996;**11**:438–43.
13 **Gregorini G**, Ferioli A, Donato F, et al. Association between silica exposure and necrotizing crescentic glomerulonephritis with p-ANCA and anti-MPO antibodies: a hospital- based case-control study. Adv Exp Med Biol 1993;**336**:435–40.
14 **Hogan SL**, Satterly KK, Dooley MA, et al. Silica exposure in anti-neutrophil cytoplasmic autoantibody-associated glomerulonephritis and lupus nephritis. J Am Soc Nephrol 2001;**12**:134–42.
15 **Nuyts GD**, Van Vlem E, De Vos A, et al. Wegener granulomatosis is associated to exposure to silicon compounds: a case-control study. Nephrol Dial Transplant 1995;**10**:1162–5.
16 **Devogelaer JP**, Pirson Y, Vandenbroucke JM, et al. D-penicillamine induced crescentic glomerulonephritis: report and review of the literature. J Rheumatol 1987;**14**:1036–41.
17 **Finkel TH**, Torok TJ, Ferguson PJ, et al. Chronic parvovirus B19 infection and systemic necrotising vasculitis: opportunistic infection or aetiological agent? Lancet 1994;**343**:1255–8.
18 **Mandell BF**, Calabrese LH. Infections and systemic vasculitis. Curr Opin Rheumatol 1998;**10**:51–7.
19 **Guillevin L**, Visser H, Noel LH, et al. Antineutrophil cytoplasm antibodies in systemic polyarteritis nodosa with and without hepatitis B virus infection and Churg-Strauss syndrome: 62 patients. J Rheumatol 1993;**20**:1345–9.
20 **Schwarz MI**, Mortenson RL, Colby TV, et al. Pulmonary capillaritis. The association with progressive irreversible airflow limitation and hyperinflation. Am Rev Respir Dis 1993;**148**:507–11.
21 **Schwarz MI**, Brown KK. Small vessel vasculitis of the lung. Thorax 2000;**55**:502–10.
22 **Macnaughton PD**, Morgan CJ, Denison DM, et al. Measurement of carbon monoxide transfer and lung volume in ventilated subjects. Eur Respir J 1993;**6**:231–6.
23 **Macnaughton PD**, Evans TW. Measurement of lung volume and DLCO in acute respiratory failure. Am J Respir Crit Care Med 1994;**150**:770–5.
24 **Cohen BA**, Clark WF. Pauci-immune renal vasculitis: natural history, prognostic factors, and impact of therapy. Am J Kidney Dis 2000;**36**:914–24.
25 **Lauque D**, Cadranel J, Lazor R, et al. Microscopic polyangiitis with alveolar hemorrhage. A study of 29 cases and review of the literature. Groupe d'Etudes et de Recherche sur les Maladies "Orphelines" Pulmonaires (GERM"O"P). Medicine (Baltimore) 2000;**79**:222–33.
26 **Davies DJ**, Moran JE, Niall JF, et al. Segmental necrotising glomerulonephritis with antineutrophil antibody: possible arbovirus aetiology? BMJ (Clin Res Ed) 1982;**285**:606.
27 **Goldschmeding R**, van der Schoot CE, ten Bokkel Huinink D, et al. Wegener's granulomatosis autoantibodies identify a novel diisopropylfluorophosphate-binding protein in the lysosomes of normal human neutrophils. J Clin Invest 1989;**84**:1577–87.
28 **Jenne DE**, Tschopp J, Ludemann J, et al. Wegener's autoantigen decoded. Nature 1990;**346**:520.
29 **Jennette JC**, Hoidal JR, Falk RJ. Specificity of anti-neutrophil cytoplasmic autoantibodies for proteinase 3. Blood 1990;**75**:2263–4.
30 **Niles JL**, McCluskey RT, Ahmad MF, et al. Wegener's granulomatosis autoantigen is a novel neutrophil serine proteinase. Blood 1989;**74**:1888–93.
31 **Falk RJ**, Jennette JC. Anti-neutrophil cytoplasmic autoantibodies with specificity for myeloperoxidase in patients with systemic vasculitis and idiopathic necrotizing and crescentic glomerulonephritis. N Engl J Med 1988;**318**:1651–7.
32 **Savige J**, Gillis D, Benson E, et al. International Consensus Statement on Testing and Reporting of Antineutrophil Cytoplasmic Antibodies (ANCA). Am J Clin Pathol 1999;**111**:507–13.
33 **Hagen EC**. Development of solid-phase assays for the detection of anti-neutrophil cytoplasmic antibodies (ANCA) for clinical application: report of a large clinical evaluation study. Clin Exp Immunol 1995;**101**(Suppl 1):29.
34 **Adu D**, Savage COS, Lockwood CM, et al. ANCA positive and ANCA negative microscopic polyarteritis. Clin Exp Immunol 1995;**101**(Suppl 1):62.
35 **Bindi P**, Mougenot B, Mentre F, et al. Necrotizing crescentic glomerulonephritis without significant immune deposits: a clinical and serological study. Q J Med 1993;**86**:55–68.
36 **Fauci AS**, Haynes BF, Katz P, et al. Wegener's granulomatosis: prospective clinical and therapeutic experience with 85 patients for 21 years. Ann Intern Med 1983;**98**:76–85.
37 **Hoffman GS**, Kerr GS, Leavitt RY, et al. Wegener granulomatosis: an analysis of 158 patients. Ann Intern Med 1992;**116**:488–98.
38 **Jayne D**. Update on the European Vasculitis Study Group trials. Curr Opin Rheumatol 2001;**13**:48–55.
39 **Kallenberg CG**, Cohen Tervaert JW. New treatments of ANCA-associated vasculitis. Sarcoid Vasc Diffuse Lung Dis 2000;**17**:125–9.
40 **Levy JB**, Winearls CG. Rapidly progressive glomerulonephritis: what should be first-line therapy? Nephron 1994;**67**:402–7.
41 **Pusey CD**, Rees AJ, Evans DJ, et al. Plasma exchange in focal necrotizing glomerulonephritis without anti-GBM antibodies. Kidney Int 1991;**40**:757–63.
42 **Matic G**, Michelsen A, Hofmann D, et al. Three cases of C-ANCA-positive vasculitis treated with immunoadsorption: possible benefit in early treatment. Ther Apher 2001;**5**:68–72.
43 **Palmer A**, Cairns T, Dische F, et al. Treatment of rapidly progressive glomerulonephritis by extracorporeal immunoadsorption, prednisolone and cyclophosphamide. Nephrol Dial Transplant 1991;**6**:536–42.
44 **Jordan SC**, Toyoda M. Treatment of autoimmune diseases and systemic vasculitis with pooled human intravenous immune globulin. Clin Exp Immunol 1994;**1**:31–8.
45 **Jayne DR**, Chapel H, Adu D, et al. Intravenous immunoglobulin for ANCA-associated systemic vasculitis with persistent disease activity. Q J Med 2000;**93**:433–9.
46 **Lockwood CM**, Thiru S, Stewart S, et al. Treatment of refractory Wegener's granulomatosis with humanized monoclonal antibodies. Q J Med 1996;**89**:903–12.
47 **Matsumoto T**, Ueki K, Tamura S, et al. Extracorporeal membrane oxygenation for the management of respiratory failure due to ANCA-associated vasculitis. Scand J Rheumatol 2000;**29**:195–7.

19 Illustrative case 4: neuromusculoskeletal disorders

N Hart, A K Simonds

Congenital or acquired disorders affecting the respiratory muscles and/or causing chest wall deformity can precipitate ventilatory insufficiency either through the development of inspiratory muscle weakness or by a marked increase in the work of breathing due to low thoracic compliance. In some congenital disorders such as Duchenne muscular dystrophy and intermediate spinal muscular atrophy respiratory muscle involvement is almost inevitable; in others such as limb girdle muscular dystrophy and facioscapulohumeral muscular dystrophy respiratory muscle weakness is highly variable. Expiratory muscle weakness reduces cough efficiency and increases the tendency to atelectasis. Bulbar muscle involvement predisposes the individual to aspiration. Risk factors for ventilatory decompensation in patients with idiopathic scoliosis include early onset scoliosis (before the age of 5 years), a high (cephalad) thoracic curve, and a vital capacity of less than 30% predicted. Some acquired neuromuscular disorders—for example, motor neurone disease, Guilllain Barré syndrome—may present with ventilatory failure due to respiratory muscle weakness; other patients with a precarious balance between ventilatory load and capacity may decompensate during a chest infection or after surgical intervention. In some neuromuscular disorders—for example, Duchenne muscular dystrophy and acid maltase deficiency—cardiomyopathy may complicate the picture. In addition, it should be remembered that congenital scoliosis is associated with an increased incidence of congenital heart disease. Intensivists should be able to identify patients at high risk of ventilatory failure from neuromusculoskeletal disorders and be prepared for weaning problems. They should also be aware of advances in non-invasive ventilation (NIV) that may be of value in avoiding the need for endotracheal intubation and conventional ventilation, and help facilitate early discharge from the intensive care unit (ICU).

CASE REPORT

A 40 year old woman was found to be anaemic at a routine blood donor session. Shortly after she developed joint pains and pruritus, and autoimmune haemolytic anaemia was diagnosed. A mediastinal mass was observed on her chest radiograph which was shown to be a thymoma on needle biopsy. The autoimmune haemolytic anaemia was complicated by red cell aplasia. Following prednisolone therapy the haemoglobin rose from 6.2 to 12.8 g/dl. There were no symptoms of myasthenia such as diplopia, limb weakness or dyspnoea, and the FEV_1/FVC was 2.39/2.98 litres. The patient underwent a thoracotomy during which the thymic tumour was found to be adherent to the right hilum, right phrenic nerve, and pericardium. The tumour was resected with strips of the right lung at the hilum. Histologically, the

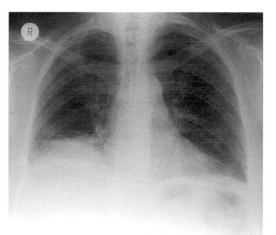

Figure 19.1 Chest radiograph showing elevated right hemidiaphragm and bibasal atelectasis, more marked at the right lung base.

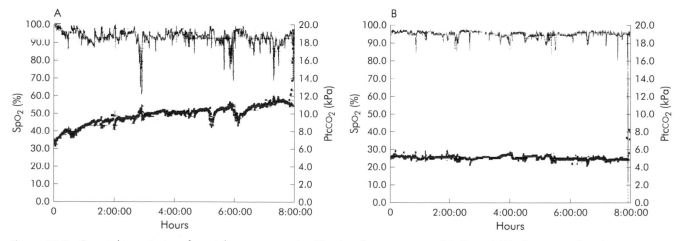

Figure 19.2 Overnight monitoring of arterial oxygen saturation (SpO_2) and transcutaneous CO_2 ($PtcCO_2$) (A) after surgery breathing spontaneously and (B) during NIV.

Table 19.1 Respiratory muscle strength results

Tests of respiratory muscle strength	Predicted value (cm H₂O)	Baseline (cm H₂O)	6 months (cm H₂O)
Sniff Poes	>70	20.6	29.8
Sniff Pdi	>70	2.4	13.8
Cough Pgas	>120	77.3	143.1
Bilateral TwPdi	>20	0.0	5.0
Right TwPdi	>7	0.0	0.0
Left TwPdi	>8	0.0	5.0

Sniff Poes=maximum sniff oesphageal pressure; sniff Pdi=maximum sniff trandiaphragmatic pressure; cough Pgas=maximum cough gastric pressure; TwPdi=twitch transdiagphragmatic pressure following unilateral and bilateral magnetic stimulation of the phrenic nerve.

tumour was a cortical thymoma. Initially the patient made a good recovery on the ICU and was rapidly extubated. However, over the following 2 weeks she became progressively more breathless and orthopnoeic. The chest radiograph showed elevation of the right hemidiaphragm and bibasal consolidation (fig 19.1). A ventilation-perfusion scan confirmed matched defects at both lung bases. Little response was seen to several courses of antibiotics and physiotherapy, and the patient reported continued orthopnoea and fragmented sleep. She was therefore referred to the weaning programme at the Royal Brompton Hospital for further assessment.

On arrival, breathing spontaneously she was unable to lie flat and the FEV_1/FVC while sitting was 1.05/1.2 litres. Arterial blood gas tensions on air were Po_2 10.6 kPa, Pco_2 5.9 kPa, HCO_3 30.3 mmol/l. Overnight monitoring during which the patient slept very lightly showed a rise in transcutaneous (Tc) CO_2 to 12 kPa with dips in arterial oxygen saturation (Sao_2) to 60% breathing air (fig 19.2A). A CT scan showed patchy subsegmental atelectasis affecting the right and left lower lobes with marked elevation of the right hemidiaphragm. There was no evidence of thromboembolism. Baseline respiratory muscle test results are shown in table 19.1 and indicate a marked reduction in inspiratory muscle strength with a modest reduction in expiratory muscle strength. Stimulation of the phrenic nerves generated no transdiaphragmatic pressure spike bilaterally. A tensilon test using the diaphragm as the test muscle was negative (fig 19.3).

Thyroid function tests demonstrated hypothyroidism (free thyroxine 7.6 pmol/l (NR 9–23), thyroid stimulating hormone 17.7 mU/l (NR 0.32–5)).

Diagnosis

The patient had developed bilateral basal atelectasis and consolidation after thoracotomy for thymic resection because of marked diaphragmatic weakness. Ventilatory decompensation occurred during sleep due to loss of intercostal muscle tone in REM sleep leaving ventilation dependent on the already weak diaphragm. Ventilation is further compromised during sleep by a reduction in central drive and basal ventilation-perfusion mismatch. In this patient the differential diagnosis of respiratory muscle weakness lies between:

- myasthenia gravis;

- phrenic nerve injury caused by thymic tumour involvement and/or surgery;

- a combination of myasthenia and phrenic palsy;

- respiratory muscle weakness associated with hypothyroidism.[1]

The tensilon test was negative and respiratory muscle tests showed absent conduction down both phrenic nerves indicating that the main problem was phrenic nerve injury. The situation was probably exacerbated by hypothyroidism induced myopathy. Acetylcholinesterase (Ach) antibody was subsequently shown to be positive in this patient, but the combina-

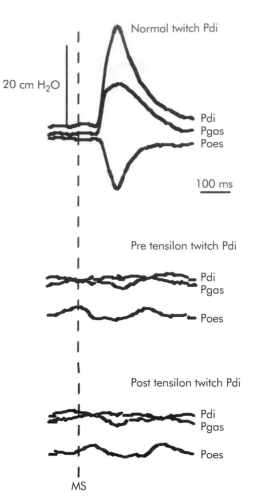

Figure 19.3 Twitch transdiaphragmatic pressure before and after the tensilon test. Pdi=transdiaphragmatic pressure; Pgas=gastric pressure; MS=magnetic stimulation. A normal twitch Pdi is given above for reference.

tion of red cell aplasia, thymoma and Ach antibodies *without* clinical features of myasthenia has been reported previously. In a Japanese series of 17 cases of red cell aplasia and thymoma, only two patients had myasthenia.[2]

Management

The patient was started on nocturnal NIV via a nasal mask and thyroxine replacement therapy. She also received physiotherapy during NIV to facilitate coughing and secretion clearance. Theoretically, in this situation bilevel non-invasive positive pressure support may be more beneficial in addressing atelectasis than volume preset ventilation or inspiratory pressure support alone.[3] The patient's sleep quality improved, and overnight monitoring on NIV showed improvements in Sao_2 and $Tcco_2$ (fig 19.2B). Persistent anaemia was treated by transfusion to raise the haemoglobin above 8 g/dl. Basal atelectasis resolved over 1 week but the right hemidiaphragm remained elevated. The patient was discharged home after 16 days and continued to use nocturnal NIV.

Two months later the sniff inspiratory pressure was 27.6 cm H_2O compared with a value of 16.2 cm H_2O on arrival, and the patient had returned to work having completed a course of radiotherapy. Respiratory muscle test results obtained 6 months after surgery are given in table 19.1. These show a further improvement in inspiratory muscle strength with some recovery in conduction down the left phrenic nerve (fig 19.4), indicating that it was probably traumatised during the difficult surgical resection. There was no recovery in right phrenic nerve function, presumably because of partial

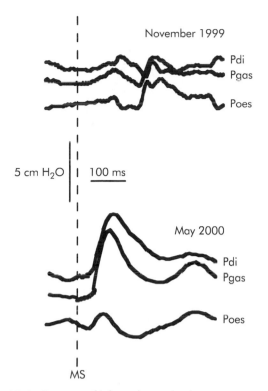

Figure 19.4 Recovery of left twitch transdiaphragmatic pressure after 6 months. Pdi=transdiaphragmatic pressure; Poes=oesophageal pressure; Pgas=gastric pressure; MS=magnetic stimulation.

resection. A sleep study with the patient breathing spontaneously showed normal Tcco$_2$ and Sao$_2$ values, so the patient was weaned from nocturnal ventilatory support.

DISCUSSION

Phrenic nerve injury occurs variably after cardiothoracic surgery[4] and ranges from complete nerve ablation to the "frostbitten phrenic" seen after procedures involving topical cooling to produce cardioplegia.[5] If the nerve is not irretrievably damaged, recovery is usually seen over a number of months.[6] Patients with bilateral phrenic nerve injury often present with bibasal atelectasis. In those with underlying respiratory compromise overt ventilatory failure is precipitated.[7]

In this non-smoker, ventilatory decompensation only occurred at night due to the effects of sleep on respiration, but sleep fragmentation exacerbated her daytime symptoms. Respiratory muscle tests[8] were used to help differentiate a true myasthenic syndrome from phrenic nerve damage.

NIV is a useful weaning tool. A randomised trial comparing rapid extubation on to NIV with continued intubation and pressure support ventilation in COPD patients showed more rapid weaning with fewer complications in the NIV group.[9] In patients with restrictive ventilatory defects due to neuromuscular or chest wall disease, case series data[10] suggest that NIV can shorten weaning and reduce the time spent on the ICU. NIV can also be used to prevent the need for reintubation if ventilatory failure recurs after extubation.[11] In the case presented here, reintroduction of invasive ventilation following extubation was not indicated but NIV is likely to have facilitated recovery from basal atelectasis. NIV was successfully carried out on a high dependency unit and subsequently on a general respiratory ward, thereby eliminating the need for continued ICU bed occupancy.

REFERENCES

1 **Siafakas NM**, Salesiotou V, Filaditaki V, *et al.* Respiratory muscle strength in hypothyroidism. *Chest* 1992;**102**:189–94.

2 **Masaoka A**, Hashimoto I, Yamakawa Y, *et al.* Thymomas associated with pure red cell aplasia. Histologic and follow-up studies. *Cancer* 1989;**64**:1872–8.

3 **Elliott MW**, Simonds AK. Nocturnal assisted ventilation using bilevel positive airway pressure: the effect of expiratory positive airway pressure. *Eur Respir J* 1995;**8**:436–40.

4 **Tripp HF**, Bolton JW. Phrenic nerve injury following cardiac surgery: a review. *J Cardiac Surg* 1998;**13**:218–23.

5 **Mills GH**, Khan ZP, Moxham J, *et al.* Effects of temperature on phrenic nerve and diapragmatic function during cardiac surgery. *Br J Anaesth* 1997;**79**:726–32.

6 **Olopade CO**, Staats BA. Time course of recovery from frostbitten phrenics after coronary artery bypass. *Chest* 1991;**99**:1112–5.

7 **Burgess RW**, Boyd AF, Moore PG, *et al.* Post-operative respiratory failure due to bilateral phrenic nerve palsy. *Postgrad Med J* 1989;**65**:39–41.

8 **Polkey MI**, Moxham J. Clinical aspects of respiratory muscle dysfunction in the critically ill. *Chest* 2001;**119**:926–9.

9 **Nava S**, Ambrosino N, Clini E, *et al.* Non-invasive mechanical ventilation in the weaning of patients with respiratory failure due to chronic obstructive pulmonary disease. A randomized controlled trial. *Ann Intern Med* 1998;**128**:721–8.

10 **Udwadia ZF**, Santis GK, Steven MH, *et al.* Nasal ventilation to facilitate weaning in patients with chronic respiratory insufficiency. *Thorax* 1992;**47**:715–8.

11 **Hilbert G**, Gruson D, Portel L, *et al.* Noninvasive pressure support ventilation in COPD patients with postextubation hypercapnic respiratory insufficiency. *Eur Respir J* 1998;**11**:1349–53.

20 Illustrative case 5: HIV associated pneumonia

R J Boyton, D M Mitchell, O M Kon

An estimated 36 million people worldwide are currently infected with HIV, about 1.46 million in North America and Western Europe and a further 25.3 million in sub-Saharan Africa.[1] An estimated 30 000 adults and children became infected with HIV in Western Europe during the year 2000. The rate of infection, coupled with longer survival due to primary and secondary prophylaxis against opportunistic infection and highly active antiretroviral therapy (HAART), has resulted in the prevalence continuing to increase.[1 2]

Infection with HIV is associated with increased susceptibility to opportunistic infection with more than 100 viruses, bacteria, protozoa and fungi.[3] Primary and secondary prophylaxis against opportunistic infections and HAART has led to changes in the nature, incidence, and presentation of opportunistic infections such as *Pneumocystis* pneumonia (PCP), *Mycobacterium avium intracellulare* (MAI), and cytomegalovirus (CMV) retinitis.[2 4] New challenges are presented to physicians in medical high dependency units (HDUs) and intensive care units (ICUs). We report a patient who presented with HIV associated pneumonia and discuss the issues concerning admission to HDU/ICU of HIV infected individuals in the PCP prophylaxis and post-HAART era, drawing together current views of prognostic indicators and outcomes.

CASE REPORT

A 39 year old white man presented with a 3 week history of increasing shortness of breath accompanied by a non-productive cough, fever, and 5 kg weight loss. A diagnosis of HIV infection with a low CD4 count of 30 cells/mm^3 had been made 6 months earlier. He was homosexual with no history of recreational intravenous drug use. He was not taking PCP prophylaxis or HAART but instead took homeopathic treatment. On physical examination oral candidiasis, oral herpes infection, axillary and inguinal lymphadenopathy were identified. He had fever (38°C), tachypnoea, tachycardia, and oxygen saturation on air of 85%. There were no chest signs. A plain chest radiograph showed diffuse bilateral shadowing. Arterial blood gas measurements on air were as follows: Pao$_2$ 5.8 kPa, Pco$_2$ 3.54 kPa, O$_2$ saturation 82%. The erythrocyte sedimentation ratio was raised at 119 mm/h and the C reactive protein (CRP) level was raised at 144 mg/l. Liver and renal function tests were normal. The patient was unable to tolerate a diagnostic bronchoscopy.

A clinical diagnosis of PCP/community acquired pneumonia was made and he was started on high dose intravenous co-trimoxazole with adjunctive corticosteroid therapy, oral fluconazole, and intravenous cefuroxime/oral clarithromycin. Continuous positive airway pressure (CPAP) ventilation was started. Initially there was clinical improvement. In particular, the oxygen saturation improved to 93% on air and the CRP level fell to 7 mg/l. However, on day 9 he became unwell with fever (38°C), tachypnoea, and tachycardia. A chest radiograph showed increased diffuse bilateral change with a nodular appearance and patchy consolidation. Arterial blood gas measurements on air were as follows: Pao$_2$ 4.48 kPa, Pco$_2$ 4.39 kPa, O$_2$ saturation 71%. CRP had risen to 163 mg/l. He was treated for hospital acquired pneumonia with piperacillin/tazobactam and vancomycin in addition to the PCP treatment. Ganciclovir therapy was started. He was transferred to the ICU for increased respiratory support with bilevel positive airway pressure (BiPAP) ventilation via a nasal mask and subsequently improved clinically.

DISCUSSION
Pneumonia and HIV

The case described was initially treated empirically for community acquired bacterial pneumonia and PCP. Table 20.1 outlines common HIV associated pulmonary infections. In the absence of confirmatory tests, a diagnosis of PCP was most likely based on the clinical presentation and chest radiographic appearance in this at risk patient. PCP is nowadays most commonly seen in newly diagnosed HIV infected patients with advanced disease or HIV infected individuals not taking PCP prophylaxis or HAART. In the case described the patient had recently been diagnosed with advanced disease (CD4 count 30 cells/mm^3) and was not taking PCP prophylaxis or HAART. PCP typically presents when the CD4 count falls below 200 cells/mm^3 and is one of the most common opportunistic infections precipitating admission to the HDU and ICU for respiratory support.[4 10–13] The risk of a first episode of infection below a CD4 count of 200 cells/mm^3 (in patients not taking PCP prophylaxis or HAART) is estimated to be 18% at 12 months in asymptomatic individuals, rising to 44% in those with early symptomatic disease such as oral candidiasis as in the case described.[14] PCP prophylaxis with co-trimoxazole is recommended when the CD4 count falls to 200 cells/mm^3 or below. Patients with HIV infection on HAART with a CD4 count consistently improved to >200 cells/mm^3 have had PCP primary and secondary prophylaxis stopped without significant risk of subsequent PCP.[15–20]

Methods of diagnosis range from sputum induction to open lung biopsy. The diagnostic test of choice is fibreoptic bronchoscopy with lavage, providing the patient can tolerate the procedure. Transbronchial biopsy is useful but is occasionally complicated by haemorrhage and pneumothorax. Sputum induction with nebulised saline has a lower diagnostic sensitivity and should be carried out in a negative pressure facility. Patients unable to tolerate bronchoscopy should be treated empirically, based on clinical judgement and expert advice, as was the case here. The case discussed was treated with high dose co-trimoxazole

Table 20.1 HIV associated pulmonary infections

Bacteria	Mycobacteria	Fungi	Parasites	Viruses
Streptococcus pneumoniae*	M tuberculosis**	Pneumocystis carinii†	Toxoplasma gondii,	Influenza
Haemophilus influenzae*	M avium intracellulare	Cryptococcus neoformans***	Cryptosporidium spp	Parainfluenza
Staphylococcus aureus*	M kansasii	Candida albicans	Microsporidium spp	Respiratory syncytial virus
Klebsiella pneumoniae*		Aspergillus spp	Leishmania spp	Rhinovirus
Pseudomons aeruginosa*		Penicillium marneffei	Strongyloides stercoralis	Adenovirus
Nocardia asteroides		Histoplasma capsulatum		Cytomegalovirus
Rochalimaea henselae		Coccidiodes immitis		Herpes simplex virus
		Blastomyces dermatitidis		Herpes varicella-zoster virus
Bacterial pneumonia occurs more frequently in HIV positive patients at all CD4 counts than HIV negative controls. The risk increases as the CD4 count falls below 200 cells/mm³ and in intravenous drug users[5]	HIV positive individuals are at increased risk of infection with M tuberculosis, whatever the CD4 count, and should be offered an HIV test.[7] Extrapulmonary tuberculosis tends to occur at CD4 counts <150 cells/mm³. M avium intracellulare and M kansasii both occur late in the course of HIV infection when the CD4 count falls below 50–100 cells/mm³	Pulmonary infections with Candida and Aspergillus are relatively rare. Endemic mycoses caused by Histoplasma capsulatum, Coccidiodes immitis and Blastomyces dermatitidis occur in patients who live in North America		Common respiratory viral infections occur comparably in HIV infected and non-infected people. CMV is frequently isolated in BAL, but its role in causing disease is not clear. The presence of CMV in BAL is associated with a worse prognosis in PCP[9]

*The common causes of bacterial pneumonia are shown.[5] [6] One third of the pneumonias are bacteraemic. Bacteraemia is more common in pneumococcal pneumonia. Pseudomonal pneumonia is associated with a lower CD4 count than with pneumococcal pneumonia.[6]
**Multidrug-resistant (MDR) tuberculosis (resistant to isoniazid and rifampicin) is becoming an increasing problem among HIV positive individuals in North America. Antituberculous treatment requires careful monitoring for drug interactions and toxicity, especially if the patient is on HAART. Interactions such as those between the rifamycins and protease inhibitors or non-nucleoside reverse transcriptase inhibitors can lead to lower efficacy or increased toxicity of the anti-retroviral regimen.[4]
***Cryptococcal infection presents either as a primary lung infection or as part of a disseminated infection with cryptococcaemia, pneumonia, meningitis, and cutaneous disease.[8]
†Pneumocystis organisms from different host species have different DNA sequences. It has recently been suggested that the organism that causes human Pneumo Cysitis Pneumonia (PCP) should be named Pneumocystis jiroveci Frenkel 1999. Pneumocystis carinni should now be used to describe the rat derived infection (Stringer JR, Beard CB, Miller RF, Wakefield AE. A new name (Pneumocystis jiroveci) for Pneumocystis from humans. Emerging Infect Dis 2002;8:891–6.)

and adjuvant high dose steroids, which is the most effective first line treatment for severe PCP. Table 20.2 describes first and second line treatment for PCP in mild to moderate and severe disease. Second line treatment should be used for patients intolerant of or who have not responded to co-trimoxazole. The optimal dose of steroid and preferred second line treatment has yet to be determined.

The deterioration on day 9 was probably secondary to hospital acquired pneumonia and the patient was started on appropriate antibiotic treatment for this. He was also started on intravenous gancyclovir. The role of CMV infection during PCP is controversial and difficult to evaluate. Studies carried out before the introduction of adjuvant corticosteroid treatment in severe PCP concluded that CMV co-infection did not influence the outcome of PCP.[22] [23] A more recent study showed that culture of CMV in the lavage of patients receiving adjuvant corticosteroid treatment was, independently of CD4 count, associated with a 2.7-fold increased risk of death.[9] Based on these findings, it has been proposed that survival rates for patients with severe PCP might be improved with anti-CMV therapy. The use of corticosteroids has also been related to the subsequent development of CMV retinitis and colitis in HIV infected patients.[24] Furthermore, in vitro studies have shown increased CMV replication in corticosteroid treated macrophages.[25] The mechanisms by which CMV shortens survival of patients on corticosteroid treatment are unknown. Further studies are needed to establish which patients receiving adjuvant corticosteroid therapy for severe PCP would benefit from treatment with foscarnet or gancyclovir.

Pneumocystis pneumonia (PCP) and respiratory support on HDU/ICU

Survival after a diagnosis of PCP has improved in recent years. Among 4412 patients in the USA with 5222 episodes of PCP during follow up (1992–1998), 12 month survival increased from 40% in 1992–3 to 63% in 1996–8. Early death was associated with a history of PCP, age >45 years, and CD4 count

<50 cells/mm³.[26] A recent study of 169 admissions of HIV positive individuals to the ICU found respiratory failure to be the most common reason for admission (38%).[12] PCP is the most common cause of respiratory failure leading to ICU admission in HIV infected individuals.[4] [10–13]

Outcomes of mechanical ventilation for respiratory failure from PCP have changed since the start of the HIV epidemic.[27] Before 1985 a hospital mortality of about 80% was described in this group.[28–30] Table 20.3 shows a mortality rate for ventilated HIV positive patients with PCP from 1985 to 1997 of 50–79%. These changes are difficult to compare because of changing trends over the periods of studies, including the introduction of HAART and changes in the subgroup of patients with PCP progressing to mechanical ventilation on the ICU. Nevertheless, there appears to be an overall improvement in ICU survival. Furthermore, changes with respect to PCP prophylaxis and the use of adjunctive corticosteroids have yielded an overall improvement for HIV positive patients. PCP prophylaxis has resulted in fewer episodes of PCP, and the use of adjunctive corticosteroids has resulted in a smaller proportion of patients with PCP progressing to mechanical ventilation.[35–39]

A French study of 110 cases of PCP requiring intensive care between 1989 and 1994 showed a 3 month mortality rate of 34.6% and 1 year survival estimated at 47%. Most patients only required CPAP support. One third required mechanical ventilation and, of those, 79% died.[33] In another study in 1995–7 of 1660 patients with PCP only 9% required mechanical ventilation and the hospital mortality rate was 62%.[34] A study covering the period 1993–6 correlated CD4 lymphocyte count and mortality in AIDS patients requiring mechanical ventilation due to PCP. Mortality increased from 25% for patients with CD4 cell counts >100 cells/mm³ to 100% in those with CD4 counts <10 cells/mm³.[40] A prospective study of 176 HIV positive patients with PCP identified PCP prophylaxis as predictive of progression to death, other factors being age, one or more episodes of PCP, treatment other than co-trimoxazole, and isolation of CMV from the BAL fluid.[9]

Table 20.2   Treatment of *Pneumocystis* pneumonia (PCP)[14 21]

Drug**	Duration of treatment	Side effects	Comments
First line treatment *Co-trimoxazole 120 mg/kg daily in 2–4 divided doses po/iv (480mg co-trimoxazole consists of sulfamethoxazole 400 mg and trimethoprim 80 mg)	21 days	Nausea, vomiting, fever, rash (including Stevens-Johnson's syndrome, toxic epidermal necrolysis, photosensitivity), blood disorders (including neutropenia, thrombocytopenia, rarely agranulocytosis and purpura), rarely allergic reactions, diarrhoea, glossitis, stomatitis, anorexia, arthralgia, myalgia, liver damage, pancreatitis, antibiotic associated colitis, eosinophilia, aseptic meningitis, headache, depression, convulsions, ataxia, tinnitus, megaloblastic anaemia due to trimethoprim, crystaluria, renal disorders including interstitial nephritis	Intolerance common. Initial treatment with iv preparation. Comes in ampoule containing 480 mg; these should be diluted in at least 75 ml of 5% dextrose. Infuse over 60 minutes
Severe disease: *Adjuvant high dose steroids (e.g. prednisolone 40–80 mg daily po. Alternatively, hydrocortisone may be given iv)	5 days; reduce dose over 14–21 days		Indicated in severe disease. Optimal dose not determined. Consult HIV specialist for advice
Second line treatment Mild to moderate disease: *Trimethoprim 20 mg/kg/day po/iv in 2–3 divided doses and dapsone 100 mg po daily	21 days	Trimethoprim: gastrointestinal disturbance, pruritus, rash, depression of haematopoiesis; rarely erythema multiforme, toxic epidermal necrolysis; aseptic meningitis Dapsone: haemolysis, methaemoglobinaemia, neuropathy, allergic dermatitis, anorexia, nausea, vomiting, insomnia, psychosis, agranulocytosis; dapsone syndrome (rash with fever and eosinophilia) - stop immediately (may progress to exfoliative dermatitis, hepatitis, hypoalbuminaemia, psychosis and death)	Avoid in G6PD deficiency
*Clindamycin 600 mg 6 hourly po/iv and primaquine 15 mg daily po	21 days	Clindamycin: diarrhoea, nausea and vomiting; jaundice, abnormal liver function tests; neutropenia, eosinophilia, agranulocytosis and thrombocytopenia; rash Primaquine: nausea and vomiting, abdominal pain; methaemoglobinaemia, heamolytic anaemia.	*Clostridium difficile* toxin associated diarrhoea is a complication of clindamycin therapy Primaquine: caution in G6PD deficiency
Atovaquone suspension 750 mg twice daily	21 days	Nausea, vomiting and diarrhoea; headache, insomnia; rash, fever; elevated liver enzymes and amylase; anaemia, neutropenia; hyponatraemia	Consider combination with iv pentamidine as resistance reported with monotherapy
Severe disease: *Pentamidine isethionate 4 mg/kg/day as a slow intravenous infusion	21 days	Severe reactions, sometimes fatal, due to hypotension, hypoglycaemia, pancreatitis and arrythmias; also leucopenia, thrombocytopenia, acute renal failure, hypocalcaemia; also reported azotaemia, abnormal liver function tests, anaemia, hyperkalaemia, nausea and vomiting, dizziness, syncope, flushing, hyperglycaemia, rash, taste disturbance; Stevens-Johnson's syndrome reported; on inhalation, bronchoconstriction, cough, shortness of breath and wheeze; discomfort, pain, induration, abscess formation, and muscle necrosis at injection site.	Give over at least 1 hour with patient lying flat. Monitor blood pressure closely. Important side effects include severe hypotension and hypoglycaemia. Monitor BMstix during and after infusion for 12 hours. If changing from co-trimoxazole to pentamidine due to poor clinical response, continue co-trimoxazole for 3 days. If intolerant, give nebulised pentamidine 600 mg daily for first 3 days.
*Trimetrexate 45 mg/m² iv and folinic acid 80 mg/m²	21 days	Blood disorders (thrombocytopenia, granulocytopenia and anaemia); diarrhoea and vomiting, oral and gastrointestinal mucosal ulceration; fever; confusion, rarely seizures; disturbed liver function tests, plasma calcium, potassium and magnesium reported; rash, anaphylaxis and local irritation at the injection site.	Used as an alternative for patients intolerant of co-trimoxazole and pentamidine isethionate or who do not respond to these drugs. Trimetrexate is a potent dihydrofolate reductase inhibitor and must be give with calcium folinate. Administer calcium folinate during treatment and for 72 hours after last dose (to avoid potentially serious bone marrow suppression, oral and gastrointestinal ulceration, and renal and hepatic dysfunction); suspend myelosuppressive drugs (e.g. zidovudine)

po=by mouth; iv=intravenously.
* Consult HIV specialist for advice.
**Treatment of PCP infections should be undertaken where facilities for appropriate monitoring are available; consult a microbiologist/HIV specialist and the product literature before administering these drugs.

Table 20.3 ICU admission, mechanical ventilation, and mortality in epidsodes of HIV related *Pneumocystis* pneumonia (PCP) studied between 1985 and 1997

HIV related PCP episodes studied (n)	Country of study	Period of study	% of patients admitted to ICU	% of patients requiring mechanical ventilation	Mortality (%) of patients mechanically ventilated	Reference
348	USA	1985–89	6.3	5.7	60	31
2174	USA	1987–90	18	*	62–46**	32
110	France	1989–94	100***	31	79	33
257	USA	1990–95	8.2	4.7	50	31
1660	USA	1995–97	14	9	62	34

*Data not available.
**Episodes were stratified into patients receiving care in an ICU with (first figure) or without (second figure) a prior AIDS defining illness. Data relating to mechanical ventilation status not available for this study.
***This study was limited to ICU admissions.

Table 20.4 Prognostic markers significantly associated with mortality in ICU admissions of HIV positive patients with *Pneumocystis* pneumonia (PCP) requiring mechanical ventilation

HIV related PCP episodes studied (n)	Period of study	Prognostic markers associated with ICU mortality*	Reference
110	1989–94	Respiratory status deterioration requiring delayed mechanical ventilation; mechanical ventilation for 5 days or more; nosocomial infection, pneumothorax	33
48*	1993–96	Low CD4 cell count within 2 weeks of admission**	40
176	1990–99	Low CD4 cell count; prior PCP prophylaxis, CMV in BAL fluid, age, initial anti-PCP therapy	9
155	1995–97	Prior PCP prophylaxis	34
21	1993–98	High APACHE II score >17, low serum albumin <25 g/l, ARDS, low CD4 cell count <150 cells/mm^3, arterial pH <7.35	42

*Rows cannot be directly compared since studies considered different sets of variables. In most of the studies shown here a low CD4 cell count is taken to mean <200 cells/mm^3.
**This study was limited to patients with CD4 count <200 cells/mm^3 and on ICU with mechanical ventilation. Mortality varied significantly depending on CD4 counts: >100 cells/mm^3, 25%; 51–100 cells/mm^3, 50%; 11–50 cells/mm^3, 88%; 0–10 cells/mm^3, 100%.

Attempts have been made to use staging systems to predict inpatient mortality from HIV associated PCP since the introduction of PCP prophylaxis and HAART. One such system generated from data relating to 1660 cases of PCP diagnosed between 1995 and 1997 identified an ordered five category staging system based on three predictors: wasting, alveolar-arterial oxygen gradient, and serum albumin level. The mortality rate increased with stage, ranging from 3.7% for stage 1 to 49.1% for stage 5.[41] The prognostic markers identified are summarised in table 20.4.

Impact of early HAART

Since 1996 HAART has had an enormous impact on the natural history of HIV infection. HAART usually involves triple therapy with two nucleoside reverse transcriptase inhibitors and either a protease inhibitor or a non-nucleoside reverse transcriptase inhibitor. During the first 2 years of the widespread application of HAART there was a reduction in HIV related mortality, although this has since levelled out.[1 2 43] There are problems with adherence, pharmacology, and toxicity, but 50–90% of patients on HAART achieve sustained suppression of the virus and most patients show low persistent viral replication. Unfortunately, the viral mutation rate is such that viral genomes with each possible nucleotide substitution can be generated daily in an infected host, making the speed with which drug resistant HIV mutants can arise extremely rapid.[43] This has led to predictions that about half of all patients may develop resistance to current treatments.[43 44]

The success of HAART has led to a reappraisal of the role of prophylaxis for opportunistic infections such as PCP, CMV, and *M avium*. This is due to the decreased risk of opportunistic infections in the face of a reduced viral load and sustained or increased CD4 T cell levels, and because of problems of drug interactions between HAART and prophylactic therapies.[4 15–20 45–48] The Adult/Adolescent Spectrum of HIV Dis-ease Cohort Study showed a decrease of 55% in opportunistic infections including PCP, CMV, and *M avium* between 1992 and 1997.[49] The EuroSIDA study (a prospective study involving about 7300 patients) looked at the risk of opportunistic infections or death for patients on HAART. Patients with CD4 counts that consistently rose from <200 cells/mm^3 to >200 cells/mm^3 on HAART were substantially protected against opportunistic infections compared with patients with CD4 counts persistently below 50 cells/mm^3 (3.7–8.1 v 72.9 episodes per patient year).[50] There is evidence to suggest that HAART is associated with improved early survival from PCP (odds ratio 0.2).[26] Patients with bacterial pneumonia or PCP were admitted to the ICU less frequently following the introduction of HAART in 1996.[31] The optimal timing for the introduction of HAART in patients with PCP is not known. Cases of severe acute respiratory failure have been described following the early introduction of HAART (1–16 days after the diagnosis of PCP) who recovered after HAART interruption or steroid reintroduction.[51] This phenomenon could be due to rapid recruitment of competent inflammatory cells responding to persistent *pneumocystitis* cysts.

CONCLUSION

Many studies have tried to identify prognostic markers for the survival of HIV infected patients admitted to the ICU, with relatively little consensus. The strongest single indicator seems to be the CD4 count. Identifying objective outcome predictors will help clinicians to decide when to pursue aggressive treatment and when to withhold or withdraw it. The mortality rate of HIV infected patients admitted to the ICU has improved and probably reflects improved outcome of HIV infection in general with the introduction of PCP prophylaxis, adjunctive corticosteroid use in the treatment of PCP, and HAART. For selected cases, ICU care of HIV infected individuals with respiratory failure secondary to pneumonia is associated with a positive outcome. HIV and intensive care physicians need to work in close collaboration to deliver optimal care.

ACKNOWLEDGEMENT

The authors thank Dr Daniel Altmann for his critical review of the manuscript. Department of Infectious Diseases, Hammersmith Campus, Imperial College, London, UK.

REFERENCES

1 **Piot P**, Bartos M, Ghys PD, *et al*. The global impact of HIV/AIDS. *Nature* 2001;**410**:968–73.

2 **Palella FJ**, Delaney KM, Moorman AC, *et al*. Declining mortality among patients with advanced human immunodeficiency virus infection. *N Engl J Med* 1998;**338**:853–60.

3 **Weiss RA**. Gulliver's travels in HIVland. *Nature* 2001;**410**:963–7.

4 **Kovacs JA**, Masur H. Prophylaxis against opportunistic infections in patients with human immunodeficiency virus infection. *N Engl J Med* 2000;**342**:1416–29.

5 **Hirschtick RE**, Glassroth J, Jordan MC, *et al*. Bacterial pneumonia in persons infected with the human immunodeficiency virus. *N Engl J Med* 1995;**333**:845–51.

6 **Afessa B**, Green, B. Bacterial pneumonia in hospitalized patients with HIV infection. *Chest* 2000;**117**:1017–22.

7 **Bowen EF**, Rice PS, Cooke NT, *et al*. HIV seroprevalence by anonymous testing in patients with Mycobacterium tuberculosis and in tuberculosis contacts. *Lancet* 2000;**356**:1488–9.

8 **Saag MS**, Graybill RJ, Larsen RA, *et al*. Practice guidelines for the management of cryptococcal disease. *Clin Infect Dis* 2000;**30**:710–18.

9 **Benfield TL**, Helweg-Larsen J, Bang D, *et al*. Prognostic markers of short-term mortality in AIDS-associated Pneumocystis carinii pneumonia. *Chest* 2001;**119**:844–51.

10 **De Palo VA**, Millstein BH, Mayo PH, *et al*. Outcome of intensive care in patients with HIV infection. *Chest* 1995;**107**:506–10.

11 **Casalino E**, Mendoza-Sassi G, Wolff M, *et al*. Predictors of short and long term survival in HIV infected patients admitted to the ICU. *Chest* 1998;**113**:421–9.

12 **Afessa B**, Green B. Clinical course, prognostic factors, and outcome prediction for HIV patients in ICU. *Chest* 2000;**118**:138–45.

13 **Gill JK**, Greene L, Miller R, *et al*. ICU admission in patients infected with human immunodeficiency virus: a multicentre survey. *Anaesthesia* 1999;**54**:727–32.

14 **Weller V**, Williams I. ABC of AIDS. Treatment of infections. *BMJ* 2001;**322**:1350–4.

15 **Schneider MME**, Borleffs JCC, Stolk RP, *et al*. Discontinuation of prophylaxis for Pneumocystis carinii pneumonia in HIV-1 infected patients treated with highly active antiretroviral therapy. *Lancet* 1999;**353**:201–3.

16 **Furrer H**, Egger M, Opravil M, *et al*. Discontinuation of primary prophylaxis against Pneumocystis carinii pneumonia in HIV-1 infected adults treated with combination antiretroviral therapy. *N Engl J Med* 1999;**340**:1301–6.

17 **Kirk O**, Lundgren JD, Pedersen C, *et al*. Can chemoprophylaxis against opportunistic infections be discontinued after an increase in CD4 cells induced by highly active antiretroviral therapy? *AIDS* 1999;**13**:1647–51.

18 **Weverling GJ**, Mocroft A, Ledergerber B, *et al*. Discontinuation of Pneumocystis carinii pneumonia prophylaxis after start of highly active antiretroviral therapy in HIV-1 infection. *Lancet* 1999;**353**:1293–8.

19 **Lopez Bernaldo De Quiros JC**, Miro JM, Pena JM, *et al*. A randomized trial of the discontinuation of primary and secondary prophylaxis against Pneumocystis carinii pneumonia after highly active antiretroviral therapy in patients with HIV infection. *N Engl J Med* 2001;**344**:159–67.

20 **Ledergerber B**, Mocroft A, Reiss P, *et al*. Discontinuation of secondary prophylaxis against Pneumocystis carinii pneumonia in patients with HIV infection who have a response to antiretroviral therapy. *N Engl J Med* 2001;**344**:168–74.

21 **British National Formulary**. British Medical Association and the Royal Pharmaceutical Society of Great Britain, March 2000: 39.

22 **Millar A**, Patou G, Miller R, *et al*. Cytomegalovirus in the lungs of patients with AIDS: respiratory pathogen or passenger? *Am Rev Respir Dis* 1990;**141**:1474–7.

23 **Miles P**, Baughman R, Linneman C. Cytomegalovirus in BAL fluid of patients with AIDS. *Chest* 1990;**97**:1072–6.

24 **Nelson M**, Erskine D, Hawkins D, *et al*. Treatment with corticosteroids: a risk factor for the development of clinical cytomegalovirus disease in AIDS. *AIDS* 1993;**7**:375–8.

25 **Lathey J**, Spector S. Unrestricted replication of human cytomegalovirus in hydrocortisone treated macrophages. *J Virol* 1991;**65**:6371.

26 **Dworkin M**, Hanson D, Navin T. Survival of patients with AIDS after a diagnosis of Pneumocystis carinii pneumonia in the United States. *J Infect Dis* 2001;**183**:1409–12.

27 **Curtis JR**. ICU outcomes for patients with HIV infection: a moving target (editorial). *Chest* 1998;**113**:269–70.

28 **Rosen M**, Cucco R, Teirstein A. Outcome of intensive care in patients with the acquired immunodeficiency syndrome. *J Intensive Care Med* 1986;**1**:55–60.

29 **Wachter RM**, Luce JM, Turner J, *et al*. Intensive care of patients with the acquired immunodeficiency syndrome: outcome and changing patterns of utilization. *Am Rev Respir Dis* 1986;**134**:891–6.

30 **Murry J**, Felton C, Garay M, *et al*. Pulmonary complications of the acquired immunodeficiency syndrome: report of the National Heart, Lung, and Blood Institute workshop. *N Engl J Med* 1984;**310**:1682–8.

31 **Naresh G**, Mansharamani M, Garland R, *et al*. Management and outcome patterns for adult Pneumocystis carinii pneumonia, 1985 to 1995. *Chest* 2000;**118**:704–11.

32 **Curtis J**, Randall M, Bennett C, *et al*. Variations in intensive care unit utilization for patients with human immunodeficiency virus-related Pneumocystis carinii pneumonia: Importance of hospital characteristics and geographic location. *Crit Care Med* 1998;**26**:668–75.

33 **Bedos JP**, Dumoulin JL, Gachot B, *et al*. Pneumocystis carinii pneumonia requiring intensive care management: survival and prognostic study in 110 patients with human immunodeficiency virus. *Crit Care Med* 1999;**27**:1109–15.

34 **Randall Curtis J**, Yarnold PR, Schwartz RA, *et al*. Improvements in outcomes of acute respiratory failure for patients with human immunodeficiency virus related Pneumocystis carinii pneumonia. *Am J Respir Crit Care Med* 2000;**162**:393–8.

35 **El-Sadr W**, Simberkoff MS. Survival and prognostic factors in severe Pneumocystis carinii pneumonia requiring mechanical ventilation. *Am Rev Respir Dis* 1988;**137**:1264–7.

36 **Montaner JS**, Russell JA, Lawson L, *et al*. Acute respiratory failure secondary to Pneumocystis carinii pneumonia in the acquired immunodeficiency syndrome: a potential role for corticosteroids. *Chest* 1989;**95**:881–4.

37 **Efferen LS**, Nadarajah D, Palat DS. Survival following mechanical ventilation for Pneumocystis carinii pneumonia in patients with the acquired immunodeficiency syndrome: a different perspective. *Am J Med* 1989;**87**:401–4.

38 **Friedman Y**, Franklin C, Rackow C, *et al*. Improved survival in patients with AIDS, Pneumocystis carinii pneumonia, and severe respiratory failure. *Chest* 1989;**96**:862–6.

39 **Wachter RM**, Russi MB, Bloch DA, *et al*. Pneumocystis carinii pneumonia and respiratory failure in AIDS. Improved outcomes and increased use of intensive care units. *Am Rev Respir Dis* 1991;**143**:251–6.

40 **Kumar SD**, Krieger BP. CD4 lymphocyte counts and mortality in AIDS patients requiring mechanical ventilator support due to Pneumocystis carinii pneumonia. *Chest* 1998;**113**:430–3.

41 **Arozullah AM**, Yarnold PR, Weinstein RA, *et al*. A new preadmission staging system for predicting inpatient mortality from HIV-associated Pneumocystis carinii pneumonia in the Early Highly Active Antiretroviral Therapy (HAART) era. *Am J Respir Crit Care Med* 2000;**161**:1081–6.

42 **Alves C**, Nicolas J, Miro J, *et al*. Reappraisal of the aetiology and prognostic factors of severe acute respiratory failure in HIV patients. *Eur Respir J* 2001;**17**:87–93.

43 **Richman DD**. HIV chemotherapy. *Nature* 2001;**410**:995–1001.

44 **Ledergerber B**, Egger M, Oppravil, *et al*. Clinical progression and virological failure on highly active antiretroviral therapy in HIV patients: a prospective cohort study: Swiss HIV Cohort Study. *Lancet* 1999;**353**:863–8.

45 **Whitcup SM**, Fortin E, Lindblad AS, *et al*. Discontinuation of anticytomegalovirus therapy in persons with HIV infection and cytomegalovirus retinitis. *JAMA* 1999;**282**:1633–7.

46 **Macdonald JC**, Torriani FJ, Morse LS, *et al*. Lack of reactivation of cytomegalovirus (CMV) retinitis after stopping CMV maintenance therapy in AIDS patients with sustained elevations in CD4 T cells in response to highly active antiretroviral therapy. *J Infect Dis* 1998;**177**:1182–7.

47 **Tural C**, Romeu J, Sirera G, *et al*. Long lasting remission of cytomegalovirus retinitis without maintenance therapy in human immunodeficiency virus infected patients. *J Infect Dis* 1998;**177**:1080–3.

48 **Vrabec TR**, Baldassano VF, Whitcup SM, *et al*. Discontinuation of maintenance therapy in patients with quiescent cytomegalovirus retinitis and elevated CD4+ counts. *Ophthalmology* 1998;**105**:1259–64.

49 **Jones JL**, Hanson DL, Dworkin MS, *et al*. Surveillance for AIDS-defining opportunistic illnesses, 1992–1997. *MMWR CDC Surveill Summ* 1999;**48**:1–22.

50 **Miller V**, Mocroft A, Reiss P, *et al*. Relations among CD4 lymphocyte count nadir, antiretroviral therapy, and HIV-1 disease progression: results from the EuroSIDA study. *Ann Intern Med* 1999;**130**:570–7.

51 **Wislez M**, Bergot E, Antoine M, *et al*. Acute respiratory failure following HAART introduction in patients treated for Pneumocystis carinii pneumonia. *Am J Respir Crit Care Med* 2001;**164**:847–51.

21 Illustrative case 6: acute chest syndrome of sickle cell anaemia

V Mak, S C Davies

CASE REPORT

A 21 year old Afro-Caribbean man with known sickle cell disease (SCD) was admitted to hospital with painful chest, thighs, and generalised abdominal pain. This was his second admission to hospital with a sickle cell crisis. He was on no regular medications apart from analgesia taken at home during crises. Apart from anaemia, there was nothing abnormal to find on examination. The haemoglobin (Hb) was 7.5 g/dl (normal for him), white cell count 22.5×10^9, and the electrolytes were normal apart from a slightly raised C-reactive protein (CRP) level of 30 mg/l. Radiographs of his abdomen and thighs were normal, but his chest radiograph showed a small degree of basal atelectasis bilaterally. His oxygen saturation was 96% on air. He was treated with a subcutaneous opiate infusion using a syringe pump, intravenous fluids, oxygen, and encouraged to drink.

Over the next 24 hours his pain was not well controlled and required an increasing dose of opiates. He became pyrexial (38.5°C), his oxygen saturation fell to 92% on air, and antibiotics to cover community acquired pneumonia were commenced. On the third day, however, he became more drowsy with arterial blood gases of pH 7.35, Pao_2 13.5 kPa, and $Paco_2$ 7.5 kPa on 40% oxygen. A repeat chest radiograph showed new infiltrates in both lower zones and a diagnosis of acute sickle chest syndrome (ACS) was made. Despite an exchange transfusion, he continued to deteriorate and was eventually intubated and ventilated. On intensive care his Fio_2 was reduced from the initial 50% to 28% within 24 hours. Sputum samples obtained by tracheobronchial suction showed no significant bacterial growth, but his CRP had risen to 150 mg/l so the antibiotic spectrum was broadened. After 3 days of mechanical ventilation his chest radiograph showed significant clearing of the lower zones, he was extubated without incident, and discharged from hospital after a further few days. Subsequent atypical respiratory serological examination did not show any rise in titres.

DISCUSSION

ACS consists of a combination of signs and symptoms including dyspnoea, chest pain, fever, cough, multifocal pulmonary infiltrates on the chest radiograph, and a raised white cell count. It is a form of lung injury that can progress to adult respiratory distress syndrome (ARDS). It is estimated that half of all patients with sickle cell anaemia will develop ACS at least once in their lives, and ACS is the second most common cause of admission after painful vaso-occlusive crises. The most recent statistics from the USA suggest that 13% of patients with ACS require mechanical ventilation with a mortality rate of 3%, mostly affecting adults[1]; the average length of stay was 10.5 days. ACS is the most common cause of death in these patients[2-4] and may be the cause of the chronic pulmonary abnormalities seen on high resolution CT scanning.[5]

Although this illustrative case with a typical presentation of ACS had a favourable outcome, the question is raised of whether anything could have been done to avoid respiratory failure.

Pathophysiology of the acute chest syndrome in sickle cell disease

The genetic defect in sickle cell anaemia causes a substitution of valine for glycine in the β-globin subunit of haemoglobin to form HbS.[6] HbS is less soluble than normal haemoglobin (HbA) when deoxygenated, as a result of which HbS polymerises within the cell. This stiffens the erythrocyte and changes it from its normal biconcave form to a sickle shaped cell. The sickle cell also loses the flexibility required to traverse capillary beds. Hypoxia also enhances adhesion of red cells to the vascular endothelium, a process mediated by interaction between very late activation antigen 4 (VLA-4) expressed on sickle cells and vascular cell adhesion molecule 1 (VCAM-1) on endothelial cells.[7] As a consequence, the sickle cells occlude small and sometimes larger vessels causing vascular injury, especially to organs with sluggish circulation such as the spleen and bone marrow and in atelectatic areas of lung.

There are four precipitants of ACS: infection, atelectasis, fat embolism, and true thromboembolism (fig 21.1). Each may progress to a common final pathway of reduced ventilation with hypoxia and increased sickling. The most common finding in the lung during an acute painful crisis affecting the chest wall is atelectasis from a combination of poor chest expansion caused by painful rib and vertebral infarction and suppressed respiratory drive due to opiates. Atelectasis promotes sickling locally due to hypoxia causing inflammation, intravascular coagulation, and vascular obstruction with eventual micro-infarction. In adults, particularly, vaso-occlusion in the bone marrow causes marrow infarction and fat embolism. At post mortem examination many patients have bony spicules and marrow fat in the lung, and lipid laden macrophages can be found in bronchoalveolar lavage (BAL) fluid of patients with ACS.[8] There is also increased circulating secretory phospholipase A2, a potent inflammatory mediator originating from the bone marrow, both in patients with ACS and those who are at risk of developing ACS, but not in those with uncomplicated vaso-occlusive crises.[9 10]

Nitric oxide (NO) is an endothelium derived vasodilator and a modulator of diverse inflammatory processes. Plasma concentrations of secretory VCAM-1 are raised in patients with ACS and are inversely related to plasma levels of NO

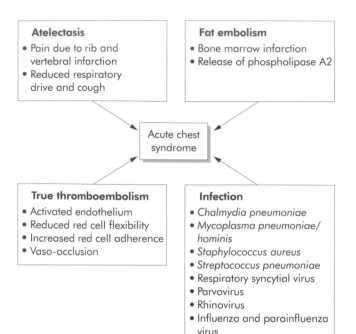

Atelectasis
- Pain due to rib and vertebral infarction
- Reduced respiratory drive and cough

Fat embolism
- Bone marrow infarction
- Release of phospholipase A2

Acute chest syndrome

True thromboembolism
- Activated endothelium
- Reduced red cell flexibility
- Increased red cell adherence
- Vaso-occlusion

Infection
- *Chalmydia pneumoniae*
- *Mycoplasma pneumoniae/ hominis*
- *Staphylococcus aureus*
- *Streptococcus pneumoniae*
- Respiratory syncytial virus
- Parvovirus
- Rhinovirus
- Influenza and parainfluenza virus

Figure 21.1 Pathophysiology of the acute chest syndrome in sickle cell disease.

metabolites.[11] NO inhibits VCAM-1 expression, thus reduced endothelial synthesis of NO during vaso-occlusive crises and hypoxia may contribute to red cell adhesion within the lung. NO binds and increases HbS avidity for oxygen both in vitro and in vivo, and hence may reduce its tendency for polymerisation[12] and thus has a potential therapeutic role in ACS.

NO is thought to play a significant role in the regulation of hypoxic pulmonary vasoconstriction. Exhaled concentrations of NO are directly related to the inhaled concentration of oxygen,[13] suggesting that oxygen may be a rate limiting substrate for NO synthesis. Normal Hb has an affinity for NO that is 3000 times that of oxygen, so Hb may act as a "biological sink" for NO[14] and rapid clearance of NO by Hb may contribute to hypoxic pulmonary vasoconstriction.[15] However, in the presence of anaemia there may be failure of hypoxic vasoconstriction due to increased local levels of NO, despite reduced local production. Failure of hypoxic vasoconstriction worsens ventilation-perfusion matching, giving ideal conditions for further sickling and eventually ACS.

Hydroxyurea has made a big impact on the management of SCD. In a double blind, placebo controlled trial in 299 adults with sickle cell anaemia who had at least three painful episodes in the preceding year, hydroxyurea reduced the frequency of painful episodes, the incidence of ACS, and reduced the need for hospitalisation and transfusion.[16] Hydroxyurea increases the concentration of fetal Hb (HbF) in erythrocytes, reducing the tendency for polymerisation of HbS.[17][18] However, some clinical improvements are seen before the HbF concentration increases.[19] In other studies hydroxyurea reduced adhesion of sickle cells to the vascular endothelium in vitro by reducing VCAM-1 expression.[20] Hydroxyurea is also oxidised by heme groups to produce NO,[21] and increased plasma NO metabolites can be detected during treatment.[22] The beneficial effects of hydroxyurea may therefore be mediated via its properties as an NO donor as well as its effects on HbF.

Management of acute chest syndrome
Most adult patients are admitted with vaso-occlusive crises and develop ACS after a few days, whereas children are more likely to have a preceding febrile illness or infection.[1][23] Once the process of lung injury has started it may be difficult to stop, and thus the aim of management should be to prevent ACS. Although the causes, clinical presentation, and outcomes

of ACS have been well documented,[1][2][23] less is known about its prevention or management.

General management
The most common cause for emergency admission of adults with SCD is a vaso-occlusive crisis. The mainstays of management are pain control, rehydration, oxygenation, and treatment of any identifiable precipitating cause. Common precipitants are infection, cold, stress, hypoxia and dehydration, but very often no obvious cause can be found. Infection—both bacterial and viral—is more common in children.

Adequate pain control usually requires initially high doses of opiates given by subcutaneous or intramuscular injection. The aim is to control pain rather than treating it as required. It is not uncommon for the doses required to suppress respiration and cough, causing atelectasis, retained secretions, and hypoxaemia. On the other hand, inadequate pain control may limit expansion and cough with the same consequences. In patients requiring opiates, intravenous rehydration is preferred aiming for 3–4 litres a day as the patient may not be able to drink adequate amounts owing to pain or drowsiness from excessive analgesia. Care should be taken not to cause fluid overload, especially in patients with impaired renal or cardiac function as a long term complication of SCD. Fluid overload will exacerbate pulmonary oedema associated with lung injury. Patients should be encouraged to drink freely.

There is a trend to give oxygen routinely to all patients with a vaso-occlusive crisis. However, if the oxygen saturations are normal (>97% on air), there is little to be gained from supplemental oxygen although it may reduce sickling in poorly ventilated areas of the lung. In patients with reduced respiratory drive or ventilation-perfusion mismatch, oxygen saturations may be reassuringly normal while the patient is on supplemental oxygen, masking the onset of acute lung injury. We recommend that pulse oximetry should be monitored regularly and all measurements should be performed after breathing room air for 10 minutes. If there is a fall of more than a few percent from normal values (patients with SCD may have low baseline levels due to chronic sickle lung disease), the cause should be sought and treated aggressively to prevent progression to ACS.

Specific management
Respiratory infection is a common precipitant of a sickle crisis but pathogens are rarely detected. In one study an identifiable pathogen was isolated in just over 30% of episodes,[1] but this figure is dependent on how hard one looks. The two most common organisms were *Chlamydia pneumoniae* and *Mycoplasma* (mostly *M pneumoniae* and occasionally *M hominis*). Children suffered more infections with respiratory syncytial virus and parvovirus. *Pneumococcus* or *Staphylococcus* were less common, even though most patients are hyposplenic. However, in the reported study patients with chlamydial infections were less likely to be taking prophylactic antibiotics. Many of the cases of infection also had evidence of marrow infarction.[1] Since atypical organisms predominate, a strong case can be made for treatment with macrolide antibiotics as the first line treatment when infection is thought to be the cause. However, caution should be exercised as the pattern of infectious agents in the UK may be different and further studies are required.

About 25% of patients with ACS wheeze and may respond to bronchodilators. Obstructive spirometry and small airways disease is not an uncommon finding in patients with SCD.[1] Thus, in patients on mechanical ventilation, high airway pressure may be due to airway obstruction rather than reduced lung compliance, and gas trapping and intrinsic positive end expiratory pressure should be monitored. Routine use of incentive spirometry has recently been recommended to prevent atelectasis and ACS in patients with SCD admitted with chest or bone pain.[24] In this randomised control study on

29 patients, 10 maximal inspirations with the incentive spirometer every 2 hours while the patient was awake significantly reduced the incidence of pulmonary complications. We prefer to use CPAP when the saturations fall below 93% on air or there is atelectasis on the chest radiograph. This is because pain and opiate sedation limits effort and compliance with active breathing techniques.

Blood transfusion and exchange transfusion are not required during uncomplicated painful episodes, but may be necessary when haemolysis is severe, if a large amount of blood is sequestrated in the spleen, or if there is an aplastic crisis caused by parvovirus infection. However, exchange transfusion can dramatically alter the course of ACS by replacing sickle cells with those containing HbA and by improving anaemia.[25] In addition, transfusion also rapidly improves oxygenation, which suggests that anaemia may lead to increased local pulmonary NO accumulation increasing shunt by counteracting hypoxic vasoconstriction.[26] Whether exchange transfusion is superior to simple transfusion is unclear, but in the US study of ACS both were effective with a low risk of alloimmunisation if phenotypically matched blood was used.[1] Our practice is to use exchange transfusion aiming for HbS <20% and a total Hb of <14.5 g/dl. Where simple transfusion is used, care must be taken not to raise blood viscosity which promotes sickling, so the total final Hb should be <10.5 g/dl.

Inhaled NO is widely used to improve oxygenation in respiratory failure.[27] Since NO downregulates endothelial adhesion molecule expression and increases the avidity of Hb for oxygen, reducing the tendency to sickling, there may be a specific role for NO supplementation in ACS. There have only been two reports of its use in three patients with ACS who have required mechanical ventilation.[28 29] Inhaled NO (20–80 ppm) was used for 2–4 days while all three cases were aggressively treated with exchange transfusion, rehydration, and ventilatory support. All showed improvements in oxygenation and a reduction in pulmonary artery pressure on administration of NO, and all three patients survived. The use of inhaled NO in ACS has not been rigorously examined and as yet cannot be recommended.

CONCLUSION

New insights into the pathogenesis of ACS have highlighted potential therapeutic strategies—for example, involving NO. However, the focus of management of a patient admitted with a painful crisis must be to prevent progression to ACS. A multidisciplinary approach involving haematologists, chest physicians, sickle cell specialist nurses, and physiotherapists is therefore required with emphasis on adequate pain control, rehydration, adequate oxygenation, treatment of atelectasis, prompt treatment of infection, and the use of bronchodilators.

REFERENCES

1 **Vichinsky EP**, Neumayr LD, Earles AN, *et al.* Causes and outcomes of the acute chest syndrome in sickle cell disease. *N Engl J Med* 2000;**342**:1855–65.
2 **Castro O**, Brambilla DJ, Thorington B, *et al.* The acute chest syndrome in sickle cell disease: incidence and risk factors. *Blood* 1994;**84**:643–9.
3 **Platt OS**, Brambilla DJ, Rosse WF, *et al.* Mortality in sickle cell disease: life expectancy and risk factors for early death. *N Engl J Med* 1994;**330**:1639–44.
4 **Platt OS**, Thorington BD, Brambilla DJ, *et al.* Pain in sickle cell disease. Rates and risk factors. *N Engl J Med* 1991;**325**:11–6.
5 **Aquino SL**, Gamsu G, Fahy JV, *et al.* Chronic pulmonary disorders in sickle cell disease: findings at thin section CT. *Radiology* 1994;**193**:807–11.
6 **Ingram VM**. Gene mutations in human hemoglobin: the chemical difference between normal and sickle cell hemoglobin. *Nature* 1957;**180**:326–8.
7 **Setty BN**, Stuart MJ. Vascular cell adhesion molecule-1 is involved in mediating hypoxia-induced sickle red blood cell adherence to endothelium: potential role in sickle cell disease. *Blood* 1996;**88**:2311–20.
8 **Vichinsky EP**, Williams R, Das M, *et al.* Pulmonary fat embolism: a distinct cause of severe acute chest syndrome in sickle cell anemia. *Blood* 1994;**83**:3107–12.
9 **Styles LA**, Schalkwijk CG, Aarsman AJ, *et al.* Phospholipase A2 levels in acute chest syndrome of sickle cell disease. *Blood* 1996;**87**:2573–8.
10 **Styles LA**, Aarsman AJ, Vichinsky EP, *et al.* Secretory phospholipase A(2) predicts impending acute chest syndrome in sickle cell disease. *Blood* 2000;**96**:3276–8.
11 **Stuart MJ**, Setty BN. Sickle cell acute chest syndrome: pathogenesis and rationale for treatment. *Blood* 1999;**94**:1555–60.
12 **Head C**, Brugnara AC, Martinez-Ruiz R, *et al.* Low concentrations of nitric oxide increase oxygen affinity of sickle erythrocytes in vitro and in vivo. *J Clin Invest* 1997;**100**:1193–8.
13 **Dweik R**, Laskowski AD, Abu-Soud HM, *et al.* Nitric oxide synthesis in the lung: regulation by oxygen through a kinetic mechanism. *J Clin Invest* 1998;**101**:660–6.
14 **Moncada S**, Higgs A. The L-arginine-nitric oxide pathway. *N Engl J Med* 1993;**329**:2002–12.
15 **Deem S**, Swenson ER, Alberts MK e, *et al.* Red-blood-cell augmentation of hypoxic pulmonary vasoconstriction: haematocrit dependence and the importance of nitric oxide. *Am J Respir Crit Care Med* 1998;**157**:1181–6.
16 **Charache S**, Terrin ML, Moore RD, *et al.* Effect of hydroxyurea on the frequency of painful crises in sickle cell anemia. *N Engl J Med* 1995;**332**:1317–22.
17 **Platt OS**, Orkin SH, Dover G, *et al.* Hydroxyurea enhances fetal hemoglobin production in sickle cell anemia. *J Clin Invest* 1984;**74**:652–6.
18 **Rodgers GP**, Dover GJ, Noguchi CT, *et al.* Hematologic responses of patients with sickle cell disease to treament with hydroxyurea. *N Engl J Med* 1990;**322**:1037–45.
19 **Styles LA**, Lubin B, Vichinsky E, *et al.* Decrease of very late activation antigen-4 and CD36 on reticulocytes in sickle cell patients treated with hydroxyurea. *Blood* 1997;**89**:2554–9.
20 **Adragna NC**, Fonseca P, Lauf PK. Hydroxyurea affects cell morphology, cation transport, and red cell adhesion in cultured vascular endothelial cells. *Blood* 1994;**83**:553–60.
21 **Pacelli R**, Taira J, Cook JA, *et al.* Hydroxyurea reacts with heme proteins to generate NO. *Lancet* 1996;**347**:900.
22 **Glover RE**, Ivy ED, Orringer EP, *et al.* Detection of nitrosyl hemoglobin in venous blood in the treatment of sickle cell anemia with hydroxyurea. *Mol Pharmacol* 1999;**55**:1006–10.
23 **Vichinsky EP**, Styles LA, Colangelo LH, *et al.* Acute chest syndrome in sickle cell disease: clinical presentation and course. *Blood* 1997;**89**:1787–92.
24 **Bellet PS**, Kalinyak KA, Shukla R, *et al.* Incentive spirometry to prevent acute pulmonary complications in sickle cell disease. *N Engl J Med* 1995;**333**:699–703.
25 **Wayne AS**, Kevy SV, Nathan D. Transfusion management of sickle cell disease. *Blood* 1993;**81**:1109–23.
26 **Emre U**, Miller ST, Gutierez M. Effect of transfusion in acute chest syndrome of sickle cell disease. *J Pediatr* 1995;**127**:901–4.
27 **Cranshaw J**, Griffiths MJD, Evans TW. The pulmonary physician in critical care—9: Non-ventilatory strategies in ARDS. *Thorax* 2002;**57**:823–9.
28 **Atz AM and Wessel DL**. Inhaled nitric oxide in sickle cell disease with acute chest syndrome. *Anesthesiology* 1997;**87**:988–90.
29 **Sullivan KJ**, Goodwin SR, Evangelist J, *et al.* Nitric oxide successfully used to treat acute chest syndrome of sickle cell disease in a young adolescent. *Crit Care Med* 1999;**27**:2563–8.

22 Illustrative case 7: assessment and management of massive haemoptysis

J L Lordan, A Gascoigne, P A Corris

Haemoptysis may be the presenting symptom of a number of diseases,[1][2] with an associated mortality ranging from 7% to 30%.[3-5] Although fewer than 5% of patients presenting with haemoptysis expectorate large volumes of blood, the explosive clinical presentation and the unpredictable course of life threatening haemoptysis demands prompt evaluation and management. We have reviewed the aetiology of massive haemoptysis and alveolar haemorrhage, with particular reference to current diagnostic and therapeutic strategies.

CASE HISTORY

A 69 year old woman was an emergency admission with large volume haemoptysis which did not settle spontaneously. She had previously undergone a left mastectomy for breast carcinoma. Alveolar shadowing was noted in the left mid zone on the chest radiograph, consistent with recent pulmonary haemorrhage (fig 22.1A). A thoracic computed thoracic (CT) scan confirmed consolidation and volume loss in the left upper lobe and lingula, but also showed a mass anteriorly eroding through the chest wall, consistent with local recurrence of the breast neoplasm (fig 22.1B). Pulmonary angiography showed no abnormality, but bronchial angiography identified a trunk that supplied a moderate pathological circulation anteriorly in the left upper lobe in the region of the abnormality on the CT scan. The artery was successfully embolised using polyvinyl alcohol (PVA) foam granules (500–700 μm in diameter, fig 22.2). The internal mammary artery was also catheterised and a pathological circulation was noted that was occluded using platinum coils (fig 22.1A) and PVA granules, with no complications and no recurrence of haemoptysis.

DEFINITION

Although there is no generally accepted definition of the volume of blood that constitutes a massive haemoptysis, studies have quoted volumes ranging from 100 ml up to or more than 1000 ml per day.[2] As the anatomical dead space of the major airways is 100–200 ml, a more relevant definition of massive haemoptysis is the volume that is life threatening by virtue of airway obstruction or blood loss.[5][6]

AETIOLOGY

It is important to establish that the lung is the source of bleeding, in part by excluding the nasopharynx or gastrointestinal tract. The most common causes of massive haemoptysis are listed in box 22.1. Haemoptysis originates from the bronchial and pulmonary circulation in 90% and 5% of cases, respectively.[7] Bleeding from the bronchial arteries has the propensity to cause massive haemoptysis as it is a circulation at systemic pressure. Alveolar haemorrhage is a recognised cause of haemoptysis, but rarely causes massive bleeding as the alveoli have the capacity to accommodate a large volume of blood.[8] A more common presentation is mild haemoptysis, pulmonary infiltrates, and anaemia.[2]

Chronic inflammatory conditions (including bronchiectasis, tuberculosis, lung abscess) and lung malignancies are the most common causes of massive haemoptysis.[9][10] Similarly, bleeding may occur from a mycetoma in the presence of cavitating lung disease.[11][12] The concurrent development of haemoptysis and menstruation points to a diagnosis of catamenial haemoptysis. The presence of haemoptysis and spontaneous pneumothorax in a woman of childbearing age with diffuse interstitial abnormalities on the chest radiograph should raise the suspicion of lymphangioleiomyomatosis.[16]

The presence of a saddle nose, rhinitis, or perforated nasal septum may suggest a diagnosis of Wegener's granulomatosis.[17] Features of Behcet's disease include oral or genital ulceration, uveitis, cutaneous nodules, and pulmonary artery aneurysm which is associated with a 30% 2 year mortality rate.[18] Although haematuria may be present in association with Goodpasture's disease, 5–10% of patients present without clinical evidence of renal disease.[8]

DIAGNOSTIC PROCEDURES

Sputum should be sent for microbiological investigation, including staining and culture for mycobacteria, and cytological examination if the patient is a smoker and over 40 years of age. Chest radiography may help to identify causative lesions or infiltrates resulting from pulmonary haemorrhage, but fails to localise the lesion in 20–46% of patients with haemoptysis.[19] A CT scan may show small bronchial carcinomas or localised bronchiectasis.[13][20][21] The use of contrast may help to identify vascular abnormalities such as arteriovenous malformations or aneurysms.[14][22] Despite all investigative procedures, the aetiology of haemoptysis is unknown in up to 5–10% of patients.[7]

MANAGEMENT OF MASSIVE HAEMOPTYSIS

The initial approach to managing life threatening haemorrhage involves resuscitation and protecting the airway (fig 22.3), the second step is directed at localising the site and cause of bleeding, and the final step involves the application of definitive and specific treatments to prevent recurrent bleeding.

Airway protection and resuscitation

All patients with massive haemoptysis should be monitored in an intensive care unit (ICU) or high dependency unit (HDU) and the patient's fitness

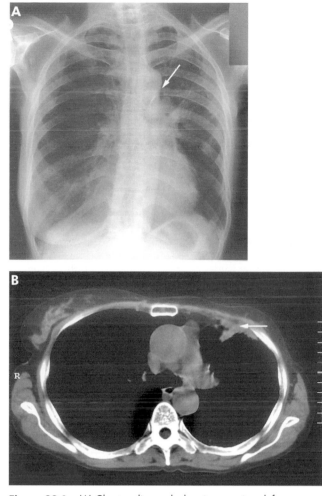

Figure 22.1 (A) Chest radiograph showing previous left mastectomy and left upper lobe and lingular infiltrates due to airway bleeding. A platinum embolisation coil is noted on this post-embolisation radiograph (arrow).(B) CT scan showing a mass lesion (arrow) involving the left anterior chest wall with associated left upper zone consolidation, consistent with recent haemoptysis and local tumour recurrence following the previous mastectomy.

for surgery established. Attempts should be made to determine the side of bleeding and the patient positioned with the bleeding side down to prevent aspiration into the unaffected lung. Blood loss should be treated with volume resuscitation, blood transfusion, and correction of coagulopathy. If large volume bleeding continues or the airway is compromised, the patient's trachea should be intubated with as large an endotracheal tube as is possible to allow adequate suctioning and access for bronchoscopy.[2] If the bleeding can only be localised to the right or left lung, unilateral lung intubation may protect the non-bleeding lung.[23] For right sided bleeding a bronchoscope may be directed into the left main bronchus which can then be selectively intubated over the bronchoscope with the patient lying in the right lateral position (fig 22.4). The left lung is then protected from aspiration and selectively ventilated. For a left sided bleeding source the patient is placed in the left lateral position and selective intubation of the right lung may be performed, but this may lead to occlusion of the right upper lobe bronchus.[2] An alternative strategy is to pass an endotracheal tube over the bronchoscope into the trachea. A Fogarty catheter (size 14 French/100 cm length) may then be passed through the vocal cords beside the endotracheal tube, directed by the bronchoscope into the left main bronchus and inflated (fig 22.5). This prevents aspiration of blood from the left lung and the endotracheal tube positioned in the trachea allows ventilation of the unaffected right lung.

An alternative strategy for unilateral bleeding is to pass a double lumen endotracheal tube, which allows isolation and ventilation of the normal lung and prevents aspiration from the side involved by bleeding (fig 22.6).[2] However, inserting double lumen tubes should only be performed by experienced operators to avoid the serious consequences of poor positioning.[24]

Identifying the site and cause of bleeding

Precise localisation of the bleeding site directs definitive treatment. Fibreoptic bronchoscopy and angiography are the modalities of choice to localise the site of bleeding and to allow therapeutic intervention, although the timing of bronchoscopy is controversial.[25 26] Early compared with delayed bronchoscopy gives a higher yield for localising the site of bleeding.[26] In contrast to mild haemoptysis, localisation of the

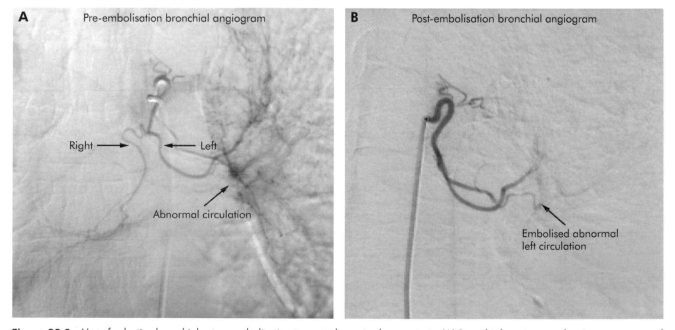

Figure 22.2 Use of selective bronchial artery embolisation to control massive haemoptysis. (A) Bronchial angiogram showing common trunk and left sided abnormal circulation pre-embolisation, and (B) post-embolisation angiogram showing the left bronchial artery and successful embolisation of abnormal vessels.

Box 22.1 Causes of massive haemoptysis and alveolar haemorrhage

Infections
- Mycobacteria, particularly tuberculosis
- Fungal infections (mycetoma)
- Lung abscess
- Necrotising pneumonia (*Klebsiella, Staphylococcus, Legionella*)

Iatrogenic
- Swan-Ganz catheterisation
- Bronchoscopy
- Transbronchial biopsy
- Transtracheal aspirate

Parasitic
- Hydatid cyst
- Paragonimiasis

Trauma
- Blunt/penetrating injury
- Suction ulcers
- Tracheoarterial fistula

Neoplasm
- Bronchogenic carcinoma
- Bronchial adenoma
- Pulmonary metastases
- Sarcoma

Haemoptysis in children
- Bronchial adenoma
- Foreign body aspiration
- Vascular anomalies

Vascular
- Pulmonary infarct, embolism
- Mitral stenosis
- Arteriobronchial fistula
- Arteriovenous malformations
- Bronchial telangiectasia
- Left ventricular failure

Coagulopathy
- Von Willebrand's disease
- Haemophilia
- Anticoagulant therapy
- Thrombocytopenia
- Platelet dysfunction
- Disseminated intravascular coagulation

Vasculitis
- Behcet's disease
- Wegener's granulomatosis

Pulmonary
- Bronchiectasis (including cystic fibrosis)
- Chronic bronchitis
- Emphysematous bullae

Miscellaneous
- Lymphangioleiomatosis
- Catamenial (endometriosis)
- Pneumoconiosis
- Broncholith
- Idiopathic

Spurious
- Epistaxis
- Haematemesis

site of bleeding is essential in the management of massive haemoptysis and urgent bronchoscopy should be considered.[7]

Fibreoptic bronchoscopy can be performed at the bedside and allows visualisation of more peripheral and upper lobe lesions, but has a limited suction capacity.[25][26] Rigid bronchoscopy provides superior suction to maintain airway patency, but it has a limited ability to identify peripheral lesions and does not permit good views of the upper lobes.[3] It is usually performed under general anaesthetic but can be performed under local anaesthesia and sedation in experienced hands.[27] The techniques can be combined when the fibreoptic bronchoscope is passed through the lumen of the rigid bronchoscope.

Bronchoscopic treatment

Instillation of epinephrine (1:20 000) is advocated to control bleeding, although its efficacy in life threatening haemoptysis is uncertain.[2] The topical application of thrombin and thrombin-fibrinogen solutions has also had some success, but further study is required before widespread use can be recommended.[28]

In massive haemoptysis, isolation of a bleeding segment with a balloon catheter may prevent aspiration of blood into the large airways, thereby maintaining airway patency and oxygenation. Having identified the segmental bronchus that is the source of bleeding, the bronchoscope is wedged in the orifice. A size 4–7 Fr 200 cm balloon catheter is passed through the working channel of the bronchoscope and the balloon is inflated in the affected segment, isolating the bleeding site (fig 7).[2] A double lumen balloon catheter (6 Fr, 170 cm long) with a detachable valve at the proximal end has recently been designed that passes through the bronchoscope channel and allows the removal of the bronchoscope without any modification of the catheter.[29] The second channel of the catheter may also be used to instil vasoactive drugs to help control bleeding. The bronchoscope can then be removed over the catheter, which is left in place for 24 hours. The balloon may be deflated under controlled conditions with bronchoscopic visualisation and the catheter removed if the bleeding has stopped. The prolonged use of balloon tamponade catheters should be avoided to prevent ischaemic mucosal injury and postobstructive pneumonia. Endobronchial tamponade should only be applied as a temporary measure until a more definitive therapeutic procedure can be deployed.

Neodymium-yttrium-aluminium-garnet (Nd-YAG) laser photocoagulation has been used with some success in the management of massive haemorrhage associated with directly visualised endobronchial lesions.[30] However, targeting the culprit vessel with the laser beam can be difficult in the presence of ongoing bleeding.

Bronchial artery embolisation (BAE)

This was first reported by Remy and colleagues in 1977[31] and is increasingly used in the management of life threatening haemoptysis.[20] The procedure involves the initial identification of the bleeding vessel by selective bronchial artery cannulation, and the subsequent injection of particles (polyvinyl alcohol foam, isobutyl-2-cyanoacrylate, Gianturco steel coils or absorbable gelatin pledgets) into the feeding vessel (fig 22.2). A number of features provide clues to the bronchial artery as the source of bleeding, including the infrequent identification of extravasated dye or the visualisation of tortuous vessels of increased calibre or aneurysmal dilatation.[32] The immediate success rates for control of massive haemoptysis is excellent, ranging from 64% to 100%, although recurrent non-massive bleeding has been reported in 16–46% of patients.[32–35] Technical failure of BAE occurs in up to 13% of cases and is largely caused by non-bronchial artery collaterals from systemic vessels such as the phrenic, intercostal, mammary, or subclavian arteries.[35] Complications of BAE include vessel perforation,

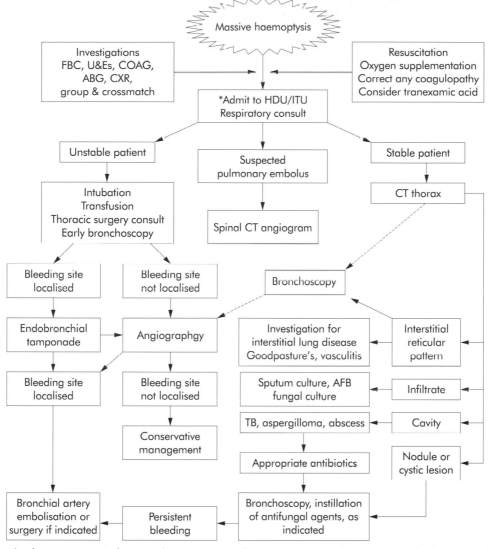

Figure 22.3 Algorithm for management of massive haemoptysis. *Palliative measures may be appropriate in the setting of advanced malignancy.

intimal tears, chest pain, pyrexia, haemoptysis, systemic embolisation, and neurological complications. When the anterior spinal artery is identified as originating from the bronchial artery, embolisation is often deferred owing to the risk of infarction and paraparesis.[32] The development and application of coaxial microcatheter systems allows more selective catheterisation and embolisation of branches of the bronchial arteries, thereby reducing the risk of occluding branches such as the anterior spinal artery.[34]

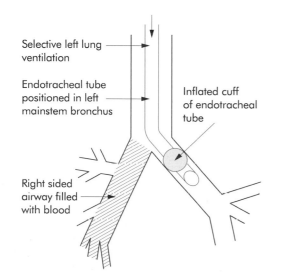

Figure 22.4 Selective intubation of left main bronchus in a case of right sided massive haemoptysis.

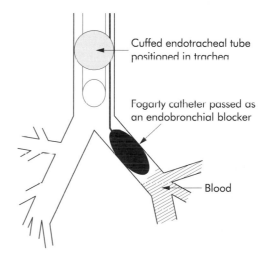

Figure 22.5 Control of left sided massive haemoptysis by tracheal intubation, placement, and inflation of a Fogarty catheter in the left main bronchus.

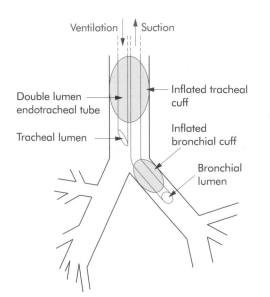

Figure 22.6 Application of a double lumen endotracheal tube for the control of massive haemorrhage. The bronchial lumen is positioned in the left main bronchus to ventilate the left lung and the tracheal lumen is positioned above the carina, allowing ventilation of the right lung while preventing occlusion of the right upper lobe orifice.

Surgical management

Surgery is considered for the management of localised lesions. Surgical mortality ranges from 1% to 50% in different series depending on selection criteria, but bias in the selection of candidates for surgery limits a direct comparison with medical treatment.[2] Surgery is contraindicated in patients with inadequate respiratory reserve or those with inoperable lung cancer due to direct thoracic spread. Surgical resection is indicated when BAE is unavailable or the bleeding is unlikely to be controlled by embolisation. It remains the treatment of choice for the management of life threatening haemoptysis due to a leaking aortic aneurysm, selected cases of arteriovenous malformations, hydatid cyst, iatrogenic pulmonary rupture, chest injuries, bronchial adenoma, or haemoptysis related to mycetoma resistant to other treatments.[7][23] Pulmonary artery rupture related to the use of pulmonary artery catheters may be temporarily controlled by withdrawing the catheter slightly and reinflating the balloon to compress the bleeding vessel more proximally.[36] However, surgical resection of the bleeding vessel is the definitive management.

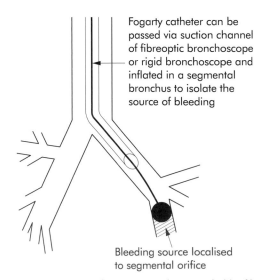

Fogarty catheter can be passed via suction channel of fibreoptic bronchoscope or rigid bronchoscope and inflated in a segmental bronchus to isolate the source of bleeding

Bleeding source localised to segmental orifice

Figure 22.7 Placement of a Fogarty catheter guided by fibreoptic bronchoscopy to control massive bleeding from a segmental bronchus.

The onset of massive haemoptysis in a patient with a tracheostomy may be associated with the development of a tracheal-arterial fistula, usually the innominate artery.[37] The prompt application of anterior and downward pressure on the tracheal cannula and overinflation of the tracheostomy balloon may help to tamponade the bleeding vessel, and immediate surgical review should be requested. Deflation of the tracheostomy balloon and removal of the tracheal cannula should be performed in a controlled environment.

Other treatment

The oral antifibrinolytic agent tranexamic acid, an inhibitor of plasminogen activation, is frequently used to control recurrent haemoptysis. Intravenous vasopressin has also been used but caution is advised in patients with coexistent coronary artery disease or hypertension. Vasoconstriction of the bronchial artery may also hamper effective BAE by obscuring the site of bleeding, leading to difficulties in cannulation of the artery.[2]

Systemic antifungal agents have been tried in the management of haemoptysis related to mycetoma, but the results have been poor. By contrast, the direct instillation of antifungal drugs such as amphotericin B with or without N-acetylcysteine or iodine by means of a percutaneous or transbronchial catheter in the cavity has resulted in satisfactory control of haemoptysis in some cases.[12][38] This technique should be considered in patients with ongoing bleeding following attempted BAE who are not otherwise fit for surgical resection.

Invasive therapeutic procedures have no role in the management of pulmonary haemorrhage related to coagulopathy, blood dyscrasias, or immunologically mediated alveolar haemorrhage. Appropriate medical treatment is usually sufficient.[39] On the rare occasion when an immunologically mediated alveolar haemorrhage leads to massive haemoptysis, the administration of systemic corticosteroids, cytotoxic agents, or plasmapheresis may be useful.[8] The long term administration of danazol or gonadotrophin releasing hormone agonists may prove useful in the management of catamenial haemoptysis.[40] Radiation therapy has been used in the management of massive haemoptysis associated with vascular tumours or mycetoma by inducing necrosis of feeding blood vessels and vascular thrombosis due to perivascular oedema.[41]

OUTCOME

Mortality has been closely correlated with the volume of blood expectorated, the rate of bleeding, the amount of blood retained within the lungs and premorbid respiratory reserve, independent of the aetiology of bleeding.[1][4] The mortality rate is 58% when the rate of blood loss exceeds 1000 ml/24 hours, compared with 9% if bleeding is less than 1000 ml/hour.[7][39] The mortality rate in patients with malignancy is 59%, which increases to 80% in the presence of a combination of malignant aetiology and a bleeding rate of more than 1000 ml/24 hours. A better outcome has been noted for massive haemorrhage due to bronchiectasis, lung abscess, or necrotising pulmonary infections, with a mortality rate of less than 1% in some series.[39]

SUMMARY

The unpredictable and potentially lethal course of massive haemoptysis requires prompt resuscitation, airway protection and correction of coagulopathy. Early investigation with bronchoscopy is recommended for localisation and control of bleeding by the application of topical adrenaline, balloon tamponade or selective lung intubation. There is increasing acceptance of bronchial artery embolisation as the treatment of choice to control acute massive haemoptysis that continues despite conservative treatment when a bronchial artery can be identified as the source of bleeding. Surgical resection remains the treatment of choice for particular conditions, where the bleeding site is localised and the patient is fit for lung resection.

ACKNOWLEDGEMENTS

The authors thank Dr Leslie Mitchell for providing the radiographic and bronchial embolisation images and Dr Stephen Cook and John Sternman for reviewing the manuscript.

REFERENCES

1 **Cahill BC**, Ingbar DH. Massive hemoptysis. Assessment and management. *Clin Chest Med* 1994;**15**:147–67.

2 **Dweik RA**, Stoller JK. Role of bronchoscopy in massive hemoptysis. *Clin Chest Med* 1999;**20**:89–105.

3 **Conlan AA**, Hurwitz SS, Krige L, *et al*. Massive hemoptysis. Review of 123 cases. *J Thorac Cardiovasc Surg* 1983;**85**:120–4.

4 **Yeoh CB**, Hubaytar RT, Ford JM, *et al*. Treatment of massive hemorrhage in pulmonary tuberculosis. *J Thorac Cardiovasc Surg* 1967;**54**:503–10.

5 **Holsclaw DS**, Grand RJ, Shwachman H. Massive hemoptysis in cystic fibrosis. *J Pediatr* 1970;**76**:829–38.

6 **Garzon AA**, Cerruti MM, Golding ME. Exsanguinating hemoptysis. *J Thorac Cardiovasc Surg* 1982;**84**:829–33.

7 **Jean-Baptiste E**. Clinical assessment and management of massive hemoptysis. *Crit Care Med* 2000;**28**:1642–7.

8 **Schwarz MI**, Brown KK. Small vessel vasculitis of the lung. *Thorax* 2000;**55**:502–10.

9 **Santiago S**, Tobias J, Williams AJ. A reappraisal of the causes of hemoptysis. *Arch Intern Med* 1991;**151**:2449–51.

10 **Hirshberg B**, Biran I, Glazer M, *et al*. Hemoptysis: etiology, evaluation, and outcome in a tertiary referral hospital. *Chest* 1997;**112**:440–4.

11 **Jewkes J**, Kay PH, Paneth M, *et al*. Pulmonary aspergilloma: analysis of prognosis in relation to haemoptysis and survey of treatment. *Thorax* 1983;**38**:572–8.

12 **Rumbak M**, Kohler G, Eastrige C, *et al*. Topical treatment of life threatening haemoptysis from aspergillomas. *Thorax* 1996;**51**:253–5.

13 **McGuinness G**, Beacher JR, Harkin TJ, *et al*. Hemoptysis: prospective high-resolution CT/bronchoscopic correlation. *Chest* 1994;**105**:1155–62.

14 **Ference BA**, Shannon TM, White RI Jr, *et al*. Life-threatening pulmonary hemorrhage with pulmonary arteriovenous malformations and hereditary hemorrhagic telangiectasia. *Chest* 1994;**106**:1387–90.

15 **Kalra S**, Bell MR, Rihal CS. Alveolar hemorrhage as a complication of treatment with abciximab. *Chest* 2001;**120**:126–31.

16 **Johnson S**. Rare diseases—1. Lymphangioleiomyomatosis: clinical features, management and basic mechanisms. *Thorax* 1999;**54**:254–64.

17 **Langford CA**, Hoffman GS. Rare diseases—3: Wegener's granulomatosis. *Thorax* 1999;**54**:629–37.

18 **Erkan F**, Gul A, Tasali E. Pulmonary manifestations of Behcet's disease. *Thorax* 2001;**56**:572–8.

19 **Marshall TJ**, Flower CD, Jackson JE. The role of radiology in the investigation and management of patients with haemoptysis. *Clin Radiol* 1996;**51**:391–400.

20 **Haponik EF**, Fein A, Chin R. Managing life-threatening hemoptysis: has anything really changed? *Chest* 2000;**118**:1431–5.

21 **Millar AB**, Boothroyd AE, Edwards D, *et al*. The role of computed tomography (CT) in the investigation of unexplained haemoptysis. *Respir Med* 1992;**86**:39–44.

22 **Pennington DW**, Gold WM, Gordon RL, *et al*. Treatment of pulmonary arteriovenous malformations by therapeutic embolization. Rest and exercise physiology in eight patients. *Am Rev Respir Dis* 1992;**145**:1047–51.

23 **Gourin A**, Garzon AA. Control of hemorrhage in emergency pulmonary resection for massive hemoptysis. *Chest* 1975;**68**:120–1.

24 **Klein U**, Karzai W, Bloos F, *et al*. Role of fiberoptic bronchoscopy in conjunction with the use of double-lumen tubes for thoracic anesthesia: a prospective study. *Anesthesiology* 1998;**88**:346–50.

25 **Gong H Jr**, Salvatierra C. Clinical efficacy of early and delayed fiberoptic bronchoscopy in patients with hemoptysis. *Am Rev Respir Dis* 1981;**124**:221–5.

26 **Saumench J**, Escarrabill J, Padro L, *et al*. Value of fiberoptic bronchoscopy and angiography for diagnosis of the bleeding site in hemoptysis. *Ann Thorac Surg* 1989;**48**:272–4.

27 **Helmers RA**, Sanderson DR. Rigid bronchoscopy. The forgotten art. *Clin Chest Med* 1995;**16**:393–9.

28 **Tsukamoto T**, Sasaki H, Nakamura H. Treatment of hemoptysis patients by thrombin and fibrinogen-thrombin infusion therapy using a fiberoptic bronchoscope. *Chest* 1989;**96**:473–6.

29 **Freitag L**, Tekolf E, Stamatis G, *et al*. Three years experience with a new balloon catheter for the management of haemoptysis. *Eur Respir J* 1994;**7**:2033–7.

30 **Edmondstone WM**, Nanson EM, Woodcock AA, *et al*. Life threatening haemoptysis controlled by laser photocoagulation. *Thorax* 1983;**38**:788–9.

31 **Remy J**, Arnaud A, Fardou H, *et al*. Treatment of hemoptysis by embolization of bronchial arteries. *Radiology* 1977;**122**:33–7.

32 **Uflacker R**, Kaemmerer A, Picon PD, *et al*. Bronchial artery embolization in the management of hemoptysis: technical aspects and long-term results. *Radiology* 1985;**157**:637–44.

33 **Brinson GM**, Noone PG, Mauro MA, *et al*. Bronchial artery embolization for the treatment of hemoptysis in patients with cystic fibrosis. *Am J Respir Crit Care Med* 1998;**157**:1951–8.

34 **Tanaka N**, Yamakado K, Murashima S, *et al*. Superselective bronchial artery embolization for hemoptysis with a coaxial microcatheter system. *J Vasc Interv Radiol* 1997;**8**:65–70.

35 **Keller FS**, Rosch J, Loflin TG, *et al*. Nonbronchial systemic collateral arteries: significance in percutaneous embolotherapy for hemoptysis. *Radiology* 1987;**164**:687–92.

36 **Thomas R**, Siproudhis L, Laurent JF, *et al*. Massive hemoptysis from iatrogenic balloon catheter rupture of pulmonary artery: successful early management by balloon tamponade. *Crit Care Med* 1987;**15**:272–3.

37 **Schaefer OP**, Irwin RS. Tracheoarterial fistula: an unusual complication of tracheostomy. *J Intensive Care Med* 1995;**10**:64–75.

38 **Shapiro MJ**, Albelda SM, Mayock RL, *et al*. Severe hemoptysis associated with pulmonary aspergilloma. Percutaneous intracavitary treatment. *Chest* 1988;**94**:1225–31.

39 **Corey R**, Hla KM. Major and massive hemoptysis: reassessment of conservative management. *Am J Med Sci* 1987;**294**:301–9.

40 **Matsubara K**, Ochi H, Ito M. Catamenial hemoptysis treated with a long-acting GnRH agonist. *Int J Gynaecol Obstet* 1998;**60**:289–90.

41 **Shneerson JM**, Emerson PA, Phillips RH. Radiotherapy for massive haemoptysis from an aspergilloma. *Thorax* 1980;**35**:953–4.

Index

Page numbers in **bold** text refer to figures in the text; those in *italics* to tables or boxed material